Malunions and Nonunions in the Forearm, Wrist, and Hand

Editors

ERIN A. MILLER
JERRY I. HUANG

HAND CLINICS

www.hand.theclinics.com

Consulting Editor
KEVIN C. CHUNG

February 2024 • Volume 40 • Number 1

ELSEVIER

1600 John F. Kennedy Boulevard • Suite 1800 • Philadelphia, Pennsylvania, 19103-2899

http://www.theclinics.com

HAND CLINICS Volume 40, Number 1
February 2024 ISSN 0749-0712, ISBN-13: 978-0-443-18209-9

Editor: Megan Ashdown
Developmental Editor: Akshay Samson

Hand Clinics (ISSN 0749-0712) is published quarterly by Elsevier Inc., 360 Park Avenue South, New York, NY 10010-1710. Months of publication are February, May, August, and November. Business and Editorial Offices: 1600 John F. Kennedy Blvd., Ste. 1800, Philadelphia, PA 19103-2899. Customer Service Office: 3251 Riverport Lane, Maryland Heights, MO 63043. Periodicals postage paid at New York, NY and at additional mailing offices. Subscription price is $457.00 per year (domestic individuals), $100.00 per year (domestic students/residents), $506.00 per year (Canadian individuals), $579.00 per year (international individuals), $256.00 (international students/residents), and $100.00 (Canadian students/residents). For institutional access pricing please contact Customer Service via the contact information below. Foreign air speed delivery is included in all *Clinics* subscription prices. All prices are subject to change without notice. **POSTMASTER:** Send address changes to *Hand Clinics*, Elsevier Health Sciences Division, Subscription Customer Service, 3251 Riverport Lane, Maryland Heights, MO 63043. Customer Service (orders, claims, online, change of address): Elsevier Health Sciences Division, Subscription **Customer Service, 3251 Riverport Lane, Maryland Heights, MO 63043. Tel: 1-800-654-2452 (U.S. and Canada); 314-447-8871 (outside U.S. and Canada). Fax: 314-447-8029. E-mail: journalscustomerservice-usa@elsevier.com (for print support); journalsonlinesupport-usa@elsevier.com (for online support).**

Reprints. For copies of 100 or more of articles in this publication, please contact the Commercial Reprints Department, Elsevier Inc., 360 Park Avenue South, New York, New York 10010-1710. Tel.: 212-633-3874; Fax: 212-633-3820; E-mail: reprints@elsevier.com.

Hand Clinics is covered in *MEDLINE/PubMed (Index Medicus), Current Contents/Clinical Medicine, EMBASE/Excerpta Medica,* and *ISI/BIOMED.*

Contributors

CONSULTING EDITOR

KEVIN C. CHUNG, MD, MS
Charles B.G. de Nancrede Professor of
Surgery, Professor of Plastic Surgery and
Orthopaedic Surgery, Chief of Hand Surgery,
Department of Surgery, Section of Plastic
Surgery, Michigan Medicine, Assistant Dean
for Faculty Affairs, Associate Director of Global
REACH, University of Michigan Medical
School, Comprehensive Hand Center,
University of Michigan, The University of
Michigan Health System, Ann Arbor, Michigan,
USA

EDITORS

ERIN A. MILLER, MD, MS, FACS
Assistant Professor, Division of Plastic
Surgery, Department of Surgery, Adjunct
Assistant Professor, Department of Orthopedic
Surgery, University of Washington Medical
Center, Division of Plastic and Reconstructive
Surgery, University of Washington, Seattle,
Washington, USA

JERRY I. HUANG, MD
Professor, Department of Orthopedics and
Sports Medicine, University of Washington
Medical Center, Department of Orthopedic
Surgery, University of Washington, Seattle,
Washington, USA

AUTHORS

**GEERT ALEXANDER BUIJZE, MD, PhD,
FEBHS**
Surgeon, Hand, Upper Limb, Peripheral Nerve,
Brachial Plexus and Microsurgery Unit,
Clinique Generale Annecy, France; Assistant
Professor, Hand and Upper Extremity Surgery
Unit, CHU Lapeyronie, University of
Montpellier, Montpellier, France; Department
of Orthopaedic Surgery, Amsterdam UMC,
University of Amsterdam, Amsterdam,
Netherlands

CHELSEA C. BOE, MD
Assistant Professor, Department of
Orthopaedics and Sports Medicine, University
of Washington, Seattle, Washington, USA

SOFIA BOUGIOUKLI, MD, PhD
Hand Fellow, Department of Plastic Surgery,
University of Michigan Medical School, Ann
Arbor, Michigan, USA

KEVIN C. CHUNG, MD, MS
Charles B.G. de Nancrede Professor of Surgery,
Professor of Plastic Surgery and Orthopaedic
Surgery, Chief of Hand Surgery, Department of
Surgery, Section of Plastic Surgery, Michigan
Medicine, Assistant Dean for Faculty Affairs,
Associate Director of Global REACH, University
of Michigan Medical School, Comprehensive
Hand Center, University of Michigan, The
University of Michigan Health System, Ann
Arbor, Michigan, USA

STEFAN CZERNIECKI, MD, MSc
Resident Physician, Department of Plastic and
Reconstructive Surgery, The Ohio State
University, Columbus, Ohio, USA

KYLE R. EBERLIN, MD
Associate Professor, Division of Plastic
Surgery, Massachusetts General Hospital,
Harvard Medical School, Boston,
Massachusetts, USA

RYOKO HAMAGUCHI, MD
Resident Physician, Division of Plastic Surgery,
Massachusetts General Hospital, Harvard
Medical School, Boston, Massachusetts, USA

WARREN C. HAMMERT, MD
Professor of Orthopaedic Surgery and Plastic Surgery, Hand, Upper Extremity and Microsurgery, Department of Orthopaedic Surgery, Duke University Medical Center, Durham, North Carolina, USA

JAMES P. HIGGINS, MD
Chief, Curtis National Hand Center, MedStar Union Memorial Hospital, Baltimore, Maryland, USA

JERRY I. HUANG, MD
Professor, Department of Orthopedics and Sports Medicine, University of Washington Medical Center, Department of Orthopedic Surgery, University of Washington, Seattle, Washington, USA

ROBIN N. KAMAL, MD, MBA
Associate Professor, Department of Orthopedic Surgery, Stanford University, Palo Alto, California, USA

STEPHEN A. KENNEDY, MD, FRCSC
Associate Professor, Department of Orthopaedics and Sports Medicine, University of Washington, Seattle, Washington, USA

ALEXANDER LAUDER, MD
Assistant Professor, Department of Orthopedics, University of Colorado School of Medicine, Aurora, Colorado, USA; Department of Orthopedics, Denver Health Medical Center, Denver, Colorado, USA

FRASER J. LEVERSEDGE, MD
Professor and Chief, Section of Hand, Wrist and Elbow Surgery, Department of Orthopedic Surgery, University of Colorado School of Medicine, Aurora, Colorado, USA

M. CLAIRE MANSKE, MD, MAS
Department of Orthopedic Surgery, Shriners Hospital for Children Northern California, Associate Professor, Department of Orthopedic Surgery, University of California, Davis, Sacramento, California, USA

JUSTIN C. MCCARTY, DO, MPH
Division of Plastic Surgery, Massachusetts General Hospital, Harvard Medical School, Boston, Massachusetts, USA

MAXIMILIAN A. MEYER, MD
Hand & Upper Extremity Fellow, Department of Orthopedic Surgery, University of Colorado School of Medicine, Aurora, Colorado, USA

ERIN A. MILLER, MD, MS, FACS
Assistant Professor, Division of Plastic Surgery, Department of Surgery, Adjunct Assistant Professor, Department of Orthopedic Surgery, University of Washington Medical Center, Division of Plastic and Reconstructive Surgery, University of Washington, Seattle, Washington, USA

MARK MISHU, MD
Clinical Instructor House Staff, Department of Plastic and Reconstructive Surgery, The Ohio State University, Columbus, Ohio, USA

JEREMY E. RADUCHA, MD
Fellow, Hand, Upper Extremity and Microsurgery, Department of Orthopaedic Surgery, Duke University Medical Center, Durham, North Carolina, USA

SHEA RAY, MD, MS
Department of Orthopedic Surgery, Shriners Hospital for Children Northern California, Sacramento, California, USA

MARC J. RICHARD, MD
Associate Professor, Director, Hand, Upper Extremity, and Microvascular Surgery Fellowship, Department of Orthopaedic Surgery, Duke University Medical Center, Morrisville, North Carolina, USA

FRANCISCO RODRIGUEZ-FONTAN, MD
Resident, Department of Orthopedics, University of Colorado School of Medicine, Aurora, Colorado, USA

TAMARA D. ROZENTAL, MD
Chief, Hand and Upper Extremity Surgery, Professor, Department of Orthopaedic Surgery, Beth Israel Deaconess Medical Center, Harvard Medical School, Boston, Massachusetts, USA

RYAN SCHMUCKER, MD
Physician, Department of Plastic and Reconstructive Surgery, The Ohio State University, Columbus, Ohio, USA

KALPIT N. SHAH, MD
Orthopedic Hand Surgeon, Department of
Orthopedic Surgery, Scripps Clinic, San Diego,
California, USA

ANDREAS VERSTREKEN, MD
Resident, Orthopedic Department, Antwerp
University Hospital, Edegem, Belgium

FREDERIK VERSTREKEN, MD, FEBHS
Hand Surgeon, Orthopedic Department,
Antwerp University Hospital, Edegem,
Belgium; Surgeon, Orthopedic Department, AZ
Monica Hospital, Antwerp, Belgium

CATPHUONG L. VU, MD, MPH
Fellow, Hand, Upper Extremity, and
Microvascular Surgery, Department of
Orthopaedics, Duke University Medical
Center, Morrisville, North Carolina,
USA

IAN T. WATKINS, MD
Resident, Harvard Combined Orthopaedic
Residency Program, Division of Hand and
Upper Extremity Surgery, Department of
Orthopedics, Beth Israel Deaconess Medical
Center, Harvard Medical School, Boston,
Massachusetts, USA

Contents

Nonunion is a common and costly problem. Unfortunately, there is no widely agreed upon and standardized definition for nonunion. The evaluation of bony union should start with a thorough history and physical examination. The clinician should consider patient-dependent as well as patient-independent characteristics that may influence the rate of healing and evaluate the patient for physical examination findings suggestive of bony union and infection. Radiographs and clinical examination can help confirm a diagnosis of union. When the diagnosis is in doubt, however, advanced imaging modalities as well as laboratory studies can help a surgeon determine when further intervention is necessary.

We examine the range of available bone graft substitutes often used in nonunion and malunion surgery of the upper extremity. Synthetic materials such as calcium sulfate, beta-calcium phosphate ceramics, hydroxyapatite, bioactive glass, and 3D printed materials are discussed. We delve into the advantages, disadvantages, and clinical applications for each, considering factors such as biocompatibility, osteoconductivity, mechanical strength, and resorption rates. This review provides upper extremity surgeons with insights into the available array of bone graft substitutes. We hope that the reviews helps in the decision-making process to achieve optimal outcomes when treating nonunion and malunion of the upper extremity.

Forearm fractures present a unique challenge due to the anatomic relationship of the radius relative to the ulna. Associated with the complexity of the treatment for these fractures is the management of nonunion and malunion of the radius and ulna. Evaluation and management of forearm nonunions require a critical evaluation of contributing factors prior to surgical intervention. Timely and precise treatment of nonunion and malunion is necessary to restore function of the forearm.

 Video content accompanies this article at http://www.hand.theclinics.com.

The aim of this article is to review the evaluation and management of pediatric forearm malunions. Acceptable parameters for nonoperative management of pediatric forearm fractures are reviewed, followed by clinical and imaging workups of malunions and decision-making points for treatment. The landscape of available technology for planning and execution of corrective osteotomy is discussed. Several cases of pediatric forearm malunion are presented, along with surgical and functional outcomes. Recommendations are given regarding the authors' preferred approach for management of pediatric forearm malunions.

Although distal radius fractures are common injuries, nonunion is extremely rare. Nonunion has been associated with increased metaphyseal comminution, concomitant distal ulna fracture, inadequate immobilization, and patient factors. Nonunion should be suspected in patients with persistent pain, limited range of motion, and worsening wrist deformity after wrist remobilization. Treatment selection depends on presence of infection, status of the radiocarpal and distal radioulnar joints, and type of prior surgical interventions. Multiple surgical techniques exist for managing distal radius nonunions including open reduction and internal fixation of the nonunion site with/without bone graft augmentation versus total wrist arthrodesis.

Distal radius fractures are common injuries. Satisfactory outcomes are typically achieved with appropriate nonoperative or operative treatment. A proportion of these injuries develop symptomatic malunions, which may be treated surgically with distal radius corrective osteotomy. A thorough understanding of the anatomy, biomechanics, radiographic parameters, and indications is needed to provide appropriate treatment. Factors, including surgical approach, osteotomy type, use of bone graft, fixation construct, management of associated tendon and/or nerve conditions, soft tissue contracture releases, and need for ulnar-sided procedures, should be considered. A comprehensive evaluation is necessary to guide understanding for when salvage procedures may be preferred.

Intra-articular malunion of the distal radius represents a difficult clinical problem. While not all patients require treatment, corrective osteotomy may significantly improve motion, grip strength, and patient-reported outcome measures. Meticulous planning and technical precision are required with the possible need for multiple surgical approaches and both volar and dorsal implants. Arthroscopic assistance may be used to visualize the joint and articular reduction. Custom 3-dimensional planning guides are helpful in addressing complex multiplanar deformities. Regardless, intervention may not change the natural history of these injuries and post-traumatic arthritis is to be expected.

 Video content accompanies this article at http://www.hand.theclinics.com.

Although its precise added value and cost-effectiveness need to be determined, three-dimensional (3D) planning and intraoperative guidance facilitate restoration of normal anatomy. The use of 3D computer planning and patient-specific intraoperative guides leads to more accurate and reproducible correction of forearm and wrist malunion. Its value augments with increasing complexity of deformities. Combined deformities and complex intra-articular malunions of the forearm and wrist benefit the most from the use of 3D techniques. New technical developments, including lower-dose scanning technology, software improvement, artificial intelligence, and in-hospital printing, may lower the associated costs and make its application more accessible.

Ulnar styloid fractures commonly occur in the setting of distal radius fractures and often progress to asymptomatic nonunion. Displaced basilar ulnar styloid fractures involving the deep radioulnar ligament attachments may cause distal radioulnar joint (DRUJ) instability. A careful clinical history, physical examination, review of imaging studies, and selected diagnostic interventions are important for confirming the relationship of the ulnar styloid nonunion with ulnar-sided wrist symptoms and/or DRUJ instability. Improved functional and symptomatic outcomes can be achieved with nonunion repair or fragment excision with or without triangular fibrocartilage complex repair, depending on the location and size of the ulnar styloid fracture.

Management of scaphoid nonunion remains challenging despite modern fixation techniques. Nonvascularized bone graft may be used to achieve union in waist and proximal pole fractures with good success rates. Technical aspects, such as adequate debridement and restoration of scaphoid length, and stable fixation are critical in achieving union and functional wrist usage. Rigid fixation can be achieved with compression screws, K-wires, and plate constructs. The surgeon has a choice of various bone graft options including corticocancellous, cancellous, and strut grafts to promote healing and correct the humpback deformity.

If untreated, scaphoid nonunions may progress to scaphoid nonunion advanced collapse in a substantial portion of cases and may require salvage procedures. Multiple different techniques have been described to address scaphoid nonunion. Vascularized bone flaps (VBFs) are associated with faster time to union compared with nonvascularized grafts. Because these are local pedicled flaps, they do not require microsurgical anastomoses and should be within the armamentarium of all hand surgeons. Appropriately chosen local VBFs, can achieve union rates up to 90% to 100% in appropriately selected patients.

The majority of phalangeal and metacarpal fractures will proceed to union when appropriately treated. However, when a nonunion does occur, it can lead to significant functional impairment for patients and societal costs. Operative intervention is

HAND CLINICS

Preface
When Things Don't Heal as Planned

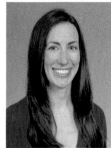
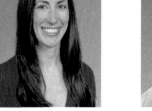

Erin A. Miller, MD, MS, FACS   Jerry I. Huang, MD
Editors

While a surgeon can reduce and stabilize a fracture perfectly, they cannot physically knit the bone back to its premorbid state. Bony healing is a complex process that is dependent on biologic, biomechanical, and environmental factors. With appropriate treatment, most fractures heal uneventfully with satisfactory function. Nonunions and symptomatic malunions are both rare. The low frequency with which we see these problems, however, makes them more difficult to treat. In this issue of *Hand Clinics*, we explore both nonunions and malunions in the upper extremity from the forearm to the fingertips.

Our goal in this issue is to provide the reader with guidance on the next steps in treatment when bones don't heal as planned. The review of bone healing at the outset of this issue is an essential foundation for the discussions that follow. This is followed by an overview of the plethora of bone graft substitutes that are available in a surgeon's armamentarium for treating bone defects. Outside the scaphoid nonunion literature, there is a paucity of evidence-based recommendations for other nonunions in the upper extremity. While the articles that follow seek to present hard data, the low frequency of nonunion makes it difficult to study in a rigorous fashion. Beginning in the forearm, we work distally into the wrist and then

fingers to discuss treatment algorithms and options for treatment of nonunions, including use of traditional bone grafting, local vascularized pedicle bone grafts, and free vascularized bone grafts. Malunion requiring surgical correction is even rarer in the upper extremity, as most patients can tolerate mild deformities without functional deficits. Despite the low volume, our authors have compiled evidence with expert opinion to provide a comprehensive resource in achieving restoration of bony anatomy. Advances in wrist arthroscopy and emerging technology of custom 3D cutting guides allow for more accurate restoration of anatomy for malunions. Each of these articles contains valuable guidance for success, and we hope it will be useful to the reader the next time you are preparing for a difficult case.

We thank the authors of each article for taking the time out of their busy surgical schedules to write; we appreciate the work that went into these articles through numerous revisions. We would also like to voice our appreciation to Hannah Lopez and Akshay Samson from Elsevier, who were essential in bringing this issue to publication. An additional thank you to Kevin Chung for the invitation and opportunity to edit this issue. Finally, both of us are indebted to our patients, who present to us with these challenging problems and

Hand Clin 40 (2024) xiii–xiv
https://doi.org/10.1016/j.hcl.2023.09.004
0749-0712/24/© 2023 Published by Elsevier Inc.

for entrusting us to come up with solutions to help them restore their hand and upper-extremity function.

Erin A. Miller, MD, MS, FACS
Division of Plastic Surgery
Department of Surgery
Department of Orthopedic Surgery
University of Washington Medical Centers
Division of Plastic and Reconstructive Surgery
University of Washington, 325 9th Avenue,
Mailstop 359796
Seattle, WA 98104, USA

Jerry I. Huang, MD
Department of Orthopedics and Sports Medicine
University of Washington Medical Centers
Department of Orthopedic Surgery
University of Washington 4245 Roosevelt Way NE
Box 357140
Seattle, WA 98105, USA

E-mail addresses:
erinmill@uw.edu (E.A. Miller)
jihuang@uw.edu (J.I. Huang)

Principles and Evaluation of Bony Unions

Tamara D. Rozental, MD[a],*, Ian T. Watkins, MD[b,c]

KEYWORDS

- Nonunion • Fracture healing • Bony union

KEY POINTS

- Nonunion is a poorly defined diagnosis.
- Bone healing is affected by patient-dependent and patient-independent factors.
- Evaluation of bony union is based on careful history and physical examination, radiographic evaluation, and further investigations include laboratory markers and advanced imaging modalities.

GOALS

How to diagnose and evaluate bony union.

INTRODUCTION

The evaluation of bone healing is a critically important skill for hand surgeons. Whether managing fractures or following postoperative fusions and osteotomies, determining when a bone is healed allows for the liberalization of immobilization and progression toward weightbearing. Conversely, understanding abnormal bone healing and when to intervene is of paramount importance in restoring function and returning patients to activities.

In 1998, the FDA wrote, "the decision that a nonunion has been established should not be made until a minimum of nine months has elapsed since the injury, and the fracture site has shown no radiographical sign of healing progression, that is, no change in the fracture callus, for the final three months (ie, six months to be considered a nonunion plus three additional months to verify that the nonunion is established)."[1] This definition, nearly 25 years old, uses a time-based distinction that does not allow diagnosis of nonunion prior to nine months, far longer than many orthopedic surgeons are willing to wait prior to intervention.

Indeed, the diagnosis of nonunion is a moving target. In a large survey of 444 orthopedic surgeons, Mohit and colleagues found little consensus in the definitions of normal fracture healing of tibial shaft fractures, with wide variation in acceptable time frames for union.[2] In an analysis of 148 prospective clinical studies on adult long-bone fracture nonunions, Wittauer and colleagues found a startling lack of agreement on the very definition of what the papers aimed to study. Of the studies, only 50% provided a definition of nonunion. Of these studies, 85% defined nonunion based on a time-related criteria, 62% on radiographic criteria, and 45% on clinical criteria. In 38% of the studies, the definition was based on a combination of time, radiographic, and clinical-related criteria. Furthermore, when analyzing time-based studies, Wittauer and colleagues reported a wide variation of cutoffs ranging from 3 to 12 months.[3]

Other, more pragmatic, definitions have been proposed. The 2020 Danish Orthopedic Trauma Society published a consensus from their fourth annual meeting on nonunion, defining the entity as "a fracture that will not heal without further intervention."[4] While there is certainly much controversy over what exactly constitutes a nonunion,

[a] Hand and Upper Extremity Surgery, Department of Orthopaedic Surgery, Beth Israel Deaconess Medical Center, Harvard Medical School, 330 Brookline Avenue - Stoneman 10, Boston, MA, 02215, USA; [b] Harvard Combined Orthopaedic Residency Program, Harvard Medical School, 55 Fruit Street, Boston, MA 02114, USA; [c] Division of Hand and Upper Extremity Surgery, Department of Orthopedics, Beth Israel Deaconess Medical Center, Harvard Medical School, Boston, MA, USA
* Corresponding author. Department of Orthopaedic Surgery, Beth Israel Deaconess Medical Center, Harvard Medical School, 330 Brookline Avenue - Stoneman 10, Boston, MA, 02215.
E-mail address: trozenta@bidmc.harvard.edu

Hand Clin 40 (2024) 1–12
https://doi.org/10.1016/j.hcl.2023.06.001

the threshold for diagnosis needs to be refined from "I know it when I see it" to a more tangible definition allowing us to compare and analyze the available evidence and to diagnose and treat afflicted patients. *It is our opinion that the diagnosis of nonunion should be made with respect to patient and fracture characteristics and specific to the bone in which it is observed. For general purposes, however, we define bony union as healing that allows for painless physiologic loading and motion.*

EPIDEMIOLOGY AND COST

Nonunion is a common problem, with 2% to 10% of all fractures developing nonunion.[5] In a large-scale demographic study of nonunions in Scotland, Mills and colleagues found an overall nonunion rate of 2%. They found that men are more likely to develop nonunion (57% vs 43% of total nonunions), with incidence peaking from age 35 to 44 years. Interestingly, they found that men were more likely to develop a nonunion at younger ages (25–34 years) compared to women, who most commonly developed nonunions from age 65 to 74 years, likely reflecting the high energy nature of fractures sustained by young men and the metabolic abnormalities of older women.[6] Other groups have found that while women had more fractures, men had a higher proportion of nonunions.[7]

It is difficult to evaluate the true impact of nonunions, including the pain and disruption of daily life caused by nonunions; however, several groups have demonstrated the significant mental health burden associated with nonunions using surveys and interviews. Brinker and colleagues found that tibial shaft nonunions were associated with a substantial burden on mental health as measured by Short Form (SF)-12 Mental Component Summary scores.[8] In evaluating the financial impacts of nonunion, a retrospective study of 99 nonunions in a cohort of 853 tibial shaft fractures, Antonova and colleagues found a mean total care cost of 25,556 USD for the nonunion group versus 11,686 USD for the routine healing group.[9] In an Australian analysis of long bone fractures over a 2 year period, admissions for nonunion were associated with a total cost of 4.9 million AUD, with a median cost of 14,957 AUD per fracture.[10] Clearly, nonunion is a financially as well as personally costly diagnosis.

Much of the literature on nonunions is focused on the lower extremity, with a significant amount of research on tibial nonunion. The upper extremity surgeon, however, also needs to be well-versed in the evaluation of nonunion. Specifically, the nonunions most likely to be encountered in the upper extremity clinic are those of the scaphoid and postoperative osteotomies. Accounting for roughly 70% of all carpal fractures, the scaphoid has a nonunion rate of 10% to 12% for all-comers, with a reported rate as high as 55% for fractures with displacement greater than 1 mm.[11] (**Fig. 1**). When treating ulnar impaction syndrome with an ulnar shortening osteotomy, 5.7% go on to delayed union, and a further 4% of all osteotomies go on to nonunion.[12] (see **Fig. 1**). Distal radial corrective osteotomies have a wide variance in reported nonunion rates, ranging from 1.8% to 21%, with risk factors including a corrective length of 5 mm or greater.[13] Likewise, when treating intra-articular distal humerus fractures with an olecranon osteotomy used for exposure, reported nonunion rates of the osteotomy site range from 3.3% to 13.3%.[14] Accurately evaluating and understanding what is normal healing is of paramount importance in the hand clinic.

It is important to understand bony union for the management of fusions as well as fractures. The "four corner" fusion of capitate, lunate, hamate, and triquetrum has a nonunion rate of between 2% and 22%.[15] These varying rates may be attributed to evolving technologies and surgical techniques. Likewise, in a metanalysis of distal interphalangeal joint arthrodesis, Dickson and colleagues found that, depending on the technique used, nearly 9% of patients can develop nonunion.[16] By understanding the biologic and mechanical necessities of fracture healing, surgeons can better understand and manage fusion procedures.

RISK FACTORS

There are several patient-dependent and patient-independent factors that can affect bone healing that are important to be aware of when managing fracture and fusion patients. Directed and thoughtful history taking in the office can identify features that can portend poor outcomes and warrant further workup or closer monitoring.

There are several patient-independent factors that can lead to delayed union or nonunion that are important to understand when evaluating patients. In a large-scale evaluation of health claims data for 309,330 appendicular skeletal fractures, Zura and colleagues found an overall nonunion rate of 4.9%, with more severe injury burden (open fracture and multiple fractures) being the highest risk factor for the development of nonunion.[7] Open fractures went on to nonunion at more than double the rate of closed fractures (10.9% to 4.7%). Open injuries are at a high risk for nonunion as both infection and disruption of the soft tissue environment creates an unfavorable

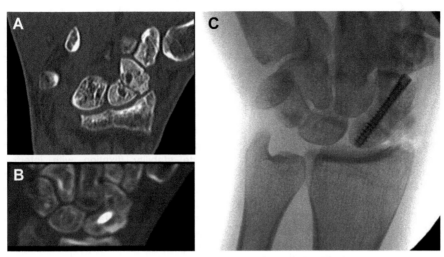

Fig. 1. 3-year-old scaphoid nonunion without callus formation, subchondral cysts (*A*), treated with bone grafting and ORIF (*C*) and healing (*B*).

environment for the complex cellular interactions required for bony healing.[17] Zura and colleagues also found that patients with more than 7 fractures went on to have at least one nonunion 24% of the time, compared to a 4.4% nonunion rate in patients with a solitary fracture. This group also found scaphoid (15.5% nonunion), tibial (14%), and femur (13.9%) fractures develop nonunion at the highest rates.[18]

Indeed, fractures in various parts of the same bone can have varying rates of nonunion.[18] Healing can take longer in certain fractures due to the bone's blood supply. For example, the retrograde blood supply of the scaphoid and fifth metatarsal base contributes to the development of nonunion or delayed union.[19] Likewise, some fractures are inherently unstable, leading to increased mechanical forces beyond which a bone can heal. Scaphoid fractures are subject to complex flexion/extension and rotational forces that predispose this fracture to nonunion.[20] By understanding the mechanism of fracture, the blood supply of the fracture, the displacing forces of a fracture, and epidemiology, a clinician can better evaluate the healing capabilities and tendencies to develop nonunion.

There are a variety of patient-dependent factors that can affect bone healing that clinicians must be aware of as well. Behavioral and social factors such as high BMI, smoking, and alcoholism are some of the highest risk factors for abnormal bone healing.[21] Smoking has a strong deleterious effect on bone healing. In a systematic review, Scolaro and colleagues found smokers had an odds ratio of nonunion of 2.32 when compared to nonsmokers.[22] Even when union is achieved at final follow-up, Hall and colleagues found that when

compared to smokers, nonsmokers had higher radiographic union scores at 3 months and better *Quick*DASH scores.[23] Markers of overall poor health, including diabetes, medications such as anticoagulants, anticonvulsants, insulin, and opioid use were all associated with an increased risk of nonunion.[7]

Much has been written about the risk of nonunion in diabetics undergoing foot and ankle surgery. Hemoglobin A1c levels and peripheral neuropathy have been shown to be independent risk factors for the development of nonunion in several studies.[24] Metabolic and endocrine anomalies such as vitamin D deficiency, thyroid disorders, and undiagnosed bone metabolism can all negatively impact the bone healing pathways.[25] Similarly, chronic inflammatory conditions impact time to bony union. In mouse models of chronic inflammatory conditions, both soft callus remodeling as well as osteoclast activity were altered, negatively affecting bony union.[26,27] These numerous markers of poor overall health can have deleterious impacts on bone healing. Some of these are modifiable while others are not, and it is important to understand these interactions to accurately interpret bony union.

Surgical techniques can impact the rate of nonunion. Inadequate fixation with insufficient stiffness creating excessive fracture mobility is a risk factor for the development of nonunion.[28] Fractures require an appropriate mechanical environment to allow for healing. As we will discuss later, complex strain-dependent signal transduction pathways guide mesenchymal cell proliferation and bony healing. Too much strain at the fracture site can lead to disruption of these complex pathways. **Fig. 2** demonstrates a nonunion related to an unfavorable mechanical environment after an inadequate orpen eduction internal fixation (ORIF) of a humerus creating too much fracture-site motion. Healing was achieved by providing a more robust mechanical environment for bone healing through a bigger limited contact dynamic compression plate (LCDC plate).

BIOLOGY OF BONE HEALING

As discussed earlier, the precise definition of nonunion is controversial. It is, therefore, important to understand normal bone healing to understand the ways that it can go wrong. Bone healing is a complex process that can be affected by intrinsic and extrinsic factors. Following a trauma, bone heals either by primary (intramembranous) or secondary (a mixture of intramembranous and endochondral) bone formation.

Fracture healing begins with an anabolic phase of tissue inflammation and hematoma formation. This hematoma acts as a temporary stabilizer for the proliferation of mesenchymal cells. This inflammatory phase is marked by several cytokines that promote cell migration and differentiation. The cellular environment and mechanical environment have a close interplay, with the mechanical environment dictating the route of bone healing. With intramembranous bone healing, the mesenchymal stem cells differentiate into osteoblasts and lay down woven bone that undergoes Haversian remodeling to form lamellar bone. In endochondral bone formation, the more unstable mechanical environment stimulates the hematoma to form a "soft callus," a cartilaginous intermediary that is then remodeled into lamellar bone via osteoblasts and osteoclasts.[29]

Primary bone healing requires an anatomic reduction, compression, and fixation limiting interfragmentary strain to less than 2%, allowing for direct remodeling of lamellar bone without callus formation.[29] Secondary bone healing, on the other hand, does not require anatomic reduction and relies on an inflammatory milieu that attracts diverse cell lines and leads to a cartilaginous intermediary and callus formation before bone remodeling. As a general rule, primary bone healing occurs with absolute stability (fixation with interfragmentary compression) and secondary bone healing with relative stability (intramedullary fixation, bridge plating, and nonoperative management).[30] It is important to understand the mode in which we expect the fracture to heal when we are evaluating patients who have suspected delayed union or nonunion. By understanding the many biologic and structural requirements for bone healing, a surgeon can understand the various ways bone healing can fail.

CLINICAL EVALUATION

In order for a bone to heal, it needs a favorable mechanical environment as well as a favorable biologic environment. It is important to identify if there is a biologic failure (see **Fig. 1**), a mechanical failure (see **Fig. 2**), or a mixed picture (**Fig. 3**). When evaluating a patient for a possible nonunion, one must consider several factors. These include biology and stability, as well as the patient-dependent and independent characteristics mentioned earlier.

First, a thorough history and physical examination is paramount to any assessment of nonunion. Establishing the injury time course, whether the

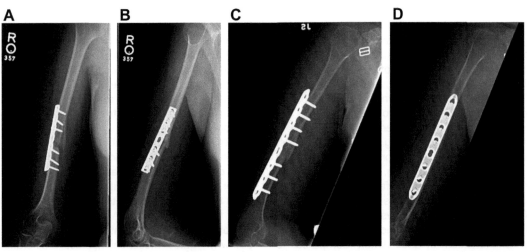

Fig. 2. Nonunion due to inadequate mechanical environment for healing (*A, B*). Treated with revision ORIF with bone graft with healing (*C, D*).

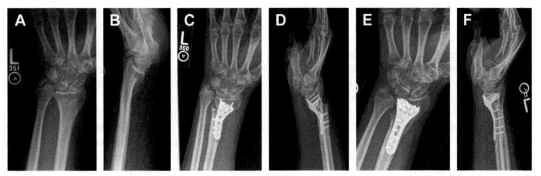

Fig. 3. Presented to clinic with malunion s/p DRF (*A, B*). Underwent fixation with allograft and developed nonunion with hardware failure (*C, D*). Treated with revision ORIF with ICBG and healed (*E, F*).

fracture was closed or open, the presence of bone loss, as well as the postoperative course, and determining the various host factors (including patient compliance) that impact union are crucial to understanding the fracture. The patient's medical history, including medical comorbidities as well as history of multiple fractures or other delayed unions or nonunions, is also critically important. Physical examination for signs of infection, overall limb alignment, signs of compensatory changes in adjacent joints, and pain with motion of the fracture are important data points to help guide diagnostics and treatment. Due to the controversy regarding the true diagnosis of nonunion, several studies have used clinical signs to define fracture union. These physical examination signs are simple to perform, require no diagnostic testing, are free, and are correlated with union. The following were the most commonly cited physical examination findings that studies used to assess for union: lack of pain with weightbearing, lack of pain with palpation at the fracture site, and the ability to bear weight.[31]

RADIOGRAPHIC ASSESSMENT
Plain Radiography

The evaluation of nonunion was traditionally based on plain radiographs and divided into *hypertrophic, oligotrophic, and atrophic* nonunions. A hypertrophic nonunion showed good biologic potential for healing with abundant callus formation but persistence of the fracture line. This was attributed to a fracture with excessive motion. An oligotrophic nonunion has less callus formation than hypertrophic nonunions, likely caused by a combination of biology and structural deficiencies. An atrophic nonunion has no callus formation, possibly indicating a biologic deficiency.[32] These broad categories have been challenged recently in the literature; however, it is important to understand that these categories were largely based on

radiographic studies of fractures managed nonoperatively. Of course, reality is more complicated than these 3 finite groups. Indeed, histologic analysis of both hypertrophic and atrophic nonunions shows no difference in the vascularity at the fracture site, challenging the idea that an atrophic nonunion is biologically deficient.[33] With further understanding of the methods of fixation and primary and secondary bone healing, these broad definitions can be informative about the etiology of nonunion.

As discussed earlier, it is important to remember the mode with which the bone is expected to heal. In fractures that are anatomically reduced and fixed in compression, you do not expect to see callus. In fractures where you expect secondary bone healing, callus should be found in a healing bone. By analyzing the formation of callus and the obliteration of fracture lines, orthogonal radiographs provide useful information related to fracture healing. Serial radiographs should show progressive callus formation and gradual blurring of the fracture line. These radiographic factors have been validated in animal models to correlate with mechanical fracture healing via measurement of torsional strength and stiffness.[34]

Unfortunately, the observation of callus, fracture lines, and other radiographic findings can be quite subjective and difficult to interpret. When evaluating scaphoid fractures with plain radiography, one of the radiographic features of poor blood flow and the possible development of nonunion is the presence of sclerosis. Sclerosis, however, may be a representation of new bone formation, dystrophic calcification, or relative osteopenia compared to the adjacent bones. It is, therefore, difficult to use sclerosis of the scaphoid as a useful predictor of healing.[35]

There have been recent pushes to standardize and categorize fracture healing. The Radiographic Union Scale of Tibia Fractures (RUST) score was developed to bring greater interobserver reliability to a subjective process. The RUST score judges the presence of callus at a fracture line on all 4 cortices using orthogonal radiographs. Each cortex (anterior, posterior, lateral, and medial) is graded on a scale of 1 to 3, with 1 being no callus and visible fracture line and 3 being bridging callus and no fracture line.[36,37] This score has been validated as a reproducible and useful way to evaluate the healing of tibia fractures.[36] Similar tools have been developed and validated to evaluate the healing of operatively treated hip fractures, using the RUSH score (radiographic union score in hip fractures).[26] When specifically applied to the upper extremity, this approach has proven useful in humeral shaft fractures, using the RHUM score, and distal radius fractures, using the RUSS score.[38,39] While evaluating distal radius fractures using the RUSS score, Patel and colleagues found strong intraobserver and interobserver reliability, and through multivariate logistical regressions that both RUSS score and time after fracture were predictors of union. These scoring systems are useful to help quantify healing, follow healing over months, and communicate with other providers. We should encourage the development of these radiographic healing scores to follow fracture healing over time to better delineate the development of a nonunion and to correlate them with computed tomography (CT) to predict fracture healing.

Computed Tomography

CT is a powerful tool to evaluate for bony union but is associated with higher doses of radiation and cost.[40] A standard chest radiograph can have 0.02 mSv of radiation, while a CT of the abdomen and pelvis has roughly 10 mSv.[41] With newer technology and methodology, CT imaging is becoming safer with less radiation dose exposure. In a study of 312 patients who underwent CT scans, Iordache and colleagues found that a CT shoulder, a CT elbow (with arm adjacent to torso), as well as a CT pelvis, all had similar radiation exposure (0.014 vs 0.015 vs 0.015 mSv/mGyXcm, respectively). Interestingly, a CT elbow with arm above the head had an equivalent dose of radiation as a CT wrist (0.0008 mSv/mGyXcm).[40] CT imaging, through new detector technology and safety standards, is becoming a less significant source of radiation exposure, especially in the upper extremities.

CT can help diagnose a radiographic union by evaluating the formation of bridging callus with secondary bone healing and identifying areas of persistent fracture line in the presence of primary bone healing. This analysis, however, is subject to metal artifact in fractures and fusions with

surrounding hardware. It may, however, have differing utility depending on the fracture.

CT is helpful in evaluating fractures that are difficult to image on plain radiographs (see **Fig. 3**), as well as fractures with equivocal radiographic findings. In an evaluation of a heterogeneous fracture database, Kleinlugtenbelt and colleagues found that when evaluating plain radiographs, 20 independent observers had fair interobserver diagnostic reliability when assessing union. Interestingly, CT scan provided no improvement in the interobserver reliability. In equivocal cases, CT scan evaluation led to more recommendations for operative rather than nonoperative treatment. This group argues that when the clinical picture is clear on radiographs, CT provides no benefit and when used in equivocal cases, leads to more aggressive treatment plans.[42]

It appears that CT has different efficacy depending on the bone that is being analyzed. Nicholson and colleagues looked at clavicle nonunions and found that CT had higher interobserver agreement for union compared to plain radiographs, and CT overall had 100% sensitivity and 82% specificity for nonunion diagnosis.[43] Like clavicles, CT can help evaluate scaphoid fracture healing (**Fig. 4**). CT can be used to detect findings such as subtle displacement and comminution, sclerosis, and give a better understanding of the fracture location that would otherwise be difficult to discern on plain radiographs (**Fig. 5**). These factors have been shown to impact time to union and predilection to develop nonunion.[44]

CT technology has been used to create virtual stress testing (VST), a computer-based biomechanical model based on inputs from a CT that converts gray-scale values to equivalent bone mineral density to determine the structural stability of the bone. By performing VST on 65 soldiers with tibia fractures being treated in external fixation, Petfield and colleagues showed that they were able to identify the patients who went on to nonunion. By focusing on the analysis of compression loading and torsional strength, VST models were 100% sensitive with a 40.9% positive predictive value of identifying the development of nonunion. Originally used to predict the risk of hip or vertebral fracture in patients with osteoporosis, VST has been adapted to provide a quantifiable way to identify patients with healing tibia fractures who can safely resume weightbearing.[45]

Nuclear Medicine

Infection is a key cause of union failure. Recently, [^{18}F]FDG PET/CT has been used to guide the diagnosis of septic nonunion. In a retrospective study of 47 patients treated for nonunion who underwent

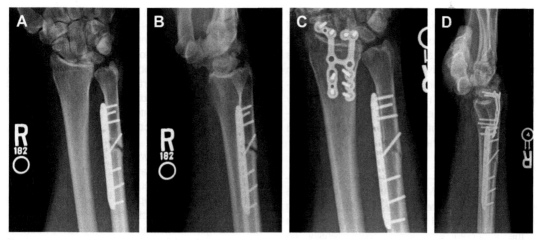

Fig. 4. Nonunion after ulnar shortening osteotomy for ulnar impaction (A, B). Healing after repeat bone grafting and radioscapholunate fusion for radiocarpal DJD (C, D).

PET/CT, Sollini and colleagues showed that PET/CT may be a promising tool for the diagnosis of septic nonunion. Of the 47 patients treated, 25 had septic nonunions as defined by positive intraoperative cultures. Of these 25 septic nonunions, 20% of them had C-reactive protein (CRP) values within normal limits. Of these 25 infected nonunions, 23 were correctly detected on PET/CT. In the final analysis, PET/CT had a sensitivity and specificity of 92% and 68%, respectively. This group found PET/CT especially helpful in the detection of these infections.[46]

Bone scans may also be used to detect the biologic activity of a fracture. These scans can be helpful for diagnosis and planning management.

Bone scintigraphy can be used to detect blood flow and new bone formation and guide treatment.[47] This can be helpful in determining the etiology of nonunion as a biologic or mechanical failure. As discussed earlier, a lack of biologic activity may necessitate a different treatment modality than robust biologic activity without union.

Ultrasound

Fracture union can also be evaluated using ultrasound. This imaging modality is inexpensive and does not use radiation. Much of the research in ultrasound evaluation of fractures has been done in pediatrics.[48] In a study of new bone formation

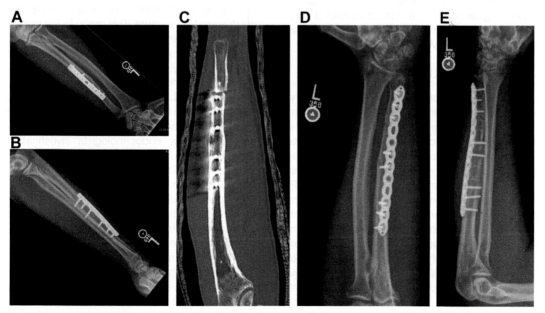

Fig. 5. Ulnar peri-implant fracture that developed a nonunion difficult to detect on plain radiographs alone (A–C), treated with revision ORIF w/autograft (D, E).

during long bone lengthening, ultrasound was able to detect new bone formation within 2 weeks of distraction, while it took 4 to 8 weeks to detect on radiographs.[49] In a study of clavicle fractures managed nonoperatively, ultrasound evaluation at 6 weeks showing bridging soft callus was a reliable predictor of union at 6 months.[50] The difficulty with ultrasonography is the subjectivity of interpretation and the lack of familiarity that most hand surgeons have with the technology.

MRI

Currently, the role of MRI for evaluation of fracture healing is limited; however, MRI with gadolinium contrast can be useful in the diagnosis of nonunion in the scaphoid with low signal intensity on T1-weighted images. In a study comparing contrast-enhanced MRI and the gold standard of intraoperative bleeding from the proximal pole, 90% of scaphoids with MRI findings consistent with Avascular Necrosis (AVN) had a confirmed intraoperative diagnosis.[51]

MRI is also excellent at evaluating and determining if there is a collection of fluid surrounding a fracture site, which is indicative of an infection. Like CT scan, using MRI while monitoring for fracture healing in the setting of an ORIF is subject to metal artifact, even with metal subtraction sequences. MRI has recently been used to evaluate the vascularity of established nonunion sites using a dynamic contrast-enhanced (DCE) sequence. This sequence was able to evaluate contrast uptake in the perifracture area compared to the surrounding muscle. Using this technique, Schoierer and colleagues found that well-vascularized nonunions fared better than less vascular ones, as determined by DCE MRI.[52]

LABORATORY EVALUATION

In coordination with physical examination, history, and imaging, laboratory evaluation can be a powerful tool to use to help evaluate bony union. Any time you suspect a nonunion, it is important to evaluate for infection. Apart from the physical examination findings as discussed earlier, infection can be investigated with a complete blood count (CBC), CRP, and erythrocyte sedimentation rate (ESR). These laboratory values can help guide management; however, they are not diagnostic of infection. Wang and colleagues found the sensitivity and specificity for identifying infected nonunion of elevated CRP values to be at 60% and 85%, respectively. This group evaluated 42 patients with CBC, CRP, ESR, and interleukin-6 (IL-6) and found that with 1, 2, 3, and 4 positive tests, the predicted probabilities of infection were 66.7%, 90%, 100%,

and 100%, respectively; however, there were very few patients with 3 or 4 positive tests. They found that IL-6 was an inferior laboratory marker to CRP.[53] It is important to be aware that septic nonunions frequently present with normal inflammatory markers, and it is important to always have them in the differential.[46] Indeed, in a cohort of 453 patients with risk factors for infection (history of surgery, infection, or open fracture) treated for nonunion, 20% had a "surprise" positive nonunion culture, meaning that infection was not anticipated preoperatively based on negative laboratory markers.[54] Positive fracture-site culture is the gold standard for the diagnosis of septic nonunion, and it takes an astute clinician to factor in the physical examination findings, the history, the radiographic information, and the laboratory findings to correctly diagnose an infection.

Seemingly healthy patients who exhibit delayed time to union or nonunion given adequate fixation or immobilization should warrant further evaluation. In addition to infection, a variety of other medical conditions can impact fracture healing, including vitamin D deficiency, diabetes, hypogonadism, and imbalances of calcium, growth hormone, and PTH.[55] From a subset of 683 patients with nonunions of the upper and lower extremities, Brinker and colleagues referred 37 patients to an endocrinologist for further evaluation. Their screening criteria were (1) unexplained nonunion that occurred despite adequate reduction and stabilization without technical error and without other obvious etiologies; (2) a history of multiple low-energy fractures with at least one progressing to nonunion; or (3) a nonunion of a nondisplaced pubic rami or sacral ala fracture. This group found that by using these screening criteria, 31 of the 37 patients were newly diagnosed with a metabolic or endocrine abnormality, with the most common being vitamin D deficiency.[25] Eight of these patients with newly diagnosed metabolic derangements were treated medically and eventually went onto union without surgical management. The basic laboratory panel ordered by endocrinologists investigating metabolic bone disorders consists of serum calcium, serum 25-hydroxyvitamin D, thyroid-stimulating hormone, phosphorus, and alkaline phosphatase levels. Clinicians managing fractures with suspected delayed union or nonunion in the setting of adequate fixation should have a high suspicion for an underlying metabolic condition and a low threshold for referral to an endocrinologist.

Like imaging, however, laboratory testing can be quite expensive. Shapiro and colleagues found that a routine endocrinology laboratory panel cost $519 in their hospital system, while an infection panel cost just under $100.[56] It is important to have a healthy appreciation for the financial impacts of routine endocrine testing, and referral to an endocrinologist for further evaluation for both diagnostic and therapeutic management can be an effective strategy.[25]

SUMMARY

Nonunion has devastating impacts on patients recovering from fusion and fracture. Nonunion patients report lower health-related quality of life scores than patients with type-1 diabetes, stroke, and HIV. With particular interest for upper extremity surgeons, nonunions of the forearm had the worst self-reported utility scores of all bones measured.[57] An overwhelming majority of fractures go onto bony union without difficulty. There are, however, high-risk features that can greatly influence the rate and time course of healing. Without a clear, universally agreed-upon definition, identifying a nonunion is a diagnostic challenge. Currently, most nonunions are diagnosed by a "I know it when I see it" philosophy. One point of agreement is that a nonunion, in the absence of metabolic derangement, will not heal without further surgical intervention. It would, therefore, be helpful to have widely agreed-upon guidelines for the diagnosis of nonunion that are specific to certain fractures, especially those that have a higher propensity to develop nonunion.

Further study is necessary to quickly identify fractures that are developing nonunion as well as research on better management strategies. It is clear that certain patients are at higher risk for the development of nonunion than others; however, it is still very much a waiting game. With recent advances in large-scale data analytics, the goal is to be able to more accurately predict incipient nonunions, allowing for quicker action. Advances in big data, combined with validated radiographic nonunion scoring systems, can help to quickly and accurately identify nonunions. Additionally, more studies on advanced imaging modalities to detect poor blood flow as well as evidence of infection are needed. Newer MRI technology, advances in ultrasound techniques, and nuclear medicine modalities may all prove to be beneficial to evaluating bony healing or identifying features at high risk for developing nonunion.

Identifying a nonunion is only part of the picture. Further research is needed on how to prevent nonunion at the index surgery or when managing fractures nonoperatively. Either through improved surgical techniques to promote bony healing or reduce the risk of infection, or through modifying patient-related risk factors, identifying interventions that minimize the rate of nonunion is paramount.

Additionally, when we do identify nonunion, we need to have better tools and techniques to manage it. Future areas of research for the management of nonunion include biologic augmentation through growth factors and refining bone grafting techniques. Additionally, there may be a future role of nonoperative treatment through medical management due to newer understandings of the complex cellular interactions of bone healing.

Upper extremity-specific nonunion research is needed. Much of the research on nonunion is focused on lower extremity, especially tibia fractures. While many of the principles are the same, it is important to validate management strategies and tailor them to the unique anatomy and mechanical environment of the upper extremity.

CLINICS CARE POINTS

- Nonunion is a common problem, representing 2% to 10% of all fractures.
- Nonunion is a controversial topic with varying definitions.
- Bones have varying rates of nonunion, with scaphoid having the highest rate in the upper extremity.
- Both patient-dependent and independent factors can influence the rate of developing a nonunion.
  - Patient dependent
    - Smoking, osteoporosis, BMI, and medical comorbidities
  - Patient independent
    - Presence of open injury, infection, bone loss, the bone involved, and appropriateness of fixation strategy
- All evaluations should begin with a thorough history and physical examination looking for signs of motion at fracture site, infection, and pain.
- X-ray is the mainstay of radiographic evaluation.
- Infection should always be considered when evaluating delayed bony union.
- CBC, CRP, and ESR are all helpful in evaluating for infection; however, up to 20% of infected nonunions have normal CRP values.
- PET-CT can be helpful in finding CRP-negative infected nonunions.
- Patients with a high pretest probability of having poor bone healing may benefit from evaluation by an endocrinologist.

DISCLOSURE

Neither author has relevant conflicts of interest to disclose.

REFERENCES

1. Food and Drug Administration. Guidance Document for Industry and CDRH Staff for the Preparation of Investigational Device Exemptions and Premarket Approval Applications for Bone Growth Stimulator Devices; Draft; Availability. Federal Register. 1998.
2. Bhandari M, Guyatt GH, Swiontkowski MF, et al. A lack of consensus in the assessment of fracture healing among orthopaedic surgeons. J Orthop Trauma 2002;16(8). https://doi.org/10.1097/00005131-200209000-00004.
3. Wittauer M, Burch MA, McNally M, et al. Definition of long-bone nonunion: A scoping review of prospective clinical trials to evaluate current practice. Injury 2021; 52(11). https://doi.org/10.1016/j.injury.2021.09.008.
4. Schmal H, Brix M, Bue M, et al. Nonunion - consensus from the 4th annual meeting of the danish orthopaedic trauma society. EFORT Open Rev 2020;5(1). https://doi.org/10.1302/2058-5241.5.190037.
5. Tzioupis C, Giannoudis PV. Prevalence of long-bone non-unions. Injury 2007;38(SUPPL. 2). https://doi.org/10.1016/j.injury.2007.02.005.
6. Mills LA, Simpson AHRW. The relative incidence of fracture non-union in the Scottish population (5.17 million): A 5-year epidemiological study. BMJ Open 2013;3(2). https://doi.org/10.1136/bmjopen-2012-002276.
7. Zura R, Xiong Z, Einhorn T, et al. Epidemiology of fracture nonunion in 18 human bones. JAMA Surg 2016;151(11). https://doi.org/10.1001/jamasurg.2016.2775.
8. Brinker MR, Hanus BD, Sen M, et al. The devastating effects of tibial nonunion on health-related quality of life. J Bone Joint Surg 2013;95(24). https://doi.org/10.2106/JBJS.L.00803.
9. Antonova E, Le TK, Burge R, et al. Tibia shaft fractures: Costly burden of nonunions. BMC Musculoskelet Disord 2013;14. https://doi.org/10.1186/1471-2474-14-42.
10. Ekegren CL, Edwards ER, de Steiger R, et al. Incidence, costs and predictors of non-union, delayed union and mal-union following long bone fracture. Int J Environ Res Public Health 2018;15(12). https://doi.org/10.3390/ijerph15122845.
11. Sgromolo NM, Rhee PC. The Role of Vascularized Bone Grafting in Scaphoid Nonunion. Hand Clin 2019;35(3). https://doi.org/10.1016/j.hcl.2019.03.004.
12. Owens J, Compton J, Day M, et al. Nonunion Rates Among Ulnar-Shortening Osteotomy for Ulnar Impaction Syndrome: A Systematic Review. J Hand Surg 2019;44(7). https://doi.org/10.1016/j.jhsa.2018.08.018.
13. Clark DM, Hoyt BW, Piscoya AS, et al. Risk factors for distal radius osteotomy nonunion. Plast Reconstr Surg 2021;148. https://doi.org/10.1097/PRS.0000000000008512.
14. Meldrum A, Kwong C, Archibold K, et al. Olecranon Osteotomy Implant Removal Rates and Associated Complications. J Orthop Trauma 2021;35(5). https://doi.org/10.1097/BOT.0000000000001979.
15. Skie MC, Gove N, Ciocanel DE, et al. Management of non-united four-corner fusions. Hand 2007;2(1). https://doi.org/10.1007/s11552-007-9021-y.
16. Dickson DR, Mehta SS, Nuttall D, et al. A Systematic Review of Distal Interphalangeal Joint Arthrodesis. J Hand Microsurg 2016;06(02). https://doi.org/10.1007/s12593-014-0163-1.
17. Al-Hourani K, Pearce O, Kelly M. Standards of open lower limb fracture care in the United Kingdom. Injury 2021;52(3). https://doi.org/10.1016/j.injury.2021.01.021.
18. Fowler JR, Hughes TB. Scaphoid Fractures. Clin Sports Med 2015;34(1). https://doi.org/10.1016/j.csm.2014.09.011.
19. Morsy M, Sabbagh MD, van Alphen NA, et al. The Vascular Anatomy of the Scaphoid: New Discoveries Using Micro–Computed Tomography Imaging. J Hand Surg 2019;44(11). https://doi.org/10.1016/j.jhsa.2019.08.001.
20. Slade JF, Dodds SD. Minimally invasive management of scaphoid nonunions. Clin Orthop Relat Res 2006;445. https://doi.org/10.1097/01.blo.0000205886.66081.9d.
21. Liska F, Haller B, Voss A, et al. Smoking and obesity influence the risk of nonunion in lateral opening wedge, closing wedge and torsional distal femoral osteotomies. Knee Surg Sports Traumatol Arthrosc 2018; 26(9). https://doi.org/10.1007/s00167-017-4754-9.
22. Scolaro JA, Schenker ML, Yannascoli S, et al. Cigarette smoking increases complications following fracture: A systematic review. J Bone Joint Surg 2014;96(8). https://doi.org/10.2106/JBJS.M.00081.
23. Hall MJ, Ostergaard PJ, Dowlatshahi AS, et al. The Impact of Obesity and Smoking on Outcomes After Volar Plate Fixation of Distal Radius Fractures. J Hand Surg 2019;44(12). https://doi.org/10.1016/j.jhsa.2019.08.017.
24. Zura R, Mehta S, Della Rocca GJ, et al. Biological risk factors for nonunion of bone fracture. JBJS Rev 2016;4(1). https://doi.org/10.2106/JBJS.RVW.O.00008.
25. Brinker MR, O'Connor DP, Monla YT, et al. Metabolic and endocrine abnormalities in patients with nonunions. J Orthop Trauma 2007;21(8). https://doi.org/10.1097/BOT.0b013e31814d4dc6.
26. Alblowi J, Kayal RA, Siqueria M, et al. High levels of tumor necrosis factor-α contribute to accelerated

loss of cartilage in diabetic fracture healing. Am J Pathol 2009;175(4). https://doi.org/10.2353/ajpath. 2009.090148.

27. Al-Sebaei MO, Daukss DM, Belkina AC, et al. Role of fas and treg cells in fracture healing as character-ized in the fas-deficient (lpr) mouse model of lupus. J Bone Miner Res 2014;29(6). https://doi.org/10. 1002/jbmr.2169.

28. dos Reis FB, Faloppa F, Fernandes HJA, et al. Outcome of diaphyseal forearm fracture-nonunions treated by autologous bone grafting and compres-sion plating. Ann Surg Innov Res 2009;3. https:// doi.org/10.1186/1750-1164-3-5.

29. Ghiasi MS, Chen J, Vaziri A, et al. Bone fracture healing in mechanobiological modeling: A review of principles and methods. Bone Rep 2017;6. https://doi.org/10.1016/j.bonr.2017.03.002.

30. Marsell R, Einhorn TA. The biology of fracture healing. Injury 2011;42(6). https://doi.org/10.1016/j.injury. 2011.03.031.

31. Corrales LA, Morshed S, Bhandari M, et al. Vari-ability in the assessment of fracture-healing in ortho-paedic trauma studies. J Bone Joint Surg 2008; 90(9). https://doi.org/10.2106/JBJS.G.01580.

32. Nicholson JA, Makaram N, Simpson AHRW, et al. Fracture nonunion in long bones: A literature review of risk factors and surgical management. Injury 2021;52. https://doi.org/10.1016/j.injury.2020.11.029.

33. Reed AAC, Joyner CJ, Brownlow HC, et al. Human atrophic fracture non-unions are not avascular. J Orthop Res 2002;20(3). https://doi.org/10.1016/ S0736-0266(01)00142-5.

34. Panjabi MM, Walter SD, Karuda M, et al. Correlations of radiographic analysis of healing fractures with strength: A statistical analysis of experimental os-teotomies. J Orthop Res 1985;3(2). https://doi.org/ 10.1002/jor.1100030211.

35. Cheema HS, Cheema AN. Radiographic evaluation of vascularity in scaphoid nonunions: A review. World J Orthop 2020;11(11). https://doi.org/10. 5312/wjo.v11.i11.475.

36. Leow JM, Clement ND, Simpson AHWR. Application of the Radiographic Union Scale for Tibial fractures (RUST): Assessment of healing rate and time of tibial fractures managed with intramedullary nailing. J Orthop Traumatol: Surgery and Research 2020; 106(1). https://doi.org/10.1016/j.otsr.2019.10.010.

37. Whelan DB, Bhandari M, Stephen D, et al. Develop-ment of the radiographic union score for tibial frac-tures for the assessment of tibial fracture healing after intramedullary fixation. J Trauma Inj Infect Crit Care 2010;68(3). https://doi.org/10.1097/TA.0b013e 3181a7c16d.

38. Christiano AV, Goch AM, Burke CJ, et al. Radio-graphic Humerus Union Measurement (RHUM) Demonstrates High Inter- and Intraobserver Reli-ability in Assessing Humeral Shaft Fracture Healing.

HSS J 2020;16. https://doi.org/10.1007/s11420-019-09680-4.

39. Patel SP, Anthony SG, Zurakowski D, et al. Radio-graphic scoring system to evaluate union of distal radius fractures. J Hand Surg 2014;39(8). https:// doi.org/10.1016/j.jhsa.2014.05.022.

40. Iordache SD, Goldberg N, Paz L, et al. Radiation exposure from computed tomography of the upper limbs. Acta Orthop Belg 2017;83(4).

41. Coakley FV, Gould R, Yeh BM, et al. CT radiation dose: What can you do right now in your practice? Am J Roentgenol 2011;196(3). https://doi.org/10. 2214/AJR.10.5043.

42. Kleinlugtenbelt YV, Scholtes VAB, Toor J, et al. Does computed tomography change our observation and management of fracture non-unions? Archives of Bone and Joint Surgery 2016;4(4).

43. Nicholson JA, Fox B, Dhir R, et al. The accuracy of computed tomography for clavicle non-union evalu-ation. Shoulder Elbow 2021;13(2). https://doi.org/10. 1177/1758573219884067.

44. Grewal R, Suh N, MacDermid JC. Use of computed tomography to predict union and time to union in acute scaphoid fractures treated nonoperatively. J Hand Surg 2013;38(5). https://doi.org/10.1016/j. jhsa.2013.01.032.

45. Petfield JL, Hayeck GT, Kopperdahl DL, et al. Virtual stress testing of fracture stability in soldiers with severely comminuted tibial fractures. J Orthop Res 2017;35(4). https://doi.org/10.1002/jor.23335.

46. Sollini M, Trenti N, Malagoli E, et al. [18F]FDG PET/ CT in non-union: improving the diagnostic perfor-mances by using both PET and CT criteria. Eur J Nucl Med Mol Imaging 2019;46(8). https://doi.org/ 10.1007/s00259-019-04336-1.

47. Gandhi SJ, Rabadiya B. Bone scan in detection of biological activity in nonhypertrophic fracture nonunion. Indian J Nucl Med 2017;32(4). https:// doi.org/10.4103/ijnm.IJNM_50_17.

48. Nicholson JA, Yapp LZ, Keating JF, et al. Monitoring of fracture healing. Update on current and future im-aging modalities to predict union. Injury 2021;52. https://doi.org/10.1016/j.injury.2020.08.016.

49. Eyres KS, Bell MJ, Kanis JA. Methods of assessing new bone formation during limb lengthening. Ultra-sonography, dual energy x-ray absorptiometry and radiography compared. Journal of Bone and Joint Surgery - Series B 1993;75(3). https://doi.org/10. 1302/0301-620x.75b3.8496200.

50. Nicholson JA, Oliver WM, LizHang J, et al. Sono-graphic bridging callus: An early predictor of frac-ture union. Injury 2019;50(12). https://doi.org/10. 1016/j.injury.2019.09.027.

51. Bervian MR, Ribak S, Livani B. Scaphoid fracture nonunion: correlation of radiographic imaging, prox-imal fragment histologic viability evaluation, and estimation of viability at surgery: Diagnosis of

scaphoid pseudarthrosis. Int Orthop 2015;39(1). https://doi.org/10.1007/s00264-014-2579-4.

52. Schoierer O, Bloess K, Bender D, et al. Dynamic contrast-enhanced magnetic resonance imaging can assess vascularity within fracture non-unions and predicts good outcome. Eur Radiol 2014; 24(2). https://doi.org/10.1007/s00330-013-3043-3.

53. Wang S, Yin P, Quan C, et al. Evaluating the use of serum inflammatory markers for preoperative diagnosis of infection in patients with nonunions. BioMed Res Int 2017;2017. https://doi.org/10.1155/2017/9146317.

54. Olszewski D, Streubel PN, Stucken C, et al. Fate of patients with a "Surprise" positive culture after nonunion surgery. J Orthop Trauma 2016;30. https://doi.org/10.1097/BOT.0000000000000417.

55. Nauth A, Lee M, Gardner MJ, et al. Principles of Nonunion Management: State of the Art. J Orthop Trauma 2018;32. https://doi.org/10.1097/BOT.0000000000001122.

56. Shapiro JA, Stillwagon MR, Tornetta P, et al. Serology and Comorbidities in Patients With Fracture Nonunion: A Multicenter Evaluation of 640 Patients. J Am Acad Orthop Surg 2022;30(18):e1179–87. https://doi.org/10.5435/JAAOS-D-21-00366.

57. Schottel PC, O'Connor DP, Brinker MR. Time trade-off as a measure of health-related quality of life: Long bone nonunions have a devastating impact. Journal of Bone and Joint Surgery - American 2014;97(17). https://doi.org/10.2106/JBJS.N.01090.

Bone Graft Substitutes— What Are My Options?

Kalpit N. Shah, MD[a],*, Robin N. Kamal, MD, MBA[b]

KEYWORDS

- Bone graft substitutes • Nonunion • Malunion • Hand and upper extremity surgery
- Synthetic bone graft

KEY POINTS

- A variety of synthetic bone graft substitutes have been developed to address the challenges of treating bone voids in the setting of nonunion and malunion surgery.
- Most synthetic bone grafts have varying strengths and resorption rates but all tend to be osteoconductive and lack osteoinductive or osteogenic potential.
- Combining bone graft substitutes with growth factors, other osteogenic molecules may help address the current limitations of available bone graft substitutes.

INTRODUCTION

Although bone regeneration occurs naturally in the healing of most fractures, nonunions and malunions present a unique challenge to the hand and upper extremity surgeon. Before embarking on a discussion on bone grafting, we must establish certain properties that are important for bone healing and consideration for bone graft use.[1–4]

For bones to heal, either in the setting of an acute fracture, nonunion or malunion, 4 well-defined prerequisites must be achieved as described by Giannoudis and colleagues, in the "diamond model" of bone healing.[3]

- Osteogenic cells: necessary cellular mechanism and machinery to produce new bone.
- Osteoconductive scaffold: mechanical matrix that allows for host fibrovascular ingrowth, osteoblast and other progenitor cell migration and attachment with eventual new bone formation.
- Osteoinductive environment: necessary growth proteins to induce differentiation of host progenitor cells to osteogenic cells; usually mediated by members of the transforming growth factor-β superfamily.
- Stabilized environment: rigid fixation permitting undisrupted incorporation of the graft by the host allowing for osteointegration.

Autologous bone graft remains the "gold standard" for addressing bone defects following debridement of a nonunion site or after corrective osteotomy of a malunion because it satisfies the needs set forth in the diamond model.[1,5–7] For defects in the upper extremity, common sites of autograft harvest include the iliac crest when cortical or cancellous graft is desired. For cancellous only bone autograft, proximal ulna, dorsal distal radius via Lister tubercle and proximal tibia via Gerdy tubercle are all commonly used bone graft sites.

However, autologous bone graft does have limited supply and is often associated with significant donor site morbidity. These include pain, wound healing issues, fracture of donor bone, injury to sensory nerves, hematoma formation, abdominal injury from iliac crest autograft harvest to name a few. Younger and colleagues reported their rate of 8.6% for major complications and 20.6% for minor complications.[8] Hartigan and colleagues showed that the use of bone autograft was associated with longer operative time, hospital stay, and higher cost.[4]

---

[a] Department of Orthopedic Surgery, Scripps Clinic, San Diego, CA, USA; [b] Department of Orthopedic Surgery, Stanford University, Palo Alto, CA, USA
* Corresponding author. 2205 Vista Way, Suite 210, Oceanside, CA 92054.
E-mail address: kalpit210@gmail.com

Hand Clin 40 (2024) 13–23
https://doi.org/10.1016/j.hcl.2023.09.001

To obviate the potential complications associated with autograft, allograft cortical or cancellous bone, as well as demineralized bone matrix (DBM) have been used. These grafts have osteoconductive and osteoinductive capabilities; however, due to the processing required (ethylene oxide or gamma irradiation) to reduce immunogenicity and viral transmission, the graft does lose a significant portion of its osteogenic capabilities.[1] Moreover, despite the processing, a small risk of immune response and viral transmission does exist with the use of bone allograft or DBM.

Bone graft substitutes have been developed to eliminate donor site morbidity, are readily available at volumes desired, and have no immunogenicity or potential for disease transmission. They are designed to be biocompatible and osteoconductive, creating a scaffold for host cells to migrate and produce bone.[6] They are usually osteointegrative and are resorbable or possess a bioreplaceable substrate design. They are pliable and malleable and can be used for defects of varying sizes and locations.[7] However, they all lack osteoinductive signaling growth factors and osteogenic bone-producing capability unless mixed with bone morphogenic proteins (BMPs), autograft bone, or bone marrow aspirate.

In this review, we will try to outline the available bone graft substitutes in the United States, their characteristics, potential use, benefits, and disadvantages.

CALCIUM SULFATE

Calcium sulfate, also known as plaster of Paris, has been used for fractures for more than 200 years. Pieter Hendriksz first described its use for fracture immobilization in 1814. The first reported use of calcium sulfate for in vivo use was by Dreesman in 1892 for filling bone voids in 1892.[9,10] A powder form of the substrate is derived from heated gypsum. Exposure to water begins the curing process, and the amount of water available during the curing process dictates the final crystalline pore structure; higher water content leads to increased porosity. Calcium sulfate is known to have better compressive strength than cancellous bone but poor tensile strength.[1,7]

Calcium sulfate provides excellent osteoconductive properties by providing a scaffold for new bone growth via vascularization and osteogenic cellular infiltration within the defect site. Additionally, calcium sulfate is biocompatible and resorbs gradually over time because it is absorbed by the infiltrating osteoclasts and replaced with new osseous growth.[11] Several studies have demonstrated successful bone healing after using calcium sulfate as a bone graft substitute for fracture surgery.[12,13]

Calcium sulfate is readily available, can be stored at room temperature, and is cost-effective compared with other bone graft substitutes. It can be obtained as pellets, blocks, or powders that can be converted into injectable paste to suit the specific defect size and shape. Additionally, products such as Stimulan (Biocomposites, Inc., Wilmington, NC) allow for addition of antibiotics to the mixture before curing when slow elution of the antibiotic into the bone defect is desired when concern for an infected nonunion, osteomyelitis, or potential postoperative infection remains high. One consideration for the surgeon when using calcium sulfate is that the curing process is exothermic and can reach temperatures of 48°C (118°F), which can cause thermal injury to surround tissues.[10]

Some limitations of calcium sulfate as a bone graft substitute include the relatively low mechanical strength compared with cortical bone where calcium sulfate was found to be 7 times weaker.[14] Additionally, calcium sulfate rapidly degrades within 4 to 12 weeks of insertion, making it the most rapidly dissolving bone graft.[6,15,16] Jepegnanam and colleagues described hardware failure in 2 elderly patients where calcium sulfate was used as bone graft after corrective osteotomy for malunion of a distal radius fracture. Although the cause for failure in those types of cases can often be multifactorial, it is recommended that calcium sulfate be used for bone defects that do not require significant structural support.[17] Another consideration is that there are no growth factors that are part of calcium sulfate so it has no intrinsic osteoinductive properties. However, it can be combined with DBM or BMPs to enhance its osteoinductive potential. Allomatrix (Wright Medical Technology, Inc., Memphis, TN) are examples of composite bone graft that include DBM and calcium sulfate.

Some commercially available calcium sulfate bone grafts in the United States include the following:

- OsteoSet (Stryker, Kalamazoo, MI)
- Ceraform (Exactech, Inc., Gainesville, FL)
- Stimulan (Biocomposites, Inc., Wilmington, NC)
- Osseotite (Zimmer Biomet, Warsaw, IN)
- BoneSave (Baxter International Inc., Deerfield, IL)

MINERAL-BASED CERAMICS

Hydroxyapatite is the basic mineral phase of bone, fluctuating between calcium phosphate and tricalcium phosphate based on exchange of ions in vivo.[1] These calcium phosphate salts were first introduced in the 1980s for bone substitution because they resemble bone precursors.[18] Their porous nature facilitates osteoconductivity by acting as scaffolds for inducing fibrovascular growth, migration of osteoblasts, and subsequent deposition of osteoid, which is later mineralized and remodeled as mature bone. These mineral-based ceramics exhibit gradual biodegradation, allowing for the gradual transfer of mechanical load from the graft used to the newly remodeled bone. This helps minimize stress shielding, thereby reducing the risk of implant failure or fracture. The rate of biodegradation can be tailored by modifying the composition and structure of the ceramic material.[19]

Coral Hydroxyapatite

Marine coral can be processed using hydrothermal techniques to remove organic matter. Further treatment of the calcium carbonate backbone with ammonium phosphate converts it to crystalline hydroxyapatite. The treated coralline hydroxyapatite structure is highly porous and found to be similar to regular skeletal bone. Its porous nature allows for cellular ingrowth and has good compressive strength making it useful when addressing metaphyseal defects.

Studies have found favorable results when used for posterolateral lumbar spine fusions, displaced tibial plateau fractures, bone voids after benign bone tumor excision, and distal radius fractures.[20–24]

Despite some clinical success, its application in clinical use remains limited. Coral hydroxyapatite exhibits low tensile strength and is relatively poorly bioabsorbed. Resorption rate of 5% to 10% per year has been reported and remains visible on the radiographs.[25,26] In addition, there is a high cost associated with its sourcing and treatment.

Commercially available coralline hydroxyapatite bone grafts in the United States include the following:

- ProOsteon (Interpore International, Irvine, CA)

Calcium Phosphate-Based Ceramics

Synthetic mineral bone substitutes have recently gained popularity. One such bone substitute is produced by precipitating ammonium dihydrogen phosphate and calcium nitrate at extremely high temperatures of 700°C and 1300°C to form the crystalline structure of hydroxyapatite ($Ca_{10}(PO_4)_6(OH)_2$).[1,26] This structure is very close in composition and form to mineral bone and has

similar osteoconductive properties. Comparatively, synthetic hydroxyapatite has been known to have a slow rate of resorption and is brittle in tensile strength.[27]

Clinically, it is often used in coatings of implants (femoral stems and acetabular cups, external fixation pins, radial head stems, and wrist and finger joint replacement stems) to assist in osseous integration. Free synthetic hydroxyapatite has also been successfully used in the upper extremity. Baer and colleagues used Endobon (Biomet, Warsaw, IN) for filling in the osseous defect left after enchondroma or cyst curettage in the upper extremity with excellent 5-year follow-up data.[28] Similarly, Werber and colleagues used ceramic hydroxyapatite as structural bone graft to fill bony defects left after a distal radius fracture.[29] Follow-up MRI and biopsy concluded that the hydroxyapatite was well integrated into skeletal bone.

Some commercially available hydroxyapatite bone grafts in the United States include the following:

- Endobon (Zimmer Biomet, Warsaw, IN)
- ProOsteon 500 (Zimmer Biomet, Warsaw, IN)

Another commercially available calcium phosphate ceramic bone substitute is β-tricalcium phosphate (TCP; $Ca_3[PO_4]_2$). Its structure is similar to hydroxyapatite; it is porous allowing for fibrovascular invasion and eventual osteointegration. Because it is more porous than synthetic hydroxyapatite and given its chemical composition, β-TCP resorbs at a quicker rate than hydroxyapatite (6–24 months) and is mechanically weaker in compression than hydroxyapatite.[27,30] Given its less porous structure, β-TCP is often combined with synthetic hydroxyapatite to improve its strength and reduce the resorption rate.

Some advantages of the calcium phosphate-based bone substitutes are realized by their relatively low cost and their synthetic design, which eliminates the risk for disease transmission.[7] Although these bone substitutes are solely osteoconductive, its combination with osteoinductive proteins such as bone morphogenic proteins (BMPs) or autograft can augment its success. Because these bone substitutes rely on fibrovascular ingrowth, they are relatively contraindicated in areas of poor vascular perfusion and ongoing infection.

Some commercially available β-TCP bone grafts in the United States include the following:

- ChronOS (Depuy Synthes, Warsaw, IN)
- Norian (Depuy Synthes, Warsaw, IN)
- Vitoss (Stryker, Portage, MI)

- Bonesync, Quickset and Osferion (Arthrex, Naples, FL)
- Hydroset (Stryker, Kalamazoo, MI)

COMPOSITES

A variety of composite bone substitutes involving differing combinations of the ones discussed above are commercially available and listed in **Table 1**.

BONE CEMENT

Polymethylmethacrylate (PMMA) bone cement was first used in orthopedic surgery for fixation of total hip arthroplasty components in the 1960s. A polymerized ester of acrylic acid, PMMA is formed by combining a powdered form of prepolymerized PMMA and the liquid of the monomer methyl methacrylate, causing polymerization and formation of the liquid cement product.[6,31,32] As the cement subsequently sets and hardens, its strength is comparable with that of bone.[31]

PMMA can provide immediate mechanical stability but has no osteogenic or osteoinductive properties. Given these properties, PMMA bone cement is often used to cement in metal implants to osteoporotic bone where press-fit implants risks causing periprosthetic fracture.[31,32] They can also be used as temporary bone support where immediate compressive strength is required in the construct. Additionally, because antibiotics can be mixed in during its preparation, it is often used to fill in defects in the setting of an infected nonunion or bone void to elute said antibiotics. However, it must be noted that the ability of the PMMA to elute antibiotics is highly variable based on the antibiotic used, the composition of PMMA, and its porosity, which is in turn dictated by the mixing protocol used.[7]

Although relatively rare, bone cement implantation syndrome has been described with clinical features of hypotension, cardiac arrhythmias, or cardiac arrest.[33] In upper extremity surgery, the risk is even lower with the use of a tourniquet, which minimizes the chance of systemic absorption of PMMA during implantation. Another disadvantage of PMMA cement lies in its inability to resorb and need to be replaced with autograft or allograft when the tissue beds are ready. The additional surgery carries risks to the local bone during removal.

In a study by Edwards and colleagues, 10 patients with scaphoid nonunions were treated with a composite bone graft substitute consisting of PMMA and autologous bone graft. The authors reported that all 10 patients achieved union after a mean time of 13.8 weeks. Similarly, a study by Di Matteo and colleagues found that the use of PMMA in combination with HA ceramic bone graft substitute was effective in promoting bone healing in patients with scaphoid nonunions.

Some commercially available PMMA bone cements in the United States include the following:

- Palacos R and Palacos R + G (gentamycin) (Zimmer Biomet, Warsaw, IN)
- Simplex P (Stryker, Portage, MI)

BIOACTIVE GLASS

Bioactive glass was first discovered by Larry L. Hench and his team at the University of Florida in the 1960s. They developed 45S5 Bioglass, which integrated well with bone in vivo and required the bone to be fractured for its removal.[34] Formed with varying amounts of calcium oxide, silicone dioxide, sodium oxide, and phosphorous, bioactive glass is known for its unique ability to form bonds between the silica layer and surrounding bone and soft tissues via the formation of hydroxycarbonate apatite. It is at this 3-dimensionally complex silica scaffold, that bioactive glass further stimulates osteointegration with native cell attachment and proliferation, resorption of the glass and hydroxyapatite deposition.[35,36]

Certain bioactive glass compositions have been noted to possess inherent antimicrobial properties. Because osteomyelitis often leads to bone voids where bone graft substitutes are needed, this antimicrobial property of bioactive glass can be particularly useful. Drago and colleagues discussed that bioactive can be both bactericidal and bacteriostatic against organisms commonly associated with osteomyelitis, namely methicillin-resistant *Staphylococcus aureus*, *Staphylococcus epidermidis*, *Pseudomonas aeruginosa*, and *Acinetobacter baumannii*.[37] Bioactive glass also has angiogenic properties that may play a role in their antimicrobial properties.

Bioactive glass comes as granules, putties, or scaffolds and can be tailored to match the defect's size and shape. However, its lack of mechanical strength makes it less suitable for load-bearing applications. Additionally, bioactive glass may have a slower resorption rate compared with some other bone graft substitutes, which could lead to prolonged healing times.[35,36,38]

Some commercially available bioactive glass bone graft substitutes in the United States include the following:

Fibergraft Bioactive Glass (Depuy Synthes, Warsaw, IN), Vitoss BA (Stryker, Kalamazoo, MI)

Table 1
List of some of the bone-graft substitutes that are available in the United States

Type	Advantages	Disadvantages	Brand Name
Calcium sulfate	Osteoconductive Low cost	Poor structural strength No osteoinductive potential unless mixed with other products	OsteoSet (Stryker, Kalamazoo, MI) Ceraform (Exactech, Inc., Gainesville, FL) Stimulan (Biocomposites, Inc., Wilmington, NC) Osseotite (Zimmer Biomet, Warsaw, IN) BoneSave (Baxter International Inc., Deerfield, IL) Hydroset (Stryker, Kalamazoo, MI)
β-Tricalcium phosphate	Osteoconductive Good compressive strength Variable resorption rate	Poor tensile strength No osteoinductive potential	ChronOS (Depuy Synthes, Warsaw, IN) Norian (Depuy Synthes, Warsaw, IN) Vitoss (Stryker, Portage, MI) Bonesync, Quickset and Osferion (Arthrex, Naples, FL) Hydroset (Stryker, Kalamazoo, MI)
Composites			
Calcium sulfate + DBM Calcium sulfate + calcium phosphate Calcium sulfate + calcium phosphate + DBM Hydroxyapatite + calcium phosphate Hydroxyapatite + calcium sulfate			Allomatrix (Stryker, Kalamazoo, MI) ProDense (Stryker, Kalamazoo, MI) ProStim (Stryker, Kalamazoo, MI) Osteomatrix (Bioventus, Durham, NC) Cerament (Lund, Sweden)
Bioactive glass	Osteoconductive Strong bond to bone and soft tissues Resorbs with time	Poor strength No osteoinductive potential	Fibergraft Bioactive Glass (Depuy Synthes, Warsaw, IN) Vitoss BA (Stryker, Kalamazoo, MI) S53P4 Bioactive Glass (BonAlive Biomaterials Ltd., Turku, Finland) Novabone (NovaBone, Jacksonville, FL) Bioactive Bonesync (Arthrex, Naples, FL)
3D-printed implants	Patient specific implants Osteoconductive Osteoinductive based on material used	Cost Significant preop planning required Lead time for planning and manufacturing	Ossio (Ossio, Inc., Woburn, MA) 4WEB Medical (4WEB Medical, Frisco, TX) Materialise (Materialise NV, Leuven, Belgium) Restor3d (Durham, North Carolina)

Some of their advantages and disadvantages are listed as well.

S53P4 Bioactive Glass (BonAlive Biomaterials Ltd., Turku, Finland)

Novabone (NovaBone, Jacksonville, FL)

THREE-DIMENSIONAL-PRINTED BONE GRAFT

Three-dimensional (3D) printing technology, also known as additive manufacturing, was recently introduced in the 1980s by Charles Hull in the United States.[39] Using this technique, 3D constructs can be created by sequential deposition of material in thin 2-dimensional layers as dictated by the design rendered using 3D modeling software.[40–42] The first clinical application of 3D printing was introduced by Mankovich in 1990 who printed a model of the skull using a patient's computed tomography (CT) imaging data.[43]

Data from advanced imaging techniques such as CT and MRI scans are used by computer-aided design (CAD) programs to create 3D models of the area of interest. The 3D model data from CAD programs is then converted to sterolithography files that a 3D printer then uses to produce 3D models.[39,42]

One advantage of 3D-printed bone graft is patient-specific customization. Surgeons, with the aid of 3D modeling experts, can tailor the design of the model to match the unique anatomy of the affected region. This may allow for optimal bone contact leading to improved osteointegration.[42]

Although a variety of applications for 3D models have been reported, including research, training, preoperative planning, intraoperative guides, the one germane to this article is its use as bone graft substitute.[39,41,44] To this end, bone scaffolds to fill bony defects may be created using a variety of different material but biphasic calcium phosphate (mixture of hydroxyapatite and tricalcium phosphate) and bioactive glass have shown promise. These materials have demonstrated the ability to promote osteoconductivity and osteointegration given its porous design, mechanical properties similar to that of bone and the fact that they act as substrate for resorption and osteoid formation.[45] Researchers continue to refine various production techniques, combinations of organic and inorganic compounds, and application of various growth factors to optimize osteointegration.[46–48]

Clinical application of 3D-printed bone graft substitutes remains in its infancy. Most widely used 3D-printed devices and implants are used for malunion correction with custom 3D-printed osteotomy guides to match the patient's abnormal anatomy with subsequent use of either off-the-shelf implants or custom 3D-printed implants.[49] Reports of 3D-printed bone graft substitutes for bone defects have been limited to animal models

and case reports that demonstrate their successful use.[50–54]

Disadvantages of 3D-printed bone graft substitutes include the high cost due to the expenses associated with 3D printing technology and the customization process. Additionally, the time required for design and fabrication may delay surgical interventions in urgent cases. The evolving nature of 3D printing technology also presents challenges related to regulatory approvals and standardization.[41,44]

A case example of a 38-year-old patient with a distal radius fracture malunion that was treated with custom, patient-specific osteotomy guides and a 3D printed titanium graft is shown in **Fig. 1**A–C.

Some of commercially available 3D-printed devices in the United States are as follows:

Ossio (Ossio, Inc., Woburn, MA)

4WEB Medical (4WEB Medical, Frisco, TX)

Materialise (materialise NV, Leuven, Belgium)

Restor3d (Durham, North Carolina)

CLINICAL OUTCOMES

Clinical studies comparing outcomes and efficacy of bone graft substitutes to autograft and allograft have been predominantly limited to retrospective studies, with some prospective studies and very few randomized controlled trials. In upper extremity surgery, its use has been most widely reported to for bony defects following curettage of benign tumors.

Clinical studies evaluating the use of bone graft substitutes in the upper extremity fracture surgery have been limited. Jakubietz and colleagues, performed a randomized clinical trial between 2 groups of patients, one treated with a dorsal locking plate only compared with another group treated with the same construct plus β-TCP graft to augment the fixation.[55] The authors found no difference in functional or radiographic outcomes.

A common application of bone graft substitutes in upper extremity surgery has been to fill in bony defects after curettage of benign lesions or management of large osseous defects after trauma. Nazarova and colleagues reported their randomized clinical trial on enchondroma curettage with either autograft or hydroxyapatite + collagen bone graft substitute. The bone graft substitute group had a significantly shorter operating time than the autograft group (27 vs 51 minutes). Both groups had similar functional and radiographic consolidation scores.[56] Hung and colleagues, retrospectively, compared their experience with the use of β-TCP graft to autograft for filling the defect left after enchondroma resection in the

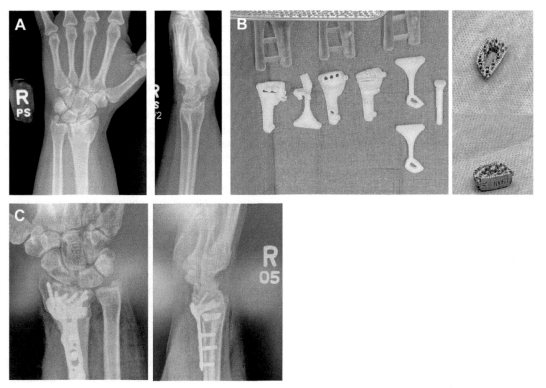

Fig. 1. (*A*) Preoperative radiographs of the right wrist of a 38-year-old woman with a distal radius malunion with an intra-articular step off, loss of radial inclination and height as well as significant dorsal angulation. (*B*) Custom patient-specific osteotomy guides used to correct her malunion and the 3D-printed titanium graft to be used to address the bone defect that resulted after malunion correction. (*C*) Postoperative radiographs of the right wrist at the 3-month follow-up visit demonstrating a healed distal radius after malunion correction with bony incorporation of the titanium bone-substitute.

phalanx or metacarpal. Patients in both groups had radiographic consolidation but the autograft group had a large portion (4 out of 11) of patients with symptomatic donor site at the last follow-up.[57] Lindfors and colleagues similarly retrospectively reviewed their patients with enchondroma of the hand during a 17-year period. A total of 190 patients were included with 116 patients who had autograft and 74 had bioactive glass used for filling the cavitary defect after curettage. Both groups had similar clinical and radiographic outcomes; however, 5 patients in the autograft required reoperation for recurrence that were treated with recurettage and either autograft or bioactive glass grafting. No patients in the bioactive glass group required a reoperation.[58]

Many authors have reported case series of their experience with bone graft substitutes for upper extremity surgery. Liodaki and colleagues used a composite calcium sulfate and hydroxyapatite injectable bone graft substitute after enchondroma curettage in 12 patients and to fill a bone defect in 4 patients with metacarpal fractures.[59] Gava and colleagues performed a systematic review to assess outcomes after benign tumor curettage and compared results between patients that did not have any form of cavity filling to those with allograft, cement, autograft, and bone substitute. The authors included 62 published articles representing 2555 patients. Although a majority of clinical outcomes (functional outcome recurrence rate and consolidation time) did not show any difference, the fracture rate was significantly higher for unfilled cavities (6.62% unfilled vs 2.12% for allograft, 4.08% for cement filling, 1.62% for autograft, and 2.07% for bone substitute).[60]

Majority of the data available today for bone graft substitutes has been reported in patients undergoing spinal surgery. Furthermore, the comparisons have been relatively heterogenous, comparing various combination of bone graft substitutes, bone marrow aspirate, local bone autograft, and iliac crest bone graft. In a systematic review evaluating the use of bone graft substitutes, Buser and colleagues gathered studies evaluating bone graft substitute use in lumbar and cervical spine, segregated by the type of bone graft used.[61] Most of the included studies reported no difference in outcome in terms of fusion achieved or for the patient-reported outcomes when bone graft substitutes were used. However, some studies did report worse outcomes after the use of bone graft substitutes when compared with autograft. Unfortunately, the authors reported significant concerns with the included studies regarding the risk of bias, unblinded evaluation, and lack of patient information that might have confounded results and unclear enrollment/inclusion methodology. More recently, Menezes and colleagues performed a randomized controlled trial on the use of a ceramic bone graft substitute vs autograft during 1-level lumbar lateral interbody fusion surgery. They reported fusion rates of 96.4% and 100% without statistical differences for the ceramic substitute and autograft groups, respectively.[62]

Some authors have evaluated the use of bone graft substitute for tibial plateau fracture defects while undergoing operative fixation.[63–66] Recently, Hofmann and colleagues reported their randomized clinical trial using either iliac crest autograft or a composite hydroxyapatite and calcium sulfate bone graft substitute for depressed tibial plateau fractures.[64] Postoperatively, they reported lower blood loss and pain scores on day 1; however, outcome scores at 26 weeks were similar between the 2 groups. Similarly, radiographic outcomes (fracture healing, defect remodeling, and articular subsidence) did not differ significantly between the groups. The authors concluded that the bone graft substitute was noninferior to iliac crest autograft.

In summary, most clinical studies reviewed suggest that bone graft substitute may represent a viable option for filling defects with potential advantages of faster operative times, lower donor-site morbidity, and lower recurrence rate for benign tumors when compared with autograft use.

DISCUSSION AND FUTURE DIRECTION

Although autograft remains the gold standard for bone replacement, advances in bone graft substitutes are important tools for helping surgeons manage bone voids. Fracture malunion and nonunion correction remain challenging surgeries where appropriate restoration of relative alignment is of utmost importance. Appropriate stabilization while respecting the soft tissue envelope to preserve vascular viability of bony stabilization is also a priority. Once accomplished, the surgeon must then carefully evaluate the need for the type of bone graft while considering the healing environment, including whether structural stability

is important, and if the bone graft needs to have osteoconductive, osteoinductive, and/or osteogenic properties.

In the upper extremity, areas with compromised vascularity such as the scaphoid, nonunion surgery often is best accomplished with the use of autograft to enhance the osteogenic potential. However, in areas such as the distal radius or after evacuating a large benign osseous tumor, bone graft substitutes with strong osteoconductive properties are generally preferred. Some of the bone graft substitutes such as calcium sulfate, calcium phosphate, hydroxyapatite, or bioactive glass are all suitable choices. Using bone graft substitutes has the inherent advantage of have no donor-site morbidity and no risk of disease transmissions as is encountered with autograft and allograft choices, respectively.

Development of bone graft substitutes for nonunion or malunion bone defects in the hand, wrist, and forearm will continue to be an area of interest and advancement. Novel biomaterials with enhanced mechanical strength, tailored resorption rates, and osteointegrative properties will likely emerge, to address the limitations of current bone graft substitutes. Unique combinations of currently available bone graft substitutes may be used to harness different strengths of each category of substitutes. Similarly, the integration of synthetic growth factors and other bioactive molecules into bone graft substitutes may enhance the lack of osteoinductive capabilities of the currently available products. Finally, the development of tissue engineering approaches, such as combining 3D-printed customization of bone graft substitutes with stem cells or other cell-based therapies, may open up new avenues for personalized and regenerative orthopedic surgery. Similarly, 3D printing to replicate bone architecture and to design custom-shaped bone graft materials may support a patient's unique needs during nonunion or malunion surgery.

CLINICS CARE POINTS

- When evaluating bone graft substitutes, surgeons must consider the substance's osteogenic, osteoconductive, or osteoinductive properties to identify the ideal bone substitute for the patient's needs.
- Calcium sulfate and mineral-based ceramic bone substitutes provide osteoconductive environment but lack strength, especially in tension or torsion.

- Bioactive glass stimulates angiogenesis and provides substrate for hydroxyapatite, conferring some osteoconductive advantages. However, this substrate also lacks strength.
- Bone cement provides immediate mechanical strength and stability but lacks osteogenic or osteoconductive potential.
- Three-dimensional-printed bone graft substrate may provide strength while conferring osteoconductive advantages. Although, these bone graft substitutes need further development and clinical testing.

DISCLOSURE

The authors have no relevant disclosures pertaining to this article.

REFERENCES

1. Bhatt RA, Rozental TD. Bone graft substitutes. Hand Clin 2012;28:457–68. Available at: https://pubmed. ncbi.nlm.nih.gov/23101596/. Accessed June 25, 2023.
2. Cypher TJ, Grossman JP. Biological principles of bone graft healing. J Foot Ankle Surg 1996;35:413–7. Available at: https://pubmed.ncbi.nlm.nih.gov/8915 864/. Accessed June 25, 2023.
3. Giannoudis PV, Einhorn TA, Marsh D. Fracture healing: The diamond concept. Injury 2007;38:S3–6.
4. Hartigan BJ, Cohen MS. Use of bone graft substitutes and bioactive materials in treatment of distal radius fractures. Hand Clin 2005;21:449–54. Available at: https://pubmed.ncbi.nlm.nih.gov/16039456/. Accessed June 25, 2023.
5. Campana V, Milano G, Pagano E, et al. Bone substitutes in orthopaedic surgery: from basic science to clinical practice. J Mater Sci Mater Med 2014;25: 2445. Available at: http://pmc/articles/PMC4169585/. Accessed June 25, 2023.
6. Gillman CE, Jayasuriya AC. FDA-approved bone grafts and bone graft substitute devices in bone regeneration. Mater Sci Eng C Mater Biol Appl 2021; 130. Available at: https://pubmed.ncbi.nlm.nih.gov/ 34702541/. Accessed June 25, 2023.
7. Lobb DC, DeGeorge BR, Chhabra AB. Bone Graft Substitutes: Current Concepts and Future Expectations. J Hand Surg Am 2019;44:497–505. e2. Available at: https://pubmed.ncbi.nlm.nih.gov/30704784/. Accessed June 25, 2023.
8. Younger EM, Chapman MW. Morbidity at bone graft donor sites. J Orthop Trauma 1989;3:192–5. Available at: https://pubmed.ncbi.nlm.nih.gov/2809818/. Accessed June 25, 2023.
9. Dreesmann H. Ueber Knochenplombirung1). DMW - Dtsch Medizinische Wochenschrift 1893;19:445–6.
   Available at: http://www.thieme-connect.de/DOI/ DOI?10.1055/s-0028-1143646. Accessed June 25, 2023.
10. Pietrzak WS, Ronk R. Calcium sulfate bone void filler: a review and a look ahead. J Craniofac Surg 2000;11:327–33. Available at: https://pubmed.ncbi. nlm.nih.gov/11314379/. Accessed June 25, 2023.
11. Stubbs D, Deakin M, Chapman-Sheath P, et al. In vivo evaluation of resorbable bone graft substitutes in a rabbit tibial defect model. Biomaterials 2004;25:5037–44.
12. Bibbo C, Patel DV. The effect of demineralized bone matrix-calcium sulfate with vancomycin on calcaneal fracture healing and infection rates: a prospective study. Foot Ankle Int 2006;27:487–93. Available at: https://pubmed.ncbi.nlm.nih.gov/16842714/. Accessed June 25, 2023.
13. Kelly CM, Wilkins RM, Gitelis S, et al. The use of a surgical grade calcium sulfate as a bone graft substitute: results of a multicenter trial. Clin Orthop Relat Res 2001;382:42–50. Available at: https:// pubmed.ncbi.nlm.nih.gov/11154003/. Accessed June 25, 2023.
14. Bucholz RW. Nonallograft osteoconductive bone graft substitutes. Clin Orthop Relat Res 2002;395: 44–52. Available at: https://pubmed.ncbi.nlm.nih. gov/11937865/. Accessed June 25, 2023.
15. Fillingham Y, Jacobs J. Bone grafts and their substitutes. Bone Joint Lett J 2016;98-B:6–9.
16. Roberts TT, Rosenbaum AJ. Bone grafts, bone substitutes and orthobiologics. https://doi.org/104161/ org23306. 2012;8:114-124. Available at: https://www. tandfonline.com/doi/abs/10.4161/org.23306 Accessed July 22, 2023.
17. Jepegnanam TS, Von Schroeder HP. Rapid Resorption of Calcium Sulfate and Hardware Failure Following Corrective Radius Osteotomy: 2 Case Reports. J Hand Surg Am 2012;37:477–80.
18. Ladd AL, Pliam NB. Bone graft substitutes in the radius and upper limb. J Am Soc Surg Hand 2003; 3:227–45.
19. Samavedi S, Whittington AR, Goldstein AS. Calcium phosphate ceramics in bone tissue engineering: A review of properties and their influence on cell behavior. Acta Biomater 2013;9:8037–45.
20. Boden SD, Martin GJ, Morone M, et al. The use of coralline hydroxyapatite with bone marrow, autogenous bone graft, or osteoinductive bone protein extract for posterolateral lumbar spine fusion. Spine (Phila Pa 1976) 1999;24:320–7. Available at: https:// pubmed.ncbi.nlm.nih.gov/10065514/. Accessed July 22, 2023.
21. Gupta AK, Kumar P, Keshav K, et al. Hydroxyapatite crystals as a bone graft substitute in benign lytic lesions of bone. Indian J Orthop 2015;49:649–55. Available at: http://www.ncbi.nlm.nih.gov/pubmed/ 26806973. Accessed July 22, 2023.

22. Mahan KT, Carey MJ. Hydroxyapatite as a bone substitute. J Am Podiatr Med Assoc 1999;89:392–7.

23. Wasielewski RC, Sheridan KC, Lubbers MA. Coralline hydroxyapatite in complex acetabular reconstruction. Orthopedics 2008;31.

24. Wolfe SW, Swigart CR, Grauer J, et al. Augmented external fixation of distal radius fractures: a biomechanical analysis. J Hand Surg Am 1998;23:127–34. Available at: https://pubmed.ncbi.nlm.nih.gov/9523966/. Accessed July 22, 2023.

25. Holmes RE. Bone regeneration within a coralline hydroxyapatite implant. Plast Reconstr Surg 1979; 63:626–33. Available at: https://pubmed.ncbi.nlm.nih.gov/432330/. Accessed July 22, 2023.

26. Van Der Stok J, Van Lieshout EMM, El-Massoudi Y, et al. Bone substitutes in the Netherlands - a systematic literature review. Acta Biomater 2011;7:739–50. Available at: https://pubmed.ncbi.nlm.nih.gov/20688196/. Accessed July 22, 2023.

27. Hing KA, Wilson LF, Buckland T. Comparative performance of three ceramic bone graft substitutes. Spine J 2007;7:475–90.

28. Baer W, Schaller P, Carl HD. Spongy hydroxyapatite in hand surgery - A five year follow-up. J Hand Surg Am 2002;27 B:101–3. Available at: https://pubmed.ncbi.nlm.nih.gov/11895356/. Accessed July 23, 2023.

29. Werber KD, Brauer RB, Weiß W, et al. Osseous integration of bovine hydroxyapatite ceramic in metaphyseal bone defects of the distal radius. J Hand Surg Am 2000;25:833–41. Available at: https://pubmed.ncbi.nlm.nih.gov/11040298/. Accessed July 23, 2023.

30. Ogose A, Kondo N, Umezu H, et al. Histological assessment in grafts of highly purified beta-tricalcium phosphate (OSferion) in human bones. Biomaterials 2006;27:1542–9. Available at: https://pubmed.ncbi.nlm.nih.gov/16165205/. Accessed July 23, 2023.

31. Kumar Ranjan R, Kumar Associate M, Kumar R, et al. Bone cement. Int J Orthop Sci 2017;3:79–82. Available at: https://www.orthopaper.com/archives/?year=2017&vol=3&issue=4&ArticleId=562. Accessed July 23, 2023.

32. Magnan B, Bondi M, Maluta T, et al. Acrylic bone cement: current concept review. Musculoskelet Surg 2013;97:93–100. Available at: https://pubmed.ncbi.nlm.nih.gov/23893506/. Accessed July 23, 2023.

33. Donaldson AJ, Thomson HE, Harper NJ, et al. Bone cement implantation syndrome. Br J Anaesth 2009; 102:12–22.

34. Jones JR. Reprint of: Review of bioactive glass: From Hench to hybrids. Acta Biomater 2015;23: S53–82.

35. Fiume E, Barberi J, Verné E, et al. Bioactive Glasses: From Parent 45S5 Composition to Scaffold-Assisted Tissue-Healing Therapies. J Funct Biomater 2018;9. Available at. http://pmc/articles/PMC5872110/. Accessed July 23, 2023.

36. Xynos ID, Hukkanen MVJ, Batten JJ, et al. Bioglass ®45S5 stimulates osteoblast turnover and enhances bone formation in vitro: Implications and applications for bone tissue engineering. Calcif Tissue Int 2000;67: 321–9. Available at: https://link.springer.com/article/10.1007/s002230001134. Accessed July 23, 2023.

37. Drago L, Toscano M, Bottagisio M. Recent Evidence on Bioactive Glass Antimicrobial and Antibiofilm Activity: A Mini-Review. Materials 2018;11. Available at. http://pmc/articles/PMC5849023/. Accessed July 23, 2023.

38. Fernandes HR, Gaddam A, Rebelo A, et al. Bioactive glasses and glass-ceramics for healthcare applications in bone regeneration and tissue engineering. Basel, Switzerland): Mater; 2018. p. 11. Available at: https://pubmed.ncbi.nlm.nih.gov/30545136/. Accessed July 23, 2023.

39. Matter-Parrat V, Liverneaux P. 3D printing in hand surgery. Hand Surg Rehabil 2019;38:338–47.

40. Skelley NW, Smith MJ, Ma R, et al. Three-dimensional Printing Technology in Orthopaedics. J Am Acad Orthop Surg 2019;27:918–25. Available at: https://journals.lww.com/jaaos/Fulltext/2019/12150/Three_dimensional_Printing_Technology_in.3.aspx. Accessed July 24, 2023.

41. Zhang D, Bauer AS, Blazar P, et al. Three-Dimensional Printing in Hand Surgery. J Hand Surg Am 2021;46: 1016–22. Available at: https://pubmed.ncbi.nlm.nih.gov/34274209/. Accessed July 24, 2023.

42. Zhang Q, Zhou J, Zhi P, et al. 3D printing method for bone tissue engineering scaffold. Med Nov Technol Devices 2023;17:100205.

43. Mankovich NJ, Cheeseman AM, Stoker NG. The display of three-dimensional anatomy with stereolithographic models. J Digit Imaging 1990;3:200–3. Available at: https://pubmed.ncbi.nlm.nih.gov/2085555/. Accessed July 24, 2023.

44. Hecker A, Tax L, Giese B, et al. Clinical Applications of Three-Dimensional Printing in Upper Extremity Surgery: A Systematic Review. J Pers Med 2023; 13:294. Available at: https://europepmc.org/articles/PMC9961947. Accessed July 24, 2023.

45. Shim KS, Kim SE, Yun YP, et al. Surface immobilization of biphasic calcium phosphate nanoparticles on 3D printed poly(caprolactone) scaffolds enhances osteogenesis and bone tissue regeneration. J Ind Eng Chem 2017;55:101–9.

46. Chen L, Deng C, Li J, et al. 3D printing of a lithium-calcium-silicate crystal bioscaffold with dual bioactivities for osteochondral interface reconstruction. Biomaterials 2019;196:138–50.

47. Kim BS, Yang SS, Kim CS. Incorporation of BMP-2 nanoparticles on the surface of a 3D-printed hydroxyapatite scaffold using an ε-polycaprolactone polymer emulsion coating method for bone tissue engineering. Colloids Surfaces B Biointerfaces 2018;170:421–9.

48. Song X, Tetik H, Jirakittsonthon T, et al. Biomimetic 3D Printing of Hierarchical and Interconnected Porous Hydroxyapatite Structures with High Mechanical Strength for Bone Cell Culture. Adv Eng Mater 2019; 21:1800678. Available at: https://onlinelibrary.wiley.com/doi/full/10.1002/adem.201800678. Accessed July 24, 2023.

49. de Muinck Keizer RJO, Lechner KM, Mulders MAM, et al. Three-dimensional virtual planning of corrective osteotomies of distal radius malunions: a systematic review and meta-analysis. Strateg Trauma Limb Reconstr 2017;12:77–89. Available at: https://link.springer.com/article/10.1007/s11751-017-0284-8. Accessed July 24, 2023.

50. Chakraborty J, Roy S, Ghosh S. 3D printed hydroxyapatite promotes congruent bone ingrowth in rat load bearing defects. Biomed Mater 2022;17:035008. Available at: https://iopscience.iop.org/article/10.1088/1748-605X/ac6471. Accessed July 25, 2023.

51. Mangano C, Giuliani A, De Tullio I, et al. Case Report: Histological and Histomorphometrical Results of a 3-D Printed Biphasic Calcium Phosphate Ceramic 7 Years After Insertion in a Human Maxillary Alveolar Ridge. Front Bioeng Biotechnol 2021;9:614325.

52. Maroulakos M, Kamperos G, Tayebi L, et al. Applications of 3D printing on craniofacial bone repair: A systematic review. J Dent 2019;80:1–14.

53. Peng Z, Wang C, Liu C, et al. 3D printed polycaprolactone/beta-tricalcium phosphate/magnesium peroxide oxygen releasing scaffold enhances osteogenesis and implanted BMSCs survival in repairing the large bone defect. J Mater Chem B 2021;9:5698–710. Available at: https://pubs.rsc.org/en/content/articlehtml/2021/tb/d1tb00178g. Accessed July 25, 2023.

54. Tovar N, Witek L, Atria P, et al. Form and functional repair of long bone using 3D-printed bioactive scaffolds. J Tissue Eng Regen Med 2018;12:1986–99. Available at: https://onlinelibrary.wiley.com/doi/full/10.1002/term.2733. Accessed July 25, 2023.

55. Jakubietz MG, Gruenert JG, Jakubietz RG. The use of beta-tricalcium phosphate bone graft substitute in dorsally plated, comminuted distal radius fractures. J Orthop Surg Res 2011;6:1–5. Available at: https://josr-online.biomedcentral.com/articles/10.1186/1749-799X-6-24. Accessed August 20, 2023.

56. Nazarova NZ, Umarova GS, Vaiman M, et al. The surgical management of the cavity and bone defects in enchondroma cases: A prospective randomized trial. Surg Oncol 2021;37. Available at: https://pubmed.ncbi.nlm.nih.gov/33848764/. Accessed August 20, 2023.

57. Hung YW, Ko WS, Liu WH, et al. Local review of treatment of hand enchondroma (artificial bone substitute versus autologous bone graft) in a tertiary referral centre: 13 years' experience. Hong Kong Med J 2015;21:217–23.

58. Lindfors N, Kukkonen E, Stenroos A, et al. Enchondromas of the Hand: Curettage With Autogenous Bone vs. Bioactive Glass S53P4 for Void Augmentation. In Vivo 2022;36:1267–73. Available at: https://pubmed.ncbi.nlm.nih.gov/35478146/. Accessed August 18, 2023.

59. Liodaki E, Kraemer R, Mailaender P, et al. The Use of Bone Graft Substitute in Hand Surgery: A Prospective Observational Study. Medicine (Baltim) 2016;95: e3631. Available at: https://europepmc.org/articles/PMC4998432. Accessed August 20, 2023.

60. Gava NF, Engel EE. Treatment alternatives and clinical outcomes of bone filling after benign tumour curettage. A systematic review. Orthop Traumatol Surg Res 2022;108. Available at: https://pubmed.ncbi.nlm.nih.gov/34033919/. Accessed August 20, 2023.

61. Buser Z, Brodke DS, Youssef JA, et al. Synthetic bone graft versus autograft or allograft for spinal fusion: a systematic review. J Neurosurg Spine 2016;25:509–16. Available at: https://thejns.org/spine/view/journals/j-neurosurg-spine/25/4/article-p509.xml. Accessed August 18, 2023.

62. Menezes CM, Lacerda GC, do Valle GSO, et al. Ceramic bone graft substitute vs autograft in XLIF: a prospective randomized single-center evaluation of radiographic and clinical outcomes. Eur Spine J 2022;31:2262–9. Available at: https://pubmed.ncbi.nlm.nih.gov/35723748/. Accessed August 18, 2023.

63. Heikkilä JT, Kukkonen J, Aho AJ, et al. Bioactive glass granules: a suitable bone substitute material in the operative treatment of depressed lateral tibial plateau fractures: a prospective, randomized 1 year follow-up study. J Mater Sci Mater Med 2011;22:1073–80. Available at: https://pubmed.ncbi.nlm.nih.gov/21431354/. Accessed August 18, 2023.

64. Hofmann A, Gorbulev S, Guehring T, et al, CERTiFy Study Group. Autologous Iliac Bone Graft Compared with Biphasic Hydroxyapatite and Calcium Sulfate Cement for the Treatment of Bone Defects in Tibial Plateau Fractures: A Prospective, Randomized, Open-Label, Multicenter Study. J Bone Joint Surg Am 2020;102:179. Available at. http://pmc/articles/PMC7508276/. Accessed August 18, 2023.

65. Pernaa K, Koski I, Mattila K, et al. Bioactive glass S53P4 and autograft bone in treatment of depressed tibial plateau fractures - a prospective randomized 11-year follow-up. J Long Term Eff Med Implants 2011;21:139–48. Available at: https://pubmed.ncbi.nlm.nih.gov/22043972/. Accessed August 18, 2023.

66. Russell TA, Leighton RK, Alpha-BSM Tibial Plateau Fracture Study Group. Comparison of autogenous bone graft and endothermic calcium phosphate cement for defect augmentation in tibial plateau fractures. A multicenter, prospective, randomized study. J Bone Joint Surg Am 2008;90:2057–61. Available at: https://pubmed.ncbi.nlm.nih.gov/18829901/. Accessed August 18, 2023.

Forearm Nonunions—From Masquelet to Free Vascularized Bone Grafting

Marc J. Richard, MD, Catphuong L. Vu, MD, MPH*

KEYWORDS

• Radius • Ulna • Forearm • Nonunion • Vascularized bone graft

KEY POINTS

- Forearm nonunions require a thorough workup to rule out infection and possible endocrine and metabolic contribution.
- Infected nonunions need a staged revision with thorough debridement and placement of an antibiotic spacer to induce a pseudomembrane for subsequent bone autograft.
- Selection of bone graft for nonunion depends on the size of the defect, the need for structural support, and/or vascularity.

BACKGROUND

Forearm fractures present a unique challenge due to the close relationship of the radius relative to the ulna. Associated with the complexity of treatment for these fractures is the management of nonunion and malunion of the radius and ulna. The incidence of nonunion in forearm fractures ranges from 2% to 10%.[1] Given the importance of the forearm in positioning the hand in space, timely and precise treatment of forearm nonunion and malunion is necessary to restore function. An understanding of the anatomy is the first step to developing a successful approach to managing forearm nonunion and malunion.

Anatomy

Functionally, the radius and ulna operate as a unit with their articulation at the proximal and distal radioulnar joints. Any change in length, alignment, or rotation of either the radius or ulna can alter the range of motion and thus function of the forearm. Proximally, the radius articulates with the ulna at the lesser sigmoid notch and is stabilized by the annular ligament, the lateral ligamentous complex, and the elbow capsule. At the distal radioulnar joint, the ulna articulates at the sigmoid notch of the radius and the joint is stabilized by the wrist joint capsule, the pronator quadratus muscle, and the triangular fibrocartilage complex. An interosseous membrane connects the 2 bones and extends from the proximal to the distal radioulnar joint. Mechanically, the forearm achieves pronation and supination motion as the radial head rotates about the proximal ulna. This range of motion depends upon the preservation of the radial bow of the forearm. This has been quantified by drawing a line from the bicipital tuberosity to the most ulnar aspect of the radius at the wrist and then a perpendicular line from the point of maximal bow to this line.[2] The height of the perpendicular line is termed maximal radial bow. In its original description, both the magnitude and the location of the maximal radial bow have been correlated to functional outcomes. Subsequent authors have not demonstrated the same association between these measurements and functional outcomes; however, there is consensus that restoration of normal anatomy is critical to optimizing function.[3]

Division of Hand, Upper Extremity, and Microvascular Surgery, Duke University, Duke University Medical Center, 5601 Arringdon Park Drive, Suite 300, Morrisville, NC 27560, USA
* Corresponding author.
E-mail address: Catphuong.vu@duke.edu

Hand Clin 40 (2024) 25–34
https://doi.org/10.1016/j.hcl.2023.08.014
0749-0712/24/© 2023 Elsevier Inc. All rights reserved.

History

Historically, when forearm fractures were treated nonoperatively, there were poor results due to loss of reduction and subsequent loss of motion.[4–8] With the advent of improved plate constructs, open reduction with internal fixation of forearm fractures with compression plating became the new standard. Early series showed union rates greater than 95% with the use of compression plates.[9–13] While intramedullary nailing has been described as an alternative option, high rates of nonunion and malunion have been reported in the literature.[14]

Epidemiology/Definition

Even with operative fixation, there is a risk of nonunion averaging about 4%. While there is a spectrum of definitions for nonunion, the common defining terms include failure to have progressive radiographic changes for 3 months, persistent pain at the fracture site, and hardware failure. The common location for nonunion in the forearm occurs at the junction of the middle and distal thirds of the shaft due to the paucity of blood supply as the descending branch of the nutrient artery terminates there, resulting in a watershed area.[15] Nonunion risk also increases in this area due to the torsional force from forearm supination and pronation.[16]

Nonunions can be further characterized as hypertrophic, oligotrophic, or atrophic based on the amount of bone formation and stability across the fracture site. Hypertrophic nonunions demonstrate the ability to generate new bone in the form of callus but are mechanically unstable. Atrophic nonunions, on the other hand, do not form callus due to an inherent biological deficiency. Oligotrophic nonunions have a combination of some biological deficiency and mechanical instability.

EVALUATION
Imaging

Interval radiographic images of the fracture are an important diagnostic component of nonunions. Both anteroposterior and lateral views are necessary to fully evaluate fracture alignment and the fixation construct along with planes of callus formation. Advanced imaging such as a computerized tomography (CT) scan should be obtained to more clearly define the extent of callus formation at the fracture site that may not be obvious on radiographs.

Workup

In approaching a nonunion workup, infection must first be ruled out as a contributing factor. A thorough history including mechanism of injury can reveal an open injury which increases the risk of infection. Workup for infection should include a complete blood count, erythrocyte sedimentation rate (ESR), and C-reactive protein level (CRP). Thresholds indicative of infection include white blood cell count (WBC) greater than 11,000, ESR greater than 30 mm/hr, and CRP level greater than 1.0 mg/dL. With all 3 laboratory tests above these thresholds, the positive predictive value for infection is 100%, while the negative predictive value is 81.6% when all 3 are negative.[17]

Further characterization of the nonunion according to hypertrophic, oligotrophic, and atrophic categories is a helpful starting point to determine if there is a lack of biology or a lack of mechanical stability or both. Mechanical instability may be a result of implant choice, length of construct, and/or applied technique. Mechanical stability usually accounts for only 9% of nonunion cases.[18] Biological factors that impact healing include a variety of endocrine and metabolic disorders, nicotine exposure, bone loss, and soft tissue injury compromising vascular supply to the region.[19–21] **Table 1** provides a comprehensive list of

Table 1 Laboratory evaluation for nonunion	
Infectious	**Metabolic/Endocrine**
ESR	CMP
CRP	Calcium −24 hr
CBC	Phosphorus
	Alkaline phosphatase
	Serum osmalality
	HbA1c
	Vitamin D
	• 1,25 dihydroxyvitamin D3 (calcitriol)
	• 25-hydroxyvitamin D (Calciferol)
	Thyroid/Parathyroid
	• Thyroid stimulating hormone
	• Thyroxine (T4)
	• Parathyroid hormone
	Hypothalamic-Pituitary-Adrenal axis
	• Cortisol
	• Adrenocorticotropic hormone
	• Renin
	• Testosterone, total
	• Estradiol
	• Follicle stimulating hormone
	• Luteinizing hormone
	Random urine
	• Sodium
	• Osmolality

Abbreviations: CBC, complete blood count; CMP, comprehensive metabolic panel; CRP, C-reactive protein leve; ESR, erythrocyte sedimentation rate; HbA1c, hemoglobin A1C.

laboratory tests which should be considered in a workup for nonunion. Any identified laboratory abnormalities should be corrected prior to the revision surgery.

TREATMENT

Once a nonunion workup has been performed, treatment for nonunion of forearm fractures should aim to address the identified biology or stability factors that may have contributed. Treatment can also follow a general algorithm similar to the diagnostic workup for nonunion as exemplified in **Fig. 1**.

Infected nonunions should first be treated with debridement and collection of tissue samples for cultures to guide antibiotic management. A series of debridements to effectively remove all devitalized tissue along with a prolonged course of antibiotics may be required to clear the infection before a revision surgery can be performed. Timing of the revision surgery will depend on normalization of laboratory values (ESR, CRP, WBC) as well as intraoperative findings confirming eradication of infection.

In a noninfected nonunion, the nonunion site should be prepared by removing fibrous tissue and callus as well as debriding sclerotic edges until healthy bleeding bone is encountered. Careful attention should be paid to the amount of bone being resected at the nonunion site as the size of defect can affect reconstruction options and bone graft choices. Preparation of the site should

also include re-establishing the medullary canals in each segment of the bone. Intraoperatively, the use of a tool such as a Hintermann device can help maintain compression at the nonunion site (**Fig. 2**).

Options of Fixation

Compression plating results in the highest rate of union in forearm fractures.[10,11] Similarly, in the nonunion setting, studies have shown that revision with compression plating with adequate fixation on either side of the nonunion site with use of autograft leads to successful osseous healing.[1,18,22] The main disadvantage of plate fixation is the need for more soft tissue exposure and thus stripping of the periosteum. Moreover, there is a risk of synostosis that is greatest for both bone fractures at the same level.

Intramedullary nails have been used for forearm fractures due to their less invasive technique that limits soft tissue disruption. However, early studies have shown higher nonunion rates and reduced stability compared to plating. An early study by Christensen and colleagues showed only a 75% union rate with intramedullary nailing of forearm fractures.[23] A biomechanical study done by Schemitsch showed that in both bone forearm fractures, intramedullary nailing of both radius and ulna resulted in a construct that is less able to resist torsion, distraction, and compression loading compared to compression plating.[24] However, these studies evaluated early generation

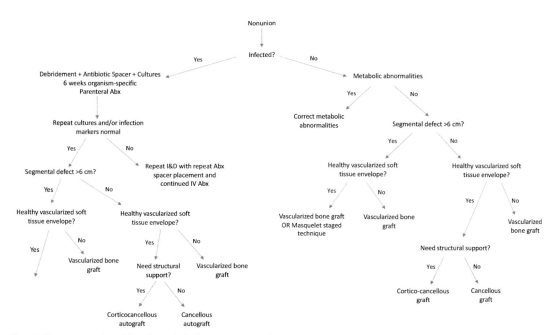

Fig. 1. Treatment algorithm for adult forearm nonunion.

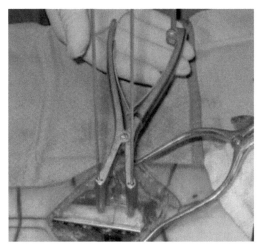

Fig. 2. Use of the Hintermann compression device to achieve and maintain compression at the nonunion site before plate fixation. (Photo courtesy of Marc Richard, MD.)

intramedullary nails that did not have the ability to control rotation like newer generation nails. Newer generation intramedullary forearm nails with pre-contoured and interlocking systems have shown improvement in union rates and faster time to mobilization. Lee and colleagues applied intramedullary nails in 38 patients with either radius or ulna or both bone fractures with reported healing within 14 weeks with 97.5% union rate at 4.4 months and average Disabilities of the Arm, Shoulder, and Hand (DASH) scores of 15 points.[25] Another study by Saka and colleagues had 59 forearm fractures treated with intramedullary nailing that all went onto union with average outcome DASH scores of 6.[26,27] New intramedullary nail options may offer an option for additive or combined use with compression plating in nonunion revisions.

Another technique described by Jewell and Merrell uses the patient's own bone for bridging large cortical defects.[28] The technique involves harvesting one-third cross section of the longer segment of bone and sliding this fragment to bridge across the nonunion site and held in place with lag screws and bridging plate.[28]

Bone Grafting

Selection of bone graft for use in nonunion depends on the size of the defect as well as the need for structural support. Cancellous grafts are used in smaller defects that do not require structural support to restore the anatomic relationship of the radius and ulna. Options include iliac crest, distal radius, lateral epicondyle, proximal tibia, olecranon, and femur cancellous aspirate.

Corticocancellous grafts are necessary in nonunion settings with large bone defects requiring structural support and include tricortical iliac crest, medial femoral condyle and trochlea, and free fibula grafts. When defects are greater than 6 cm, vascularized cortical grafts such as the free vascularized fibula graft (FVFG) offers the best healing potential.[29]

Allograft

Allograft bone grafting offers the benefit of reducing donor site morbidity; however, its efficacy in nonunion has been less studied compared to autograft. One study by Davis and colleagues evaluated the use of bulk allograft in a case series of 7 patients who had an infected nonunion with an average of 4.9 cm segmental defect.[30] Of the 7 patients, 4 patients required additional surgery with use of autologous bone grafting to achieve healing. Liu and colleagues investigated the use of bone transport in infected forearm nonunion in 21 patients and 6 patients required another surgery with autograft to achieve union.[31] Ideally, in nonunion revisions, autologous bone grafting is preferred; however, if volume is insufficient, allograft may be used to supplement.

Autograft

The gold standard bone graft in nonunion is autologous bone grafting due to its osteogenic, osteoinductive, and osteoconductive characteristics. Allografts are only osteoinductive and osteoconductive. The most common bone autografts include iliac crest bone graft (ICBG) and reamer, irrigator, aspirator (RIA) of the femur. ICBG can yield 30 cm^3 of graft compared to 60 cm^3 from RIA with similar union rates of 80% to 90%.[32,33] Drawbacks of these grafts include donor site morbidity and pain; however, RIA has lower donor site pain and faster operative time compared to ICBG.[33] Nonvascularized corticocancellous grafts such as tricortical iliac crest can restore bone defects of 3 to 5 cm. This technique was used by Prasarn and colleagues in 15 patients with an average defect of 2.1 cm (range 1–7 cm) with 100% union rate.[34] However, harvesting of corticocancellous bone grafting is more invasive with increased donor site morbidity. Multiple studies have shown that autologous cancellous graft may be sufficient to stimulate healing even in the setting of significant bone defects. Ring and colleagues demonstrated a 100% union rate in their cohort with an average 2.2 cm defect treated with cancellous autograft with compression plating.[18] Similarly, Regan and colleagues found a 91.3% healing rate with cancellous bone autograft with compression plating.[22]

Free vascularized graft

Vascularized grafts deliver nutrients for osteosynthesis that are advantageous in poorly vascularized areas including prior sites of infection and poor host biology. The disadvantages of vascularized grafts include longer operative time and the requirement of microvascular skills. In nonunion defects greater than 6 cm, vascularized bone grafting with the free fibula graft is the recommended choice with union rates demonstrated to be approximately 90%.[22,35]

FVFG also presents an alternative in recalcitrant cases where conversion to a one-bone forearm is necessary. First described in 1921 by Hey-Groves when a one-bone forearm was created from a radioulnar synostosis for failed bone-grafting in a distal radial nonunion.[36] Devandra and colleagues reported a case series of 16 patients who underwent one-bone forearm reconstruction for nonunion with achieved union in 15 patients without need for secondary procedure with a mean time to union at 6 months[37] In cases where bone loss was less than 6 cm, traditional bone grafting was performed while cases with greater than 6 cm gaps were bridged with FVFGs.

Case example for osteocutaneous free vascularized fibula graft A 25 year-old female sustained a ballistic injury to her left radius and ulna resulting in a comminuted open fracture of the radial and ulna shafts. The patient underwent temporizing stabilization with external fixation and interval debridement before reconstruction with an osteocutaneous

FVFG for the radius and intramedullary nailing of the ulna (**Fig. 3**). The ulna developed a nonunion and was revised using an ICBG with plate fixation. At 1 year postoperatively, she demonstrated union of the radius and ulna with return of functional range of motion (**Fig. 4**).

Preoperative planning

- Preoperative radiographs of the affected and contralateral forearms to determine the length of the defect and plan for the type of FVFG, if composite tissue is needed.
- Radiographs of the lower extremity from which the fibula is harvested were obtained.
- Clinical vascular examination of lower extremity to ensure adequate pulses in both posterior tibialis and dorsalis pedis arteries.
  ○ Obtain CT angiography if abnormal pulses or major previous lower extremity trauma.

Surgical approach

1. Fibula harvest
   a. Mark out the incision centered over fibula about 10 cm distal to fibula head and 10 cm proximal to lateral malleolus.
   b. If taking skin paddle, use Doppler to mark out skin perforators prior to inflation of the upper leg tourniquet.
   c. Start dissection of skin portion of fibula flap along the anterior aspect of the skin paddle over the lateral compartment muscles containing the peroneus longus and brevis muscles.

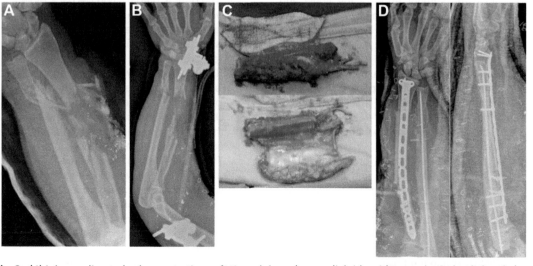

Fig. 3. (*A*) Injury radiographs demonstrating soft tissue injury along radial side with comminuted radial and ulnar shaft fractures. (*B*) Radiograph showing temporizing external fixation of forearm and subsequent debridement of radial shaft fracture with measured defect more than 6 cm. (*C*) Osteocutaneous FVFG harvested. (*D*) Inset of FVFG in radius with volar plating of radius and intramedullary nailing of ulna. FVFG, free vascularized fibula graft. (Images courtesy of Marc J. Richard, MD.)

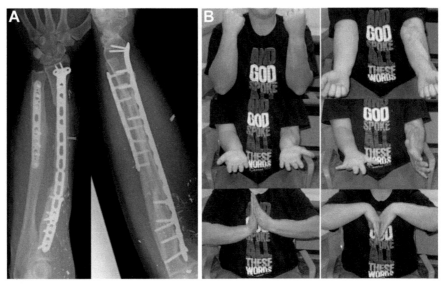

Fig. 4. (*A*) Twelve months post-op follow-up demonstrating fully healed radial shaft. Ulna shaft underwent revision with iliac crest bone graft and progressed onto union as well. (*B*) Patient demonstrated a functional arc of motion postoperatively. (Photos courtesy of Marc J. Richard, MD.)

d. Find the interval posteriorly between the peroneal and soleus muscles, usually marked by a fat stripe posterior to the peroneus longus.

e. The lateral muscle compartment is then elevated off the fibula bone leaving a small cuff of muscle to preserve periosteal blood supply until the anterior intermuscular septum is visualized.

f. Divide the anterior intermuscular septum along the anterior edge of the fibula and elevate the anterior compartment until the interosseous membrane is seen and divide that sharply adjacent to the fibular attachment.

g. At the distal end of fibula, use blunt dissection to separate the peroneal vascular bundle from bone and use a malleable retractor to protect the vessels while the distal osteotomy is made with an oscillating saw.

  i. Similarly, identify and protect the peroneal vascular bundle and the common peroneal nerve before the proximal osteotomy is made.

  ii. Harvest a longer length of fibula than the defect size to avoid the graft being too short and to increase the pedicle length.

h. Distally divide the tibialis posterior muscles to visualize the peroneal vascular bundle.

  i. Use a free tie to tie vessel bundle to fibula bone distally to prevent retraction of bundle when vessels are ligated.

  ii. Use vessel clips (2 distally and 1 proximally) and ligate the bundle.

  i. Elevate the fibula from distally to proximally until the takeoff of the anterior tibial artery from the peroneal artery is encountered.

j. Deflate the tourniquet to allow the flap to reperfuse for 15 minutes.

k. Mobilize the proximal pedicle and place vessel clips on the proximal pedicle, then remove the flap.

l. The graft is prepared on the back table and wrapped in saline soaked gauze. The final graft size is determined at the recipient site and the fibula is cut to size with an oscillating saw.

m. The artery and 2 veins from the pedicle are separated and prepared for anastomosis.

2. Preparation of the forearm

a. Under tourniquet control, the bone defect in the radius is prepared back to healthy bone edges proximally and distally.

b. The radial artery is carefully prepared along with one of the venae comitantes for an end to side artery anastomosis and an end to end vein anastomosis.

c. The FVFG is then inset with the pedicle positioned to reach the radial artery without tension.

d. Select an appropriate length metadiaphyseal radial plate to span the defect with fixation in the distal radius and the proximal radial shaft and compress through the plate using the dynamic compression holes.

e. The ulna is stabilized with an intramedullary nail.

f. The vascular anastomosis is performed under the microscope. The tourniquet is deflated to assess appropriate flow across the anastomosis.

The Masquelet Technique

In cases of infected nonunion, a staged procedure is required to help facilitate the treatment of the infection and the bone defect. The original eponymous procedure of the induced membrane technique was described by Masquelet and colleagues[38] The Masquelet technique is a staged procedure that starts with thorough debridement of the infected nonunion back to healthy bleeding bone. A cement spacer is placed in the bone gap to induce the formation of a pseudomembrane that contains growth factors including vascular endothelial growth factor, transforming growth factor-β, and other osteoconductive factors (bone morphogenic protein 2 [BMP-2]). The original description of the Masquelet technique does not utilize antibiotics in the cement; however, many surgeons will include them for the local antibiotic elution while the patient is also receiving parenteral antibiotic treatment. After repeated clinical and laboratory evaluations have verified clearance of the infection, the second stage (often planned 4–6 weeks later) involves removal of the cement spacer and placement of autograft cancellous bone within the created space. This induced membrane technique has shown efficacy in treating nonunion defects up to 25 cm in length.[38,39] On average, studies have shown success with the use of the Masquelet technique in treating forearm nonunions up to 5 cm in length.[40,41]

Case example for the Masquelet technique

A 62-year-old male with a history of an open left both bone forearm fracture previously underwent debridement and open reduction and internal fixation of radius and ulna. He subsequently developed an infection that required explantation of the hardware and a course of parenteral antibiotics. Once the infection was treated, the patient underwent revision surgery for his radius and ulna with the use of structural ICBG for the ulna. The ulna progressed to nonunion and another surgery was performed for debridement and placement of an antibiotic cement spacer for the ulna bone defect before being referred to our care (Fig. 5). Repeat laboratory tests showed no evidence of infection and he elected to proceed with a revision of the ulna nonunion utilizing the contralateral ICBG.

Preoperative planning
- Obtain nonunion laboratory tests; if there is a history of infection, obtain inflammatory markers to ensure they have returned to normal.

Surgical approach
- Preparing the ulna
  ○ The previous skin incision is used with development of the intermuscular plane between the extensor carpi ulnaris and flexor carpi ulnaris to approach the ulna shaft.
  ○ The pseudomembrane at the nonunion site is identified and divided longitudinally to access the cement spacer.
  ○ The cement spacer was removed with preservation of the induced membrane.
  ○ A 2 mm round burr was used to debride the edges of the ulnar at the site of the bone defect until healthy bleeding bone was encountered; a 2.5 mm drill bill was used to re-cannulate the ulna shaft, as needed, through the defect.
  ○ An oscillating saw was used to make oblique cuts in the proximal and distal shaft so that the defect area is a trapezoidal shape to help with compression of the bone graft. The long length of the trapezoid is placed directly below the plate to increase the inherent stability of the structural graft when compression is applied.
  ○ The final defect size was measured.
- ICBG harvest
  ○ A standard incision to the iliac crest is made and the subcutaneous tissue is bluntly dissected to expose the periosteum of the iliac crest.
  ○ Monopolar cautery is used to incise the periosteum followed by the use of a Cobb elevator to elevate the muscle off the inner and outer tables of the ilium.
  ○ The dimensions of the bone graft are marked on the iliac crest and a slightly larger piece of graft is harvested to allow reshaping as needed.
  ○ An oscillating saw is used to make the cuts with the use of an osteotome to complete the graft harvest with care to not cause a fracture of the ilium.
  ○ The bone graft block was then reshaped into a trapezoid shape to fit into the ulna defect.
- The bone block was placed into the gap at the ulna shaft and fluoroscopic imaging was obtained to ensure adequate fit.
- An appropriate small fragment dynamic compression plate was selected to achieve

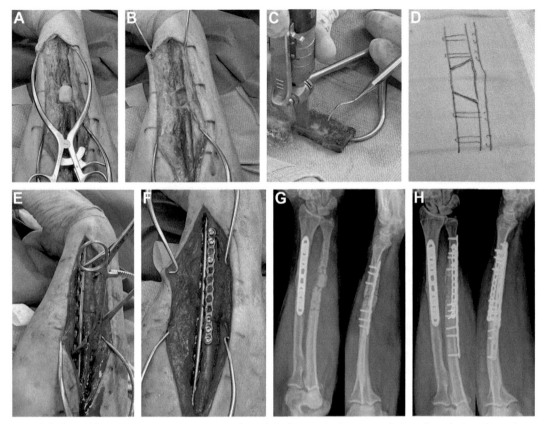

Fig. 5. (*A*) Ulna with antibiotic cement spacer in place. (*B*) After spacer is removed, there is an induced membrane along radial aspect of defect; the membrane is preserved in preparation of proximal and distal segment of ulna with burr and re-cannulation with drill. (*C, D*) ICBG is being reshaped into trapezoidal shape for better compressive fit. (*E*) ICBG in place with provisional placement of volar plate on ulna. (*F*) Final construction with addition of 2.7 mm plate orthogonally for stabilization of ICBG. (*G*) Radiograph showing preoperative imaging with antibiotic cement spacer. (*H*) Two-week postoperative radiographs. ICBG, iliac crest bone graft. (Photos courtesy of Marc J. Richard, MD.)

at least 3 points of fixation in the proximal and distal segments. The plate was positioned volar and compression was achieved through the plate with eccentric screw placement. A 2.7 mm plate was placed orthogonally for additional stabilization of the graft.

Adjunctive

BMP-7, with its osteoinductive activity, has been described as an adjunct treatment for forearm nonunions. BMPs work through inducing differentiation of osteoblasts from mesenchymal stem cells. In a study by Singh and colleagues, 25 cases of forearm and distal radius nonunions were treated with a combination of BMP-7 and autologous bone graft including iliac bone crest or RIA-achieved union.[42] Conversely, a study by von Rüden and colleagues showed that the addition of BMP in nonunion revision did not affect outcomes.[43] In a cohort of 49 patients with forearm

nonunion, 24 underwent revision with bone grafting plus BMP, while 25 underwent bone graft without BMP. Both groups had similar patient characteristics and nonunion types with the BMP group reaching osseous healing by 22 months compared to 24 months for the non-BMP group. The functional outcome evaluation based on elbow and wrist range of motion was not significantly different between the 2 groups. At this time, there is still mixed evidence for the use of BMP that may not justify its cost in revision surgeries for forearm nonunions.

SUMMARY

Forearm nonunions present a challenging and functionally limiting problem. As for all nonunions, a critical evaluation of contributing factors must occur prior to surgical intervention. Understanding that biology and stability both contribute to bone healing is critical as all potential causes must be analyzed and all reversible factors much be corrected. Furthermore, the surgical treatment of forearm nonunion requires an understanding of the unique relationship between the radius and ulna. Timing of nonunion surgery is best done within 1 year of the index injury for less soft tissue complications and better functional outcomes.

CLINICS CARE POINTS

- Nonunion can be a result of mechanical instability or biologic deficiency.
- Workup of nonunion requires evaluation of laboratory tests to rule out infection and other endocrine and/or metabolic causes before planning for revision.
- Infected nonunion requires a staged revision with initial thorough debridement, antibiotic spacer with parenteral antibiotics, and sequential negative cultures before reimplantation of hardware.
- Arbeitsgemeinschaft für Osteosynthesefragen principle of compression plating should be applied to nonunion revisions with use of autograft bone graft as the gold standard.
- Vascularized free fibula graft is the recommended choice for nonunion defects greater than 5 to 6 cm in length.

DISCLOSURE

C.L. Vu has nothing to disclose. M.J. Richard is a consultant for Acumed, DJO, Bioventus Royalties, Field Orthopedics, RTI Surgical, Acumed Stock options, and restor3d.

REFERENCES

1. Kloen P, Wiggers JK, Buijze GA. Treatment of diaphyseal non- unions of the ulna and radius. Arch Orthop Trauma Surg 2010;130(12):1439e1445.
2. Schemitsch EH, Richards RR. The effect of malunion on functional outcome after plate fixation of fractures of both bones of the forearm in adults. J Bone Joint Surg Am 1992;74(7):1068–78.
3. Goldfarb CA, Ricci WM, Tull F, et al. Functional outcome after fracture of both bones of the forearm. J Bone Joint Surg Br 2005;87:374–9.
4. Knight RA, Purvis GD. Fractures of both bones of the forearm in adults. J Bone Joint SurgAm 1949;31: 755–64.
5. Hughston JC. Fractures of the distal radial shaft. Mistakes in management. J Bone Joint Surg Am 1957;39:249–64.
6. Burwell HN, Charnley AD. Treatment of forearm fractures in adults with particular reference to plate fixation. J Bone Joint Surg Br 1964;46:404–25.
7. Matthews LS, Kaufer H, Garver DF, et al. The effect on supination-pronation of angular malalignment of fractures of both bones of the forearm. J Bone Joint Surg Am 1982;64(1):14–7.
8. Tarr RR, Garfinkel AI, Sarmiento A. The effects of angular and rotational deformities of both bones of the forearm: an in vitro study. J Bone Joint Surg Am 1984;66(1):65–70.
9. Dodge HS, Cady GW. Treatment of fractures of the radius and ulna with compression plates. J Bone Joint Surg Am 1972;54(6):1167–76.
10. Anderson LD, Sisk D, Tooms RE, et al. Compression-plate fixation in acute diaphyseal fractures of the radius and ulna. J Bone Joint Surg 1975;57(3):287–97.
11. Chapman MW, Gordon JE, Zissimos AG. Compression-plate fixation of acute fractures of the diaphyses of the radius and ulna. J Bone Joint Surg Am 1989;71(2):159–69.
12. Ross ER, Gourevitch D, Hastings GW, et al. Retrospective analysis of plate fixation of diaphyseal fractures of forearm bones. Injury 1989;20(4):211–4.
13. Teipner WA, Mast JW. Internal fixation of forearm fractures: double plating versus single compression (tension band) plating. A comparative study. Orthop Clin North Am 1980;11(3):381–91.
14. Sage FP, Smith H. Medullary fixation of forearm fractures. J Bone Joint Surg Am 1957;39(1):91–8.
15. Brakenbury PH, Corea JR, Blakemore ME. Nonunion of isolated fractures of the ulnar shaft in adults. Injury 1981;12(5):371–5.
16. Stern PJ, Drury WJ. Complications of plate fixation of forearm fractures. Clin Orthop 1983;175:25–9.
17. Stucken C, Olszewski DC, Creevy WR, et al. Preoperative diagnosis of infection in patients with nonunions. J Bone Joint Surg Am 2013;95(15): 1409e1412.
18. Ring D, Allende C, Jafarnia K, et al. Ununited diaphyseal forearm fractures with segmental defects: plate fixation and autogenous cancellous bone-grafting. J Bone Joint Surg Am 2004;86(11):2440–5.
19. Brinker MR, O Connor DP, Monla YT, et al. Metabolic and endocrine abnormalities in patients with nonunions. J Hand Surg Am 2007;21(8):557e570.
20. Buchheit T, Zura R, Wang Z, et al. Opioid exposure is associated with nonunion risk in a traumatically injured population: an inception cohort study. Injury 2018;49(7):1266e1271.
21. Raikin SM, Landsman JC, Alexander VA, et al. Effect of nicotine on the rate and strength of long bone fracture healing. Clin Orthop Relat Res 1998;353: 231–7.

22. Regan DK, Crespo AM, Konda SR, et al. Functional outcomes of compression plating and bone grafting for operative treatment of nonunions about the forearm. J Hand Surg Am 2017;43(6):564.e1–9.

23. Christensen NO. Kuntscher intramedullary reaming and nail fixation for nonunion of the forearm. Clin Orthop 1976;116:215–21.

24. Schemitsch EH, Jones D, Henley MB, et al. A comparison of malreduction after plate and intramedullary fixation of forearm fractures. J Orthop Trauma 1995;9(1):8–16.

25. Lee YH, Lee SK, Chung MS, et al. Interlocking Contoured Intramedullary Nail Fixation for Selected Diaphyseal Fractures of Forearm in Adults. JBJS 2008;90(9):1891–8.

26. Weckbach A, Blattert TR, Weisser C. Interlocking nailing of forearm fractures. Arch Orthop Trauma Surg 2006;126(5):309–15.

27. Saka G, Saglam N, Kurtulmuş T, et al. New Interlocking intramedullary radius and ulna nails for treating forearm diaphyseal fractures in adults: a retrospective study. Injury 2014;45(Suppl 1):S16–23.

28. Jewell E, Merrell G. The use of a sliding bone graft in the upper extremity for long bone nonunions. J Hand Surg Am 2015;40(5):1025e1057.

29. Adani R, Delcroix L, Innocenti M, et al. Reconstruction of large posttraumatic skeletal defects of the forearm by vascularized free fibular graft. Microsurgery 2004;24(6):423e429.

30. Davis JA, Choo A, O'Connor DP, et al. Treatment of infected forearm nonunions with large complete segmental defects using bulk allograft and intramedullary fixation. J Hand Surg Am 2016;41(9):881e887.

31. Liu T, Liu Z, Ling L, et al. Infected forearm non-union treated by bone transport after debridement. BMC Musculoskelet Disord 2013;14:273.

32. Sagi HC, Young ML, Gerstenfeld L, et al. Qualitative and quantitative differences between bone graft obtained from the medullary canal (with a reamer/irrigator/aspirator) and the iliac crest of the same patient. J Bone Joint Surg Am 2012;94(23):2128e2135.

33. Dawson J, Kiner D, Gardner W II, et al. The reamer-irrigator-aspirator as a device for harvesting bone graft compared with iliac crest bone graft: union rates and complications. J Orthop Trauma 2014;28(10):584e590.

34. Prasarn ML, Ouellette EA, Miller DR. Infected nonunions of diaphyseal fractures of the forearm. Arch Orthop Trauma Surg 2010;130(7):867e873.

35. Mattar R Jr, Azze RJ, Ferreira MC, et al. Vascularized fibular graft for management of severe osteomyelitis of the upper extremity. Microsurgery 1994;15(1):22e27.

36. Hey-Groves EW. Modern methods of treating fractures. In: Fractures of the upper limb. 2nd edition. Bristol (United Kingdom): John wright; 1921. p. 203–5.

37. Devendra A, Velmurugesan PS, Dheenadhayalan J, et al. One-bone forearm reconstruction. J Bone Joint Surg Am 2019;101(15):e74.

38. Masquelet AC, Fitoussi F, Begue T, et al. Reconstruction of the long bones by the induced membrane and spongy autograft. Ann Chir Plast Esthet 2000;45(3):346e353.

39. Pelissier P, Masquelet AC, Bareille R, et al. Induced membranes secrete growth factors including vascular and osteoinductive factors and could stimulate bone regeneration. J Orthop Res 2004;22(1):73e79.

40. Walker M, Sharareh B, Mitchell SA. Masquelet reconstruction for posttraumatic segmental bone defects in the forearm. J Hand Surg Am 2019;44(4):342. e1e342.e8.

41. Julka A, Ozer K. Infected nonunion of the upper extremity. J Hand Surg Am 2013;38(11):2244e2246.

42. Singh R, Bleibleh S, Kanakaris NK, et al. Upper limb non-unions treated with BMP-7: efficacy and clinical results. Injury 2016;47(Suppl 6):S33eS39.

43. von Rüden C, Morgenstern M, Hierholzer C, et al. The missing effect of human recombinant Bone Morphogenetic Proteins BMP-2 and BMP-7 in surgical treatment of aseptic forearm nonunion. Injury 2016;47(4):919–24.

Pediatric Forearm Malunions

Shea Ray, MD, MS[a], M. Claire Manske, MD, MAS[a,b],*

KEYWORDS

- Pediatric forearm fracture • Forearm malunion • Forearm osteotomy • 3-dimensional planning
- Patient-specific instrumentation

KEY POINTS

- Most pediatric forearm fractures can be treated nonoperatively if initial alignment or alignment after reduction falls within acceptable parameters for the patient's age and fracture type.
- Malunion of pediatric forearm fractures can lead to pain, cosmetic concerns, and functional limitations, most commonly loss of forearm rotation.
- Advances in technology have brought 3-dimensional (3-D) computer simulation and development of patient-specific instrumentation to the forefront of malunion correction.
- Preoperative planning and execution of surgical correction of pediatric forearm malunions with 3-D computer simulation and patient-specific instrumentation can be done precisely and safely with good clinical outcomes.

 Video content accompanies this article at http://www.hand.theclinics.com.

INTRODUCTION

Pediatric forearm fractures are among the most common pediatric fractures and are often successfully treated with nonoperative intervention.[1–3] Long-term malunion of these fractures is uncommon,[4–6] given the remarkable remodeling potential in skeletally immature individuals,[7–9] and symptomatic malunion is even more rare. Prevention of malunion is often possible with appropriate initial treatment of acute forearm fractures. However, when symptomatic malunions do occur, causing pain, functional limitations, or unacceptable cosmetic deformity, corrective surgery is often indicated. The purpose of this article is to review the etiology, surgical management, and outcomes of treatment of pediatric forearm malunions.

ETIOLOGY

Forearm fractures are among the most common pediatric fractures, with diaphyseal fractures of the radius and/or ulna comprising 14.9% of these injuries.[10–13] They most commonly result from falling onto an outstretched hand during activity (eg, sports, monkey bars, trampolines).

The majority of acute pediatric forearm fractures are treated appropriately and successfully with nonoperative intervention,[1–3] including closed reduction and immobilization or immobilization alone if the fracture(s) is well-aligned on initial imaging.[1,2,14,15] Unlike adult patients where anatomic reduction and rigid fixation of forearm fractures is often required, displaced pediatric forearm fractures can often be treated nonoperatively given the unique remodeling capacity of

[a] Department of Orthopedic Surgery, Shriners Hospital for Children Northern California, Sacramento, CA, USA;
[b] Department of Orthopedic Surgery, University of California Davis, 4860 Y Street, Suite 3800, Sacramento, CA 95817, USA
* Corresponding author. Department of Orthopedic Surgery, Shriners Hospital for Children Northern California, 2425 Stockton Blvd, Sacramento, CA 95817.
E-mail address: mmanske@ucdavis.edu

Hand Clin 40 (2024) 35–48
https://doi.org/10.1016/j.hcl.2023.08.016

hand.theclinics.com

skeletally immature individuals.[16] The amount of remodeling expected is dependent on several factors, including age, skeletal maturity (amount of growth remaining) and menarchal status (in females), the proximity of the fracture to the physis, and the plane of motion of the nearest joint.[9,16,17] Because the majority of longitudinal growth comes from the distal physis of the radius and ulna (75% and 80%, respectively), distal fractures have greater remodeling potential than proximal ones.[1] Johari and colleagues studied 22 children aged 3 to 15 years with midshaft forearm fractures and identified a correlation between age and capacity for remodeling in midshaft fractures, with the majority of incomplete remodeling occurring in children greater than 10 years old.[9] Another investigation of 36 children with angulated forearm fractures found a significant correlation between age and angular remodeling of the fracture and epiphyseal plate in children under 11 years old; this effect was less pronounced in midshaft fractures compared to distal fractures.[8]

While displacement and angulation may remodel in the sagittal and coronal planes, particularly in younger children, axial plane deformity (rotational malalignment) does not remodel, regardless of age.[18,19] Additional exceptions to the tremendous remodeling potential in children are Monteggia and Galeazzi fractures, in which forearm fractures are associated with dislocation of the radiocapitellar joint or distal radioulnar joint (DRUJ), respectively. In these injury patterns, regardless of the alignment of the fractured segment, the radial head joint and DRUJ must be reduced, as joint dislocations do not correct with remodeling.[17]

Acceptable radiographic parameters for closed management are based on the remodeling potential and therefore also depend on patient age, skeletal maturity, fracture location, and amount and direction of displacement.[1,2,16,18,20] **Table 1** summarizes the acceptable radiographic parameters for closed treatment of pediatric forearm fractures.[1] Even if the initial fracture alignment is acceptable or is acceptable after closed reduction, loss of reduction may occur in up to 40% of pediatric forearm fractures.[21] Failure to recognize this may lead to malunion. Fracture characteristics associated with loss of reduction include translation of 50% or more in any plane, complete fracture of the radius, radial angulation in the sagittal plane greater than 15°, and ulnar angulation greater than 10° in the coronal plate.[22] Patient characteristics associated with reduction loss include age greater than 10 years,[22–24] fractures of the nondominant arm, and obesity[25] Treatment characteristics associated with unacceptable

nonoperative management include poor quality of reduction and application of a poor quality cast as measured by the radiographic cast index.[26–29] Fractures that required a closed reduction on presentation or are at risk of displacement should be monitored with serial radiographs at 1 week intervals for at least 3 weeks following reduction and casting.[26] When it is not possible to maintain fracture alignment within acceptable parameters by nonoperative means, surgery is often indicated to prevent malunion. Operative treatment options include closed reduction or mini-open reduction with percutaneous or intramedullary fixation and open reduction internal fixation with plate and screw constructs.[2,3,30]

The optimal treatment for a malunion is prevention. Great care should be taken to ensure that fractures are reduced to within acceptable parameters, followed closely with serial radiographs through union and remodeling and particular attention given to the patient's clinical examination. Follow-up of children with serial clinical examinations until 100° of forearm motion is achieved is recommended.[17]

EVALUATION OF MALUNION

The workup of suspected forearm malunion begins with obtaining a clinical examination and appropriate imaging. It is important to synthesize the evidence from both the clinical and imaging examinations because even if radiographic malunions occur, they may not be clinically significant. Although 15% to 40% of pediatric forearm fractures result in radiographic malunion,[4–6] most fractures will continue to remodel and fewer than 1% of radiographic malunions result in symptoms or functional deficits.[4,5] However, symptomatic malunions can be disabling, resulting in pain, functional limitations, and unacceptable cosmesis.[7,31–35]

Clinical Evaluation

The evaluation of forearm fracture malunion begins with a detailed history of the patient's clinical course and symptoms, including specific activity limitations and concerns. The physical examination includes an assessment of the clinical alignment of the arm and forearm and obtaining range of motion measurements, particularly of the elbow and forearm.

Loss of forearm rotation is the most common consequence of forearm malunion.[26,36] In a study by Daruwalla and colleagues of 53 nonoperatively treated both-bone forearm fractures, 53% of which patients had a rotation limitation of at least 20°, with 75% of those occurring in patients between the ages of 9 and 15.[19] Another study by

Table 1
Summary of acceptable alignment parameters for nonoperative management of pediatric forearm fractures based on age and type of deformity

Author(s), Year	Age (years)	Displacement (%)	Angulation (degrees)	Malrotation (degrees)	Bayonet apposition
Noonan, et al.[7] 1998	0–9		<15	<45	Yes, if < 1 cm short
	10 y or older mid/distal shaft		<15	<30	None
	10 y or older proximal shaft		<10	0	None
	Approaching skeletal maturity (<2 y remaining growth)		0	0	None
Price,[15] 2010	<8 mid/distal shaft	100	< 15 (up to 20° <5 y old)	<30	-
	<8 proximal shaft	100	<10	<30	-
	>8 mid/distal shaft with >2 y growth remaining	100	<10	<30	-
	>8 proximal shaft	Anatomic reduction with internal fixation recommended			-

Colaris and colleagues prospectively followed 410 children with both-bone forearm fractures to determine the cause of limitation in forearm rotation. At a median of 205 days, 30 patients (7.3%) had a limitation in forearm pronation/supination of at least 40°. Fourteen of these were evaluated with 3-dimensional (3-D) imaging which revealed rotational malunions of the radius and ulna without bony or soft tissue impairment.[37] In a study by Price and colleagues, 47 of 79 both-bone forearm fractures treated nonoperatively progressed to malunion. Of these, 9 (23%) had loss of forearm motion.[7] The functional impact of limited forearm motion after malunion is widely varied and often depends on the patient's specific activity demands.

The accepted functional ranges of motion of the elbow and forearm in the adult population as described by Morrey and colleagues are 30° to 130° of elbow extension/flexion and a total arc of 100° of foream rotation (with 50° each of pronation and supination).[38] More recently, Valone and colleagues established functional range of motion values at the elbow in children and adolescents. They utilized motion analysis to evaluate 28 subjects aged 6 to 17 while performing 8 functional tasks (hand to top of head, hand to mouth, hand to occiput, hand to back, drinking from a glass, eating with a fork, reading a magazine, and standing from a chair pushing up on the armrests) and 4 contemporary tasks (picking up a cellular phone and placing it to the ear, typing with a keyboard, using a computer mouse, and texting on a cellular phone). They found that an elbow motion arc of 30° to 130° and a forearm arc of motion of 50° of pronation and 50° of supination were adequate for most activities. However, holding a cell phone to the ear and typing on a keyboard demanded more elbow flexion and forearm pronation.[39]

Cadaveric studies have shown that angulation as little as 20° or malrotation of 30° correlates with loss of forearm motion, with malrotation of both the radius and ulna in different directions leading to the largest limitation in forearm range of motion.[33,40,41] Kasten and colleagues showed that 40° of rotational deformity of the radius led to a loss of 20° of pronation and supination[41] and Tarr and colleagues demonstrated that 15° of angulation led to a 27% loss of forearm rotation.[42] A decrease in radial bow can also impact forearm rotation−1 study showed that children with a maximal radial bow of ≤ 6.84% can result in ≤ 70° forearm pronation.[43] In contrast, angulation of 10° or less causes minimally noticeable clinical differences in forearm rotation and may be easily addressed via small compensatory motions.[42] The specific functional consequences children have difficulty with due to loss of forearm motion, along with the radiographic findings, should inform treatment discussions.

Imaging

The imaging workup of a forearm malunion includes obtaining posteroanterior (PA) and lateral radiographs of the forearm. Dedicated radiographs of the wrist and elbow should be obtained if DRUJ or radiocapitellar joint involvement is suspected. Obtaining radiographs of the unaffected forearm is helpful for comparison. Assessment of the sagittal and coronal plane deformities tends to be easier on this imaging, but determination of rotational deformity on x-rays is more challenging.[17,44,45] Traditionally, rotational assessment is made by determining if the bicipital tuberosity and radial styloid are located 180° from each other on anteroposterior and PA radiographs and the coronoid process and ulnar styloid are oriented 180° apart on a lateral radiograph; however, this relationship may be less accurate than traditionally believed.[46] Another technique is evaluating the cortices above and below the fracture to see if they are of the same width,[44,47,48] but this may be less useful in longstanding malunions with remodeling. If axial plate deformity or multiplanar deformity is suspected, computed tomography (CT) scan of bilateral forearms for side-to-side comparison provides a more comprehensive 3-D assessment

of the deformity. Additionally, the advent of 3-D modeling has provided more accurate ways to evaluate even the most subtle deformity in all 3 planes preoperatively, as well as assist in osteotomy planning and execution of deformity correction in multiple planes intraoperatively.

TREATMENT
Nonoperative

As discussed earlier, some degree of radiographic malunion may be well-tolerated. Angular and rotational deformities of the forearm measuring 10° or less often have minimal effect on pronation and supination[33,42] and clinical appearance. Moreover, the degree of radiographic deformity may not correspond with symptoms or functional limitations.[14,19,36] Nonoperative management of radiographic malunions may be appropriate if there are no functional, cosmetic, or pain concerns (Fig. 1). Patients with mild functional limitations

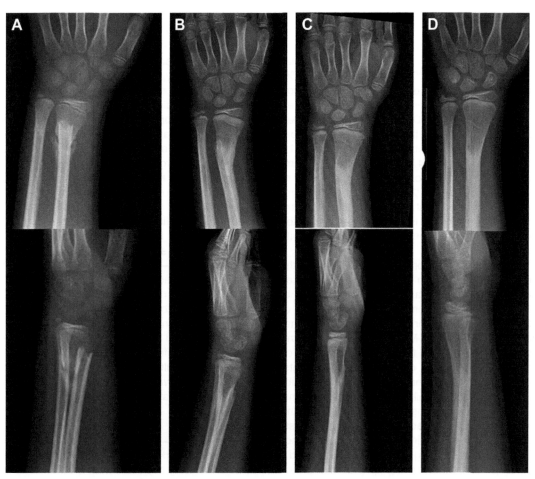

Fig. 1. Case 1: Serial radiographs showing posteroanterior and lateral projections of a remodeling distal radius metaphyseal fracture. Panel A: 2 weeks post-injury, Panel B: 3 months post-injury, Panel C: 6 months post-injury, Panel D: 12 months post-injury.

may have learned to compensate for loss of forearm rotation. For example, small losses of pronation can be compensated for by abduction of the shoulder. Although loss of supination is more difficult to compensate for, as this requires shoulder adduction across the torso, this may be better tolerated given that many contemporary tasks require forearm pronation rather than supination.[39,49] In all cases, a detailed discussion about the patient's specific limitations and functional goals should be carried out with them and their family members/caregivers to determine if surgery would benefit them.

Case 1

A 7-year-old patient who sustained closed left distal radius and ulna fractures, initially with 100% dorsal displacement, bayonet apposition, and apex volar angulation. She was treated nonoperatively with cast immobilization. At 1 year out from her injury, she has nearly completely remodeled her deformity (see **Fig. 1**). She had full pronation and supination on clinical examination.

Operative

Timing

After a decision is reached to pursue surgical correction of a forearm malunion based on the patient's clinical concerns, functional limitations, physical examination, and imaging, the timing of surgery is considered. Although debated, the optimal timing of surgical intervention is thought to be within a year of injury[34,50] to minimize the sequelae of longstanding deformity and malrotation, including soft tissue contractures[34] and degenerative joint disease of the adjacent proximal joint and DRUJ.[51] Trousdale and Linscheid found that patients who had corrective osteotomy performed within 12 months of injury gained more pronosupination than those treated after 12 months of injury (79° vs 30°) likely secondary to prevention of longstanding interosseous membrane contracture.[34] More recently, a meta-analysis of 11 observational studies found that corrective osteotomy within 12 months of injury resulted in greater improvement in forearm rotation (93° vs 61°).[52] Zlotolow and colleagues recommend surgical intervention if 100° arc of forearm motion is not achieved within 6 to 12 months of bony union, although it is important to acknowledge the relative functional importance of pronation compared to supination. Pace and colleagues recommend operative intervention if functional range of forearm rotation has not been gained by 6 months. Several studies have reported the effect of age on time of osteotomy as a predictor of outcome,[50,52] with younger age (<10 year old,[50] <13 year old[52]) having greater improvement in forearm rotation than older children.

Surgical techniques

The goal of surgical intervention is to improve forearm rotation, reduce pain, and correct cosmetic deformity, depending on the patient's and caregiver's concerns. Several techniques have been used to achieve these goals, including percutaneous osteoclasis and open corrective osteotomy with standard preoperative planning or with computer-guided technology.

Percutaneous osteoclasis Early descriptions of surgical correction for malunion include drill osteoclasis with manipulation.[32] This is indicated in impending malunions or early malunions in young children with thick periosteum that has the ability to help stabilize the osteotomy in the corrected position. This technique involves making a small incision over the center of rotational angulation (CORA) of the deformity and using a drill with drill guide to make several holes in the bone at the malunion site concentrated at the convexity of the malunion. This is followed by controlled manual manipulation of the bone to create a greenstick fracture that allows the bone to be realigned in an acceptable position. Because this technique relies on the stout periosteum to assist in maintaining the corrected alignment, it is typically only indicated in young children. The osteotomy can be held in position with a well-molded cast with or without additional stabilization, such as percutaneous crossed Kirschner wires or intramedullary fixation.

Blackburn and colleagues[32] evaluated the outcomes of this technique in 15 children aged 5 to 15 years and reported 100% angular correction within 10° of anatomic alignment with 73% of patients regaining full forearm rotation, with 67% of patients being satisfied postoperatively. They cite the absence of a large scar and no need for subsequent surgery to remove a plate as advantages of this technique.

Corrective osteotomy with conventional planning Open osteotomy is the mainstay of surgical correction of established forearm fracture malunions. The main advantage is that it can be used regardless of age or skeletal maturity. Disadvantages include the longer surgical time, more extensive surgical exposure, and the need for a second surgery in young children to remove surgical implants. Some authors have recommended concomitant release of the interosseous membrane to address the soft tissue contracture associated with limitations in forearm rotation[35]; Although there are no outcome studies, this is associated with a hypothetical risk of iatrogenic synostosis.[34]

Corrective osteotomy requires preoperative planning to identify and correct all elements of the deformity (angulation, translation, rotation, and shortening). For uniplanar and simple biplanar deformities, surgical planning involves applying the fundamental principles of deformity correction. For angular correction, the CORA method of correction, as described by Paley and colleagues, can be utilized. Lines are drawn down the mechanical or anatomic axes of the involved segments of the bone in question, and their intersection is the CORA. Location of osteotomy should be considered relative to the CORA, so secondary deformities can be avoided.[53] Using the principle of identifying the maximum plane of deformity on radiographs, Pace and colleagues describe a surgical method of deformity correction utilizing only preoperative radiographs and intraoperative fluoroscopy.[54]

The resultant osteotomies usually consist of a closing wedge osteotomy at the location of maximum angulation in the coronal and sagittal planes. Closing wedge osteotomies are preferred if possible to allow bony apposition without graft as well as to reduce tension on the soft tissue. Closing wedge osteotomies of the radius may require concomitant ulnar shortening osteotomy or epiphysiodesis if the radius osteotomy results in unacceptable ulnar positive variance (**Fig. 2**). Opening wedge osteotomies with structural autograft can also be used if needed to correct length discrepancies, but care must be taken to avoid excessive soft tissue tension and ensure bone apposition of the autograft. The osteotomies are typically stabilized with plate and screw constructs, although intramedullary fixation can be used in skeletally immature children.

Case 2 This is a 12-year-old post-menarchal right-handed female who had a fall at a trampoline park 18 months prior to presentation. She sustained a right proximal radial shaft fracture that was treated with cast immobilization. Since cast removal, she and her parents noted decreased forearm rotation, especially pronation, which has caused difficulty

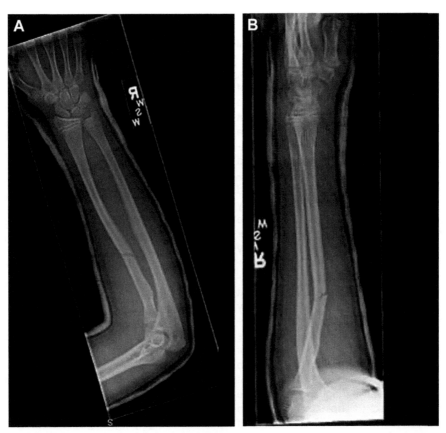

Fig. 2. Case 2: Posteroanterior (*A*) and lateral (*B*) radiographs of the right forearm at time of initial evaluation and treatment at an outside facility, demonstrating a fracture of the proximal third of the radius diaphysis, with 20° of apex volar angulation.

with school activities and playing the piano. On examination, she has full and symmetric wrist and elbow flexion and extension. In the right forearm, she has 70° of active supination (80° on the left) and active pronation to neutral (80° on the left). Injury radiographs are shown in **Fig. 2** and radiographs on presentation are shown in **Fig. 3**. Given her limitations in activities of daily living and recreational activities, she and her family elected to pursue surgical intervention with corrective osteotomy. Because that she had fractured only one bone and her deformity appeared predominantly in the sagittal plane, a uniplanar closing wedge osteotomy of the radius was performed combined with an ulnar shortening osteotomy. Radiographs at 3 months postoperatively demonstrated healing (**Fig. 4**). At the final follow-up, patient had 70° degrees of forearm supination and 75° of pronation.

Corrective Osteotomy with Computer-simulated Planning and Custom Guides For more complex deformities, including multiplanar deformity and/or deformity in the axial plane (rotational malalignment), computer-assisted planning with 3-D data is useful to simplify the planning and execution of complex multiplanar deformity correction.[51] Either MRI or, more commonly, CT scans of the affected

and unaffected forearms are obtained from the elbow joint through the carpus. The alignment and osteology of the affected forearm can then be compared to the unaffected contralateral forearm.

Computer-assisted design and computer-assisted manufacturing utilizing CT scan data have been utilized for building 3-D models to assist with preoperative planning of osteotomy,[55] simulating the osteotomy procedure preoperatively with a computer program[56] and developing patient-specific drill and cutting guides for intraoperative use for both distal radius and midshaft osteotomies.[57–59] Additionally, the plate and screw construct can be selected during the computer-simulated surgical planning, including custom contouring of the plate.

Execution of these complex osteotomies in the operating room is facilitated by the preoperative surgical simulation and use of custom drill and cutting guides which can be affixed directly to the patient's bone to create the same cuts that were planned during the surgical simulation. To ensure accurate correction, the surgeon must ensure the guides are secured to the bone exactly as planned during the simulation; this is facilitated by comparing the fit of the guides on the patient's bone with their fit on 3-D–printed models of the

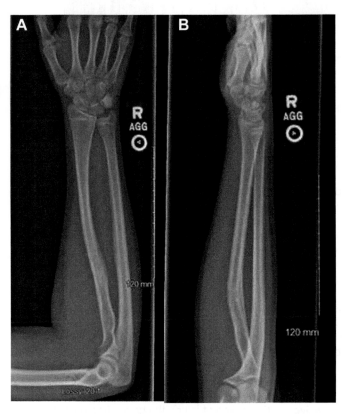

Fig. 3. Case 2: Posteroanterior (*A*) and lateral (*B*) radiographs of the right forearm 18 months after injury, demonstrating a malunion of the proximal radius diaphysis, with minimal remodeling as compared to injury radiographs.

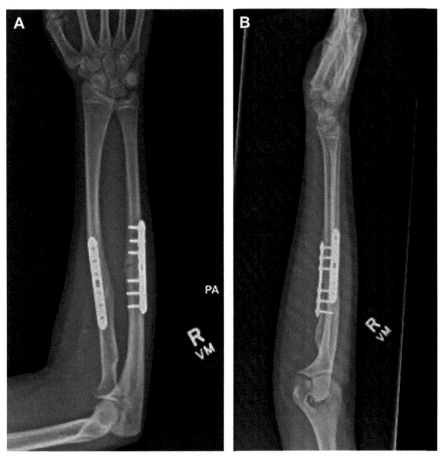

Fig. 4. Case 2: Posteroanterior (*A*) and lateral (*B*) radiographs of the right forearm 3 months postoperatively, demonstrating correction of the patient's malunion at the proximal radius. There is complete healing of the radial osteotomy and partial healing at the ulna.

affected bone intraoperatively. The drill holes for the plate are often made first, using the custom drill guide. Next, the patient-specific cutting guide is used to make the osteotomy and finally, the plate and screw construct is applied to the bone.

Case 3 The patient is a 13-year-old, postmenarchal, right hand dominant female who sustained a fall from her bike 1 year ago, resulting in fractures of the right distal radial and ulnar shafts. With forearm supination, she reports a painful clunk on the ulnar side of her wrist. Examination demonstrated volar subluxation of the distal ulna in supination (Video 1). Radiographs demonstrated malunion of both the distal radial and ulna shafts (**Fig. 5**). Given that both bones were fractured, and there is likely a rotational component to the malunion, a corrective osteotomy was planned with computer simulation (Video 2). Surgery was performed using 3-D–printed models and patient-specific drill guides and cutting jigs (**Figs. 6–8**). Intraoperatively, she had full passive

pronation and supination (**Fig. 9**). Radiographs at the final follow-up demonstrated improved radiographic alignment. (*Case provided courtesy of Lisa Lattanza, MD*)

Outcomes of Corrective Osteotomy Forearm osteotomy, when performed in the appropriately selected patient at the right time, produces satisfactory results. Trousdale and colleagues[34] presented outcomes in 20 pediatric forearm fracture malunions treated with osteotomies for loss of motion and noted greater improvement in postoperative motion if surgery was performed within 12 months of injury (gain of 79° vs 30°). Van Geenan and colleagues[50] achieved a mean gain of 85° of forearm rotation in 20 consecutive patients treated for a forearm malunion from a fracture sustained in childhood. Children who underwent surgery within 1 year of injury and those under 10 years of age at time of surgery had significantly greater gains in their motion postoperatively. Age at injury, the bones fractured, the level

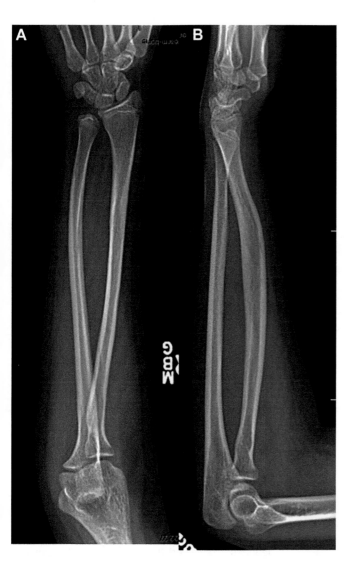

Fig. 5. Case 3: Posteroanterior (*A*) and lateral (*B*) radiographs of the right forearm at the time of presentation, 12 months after the injury, demonstrating a fracture malunion of the distal third of the radius diaphysis, with 25° of apex volar angulation and ulnar bowing in the coronal plane.

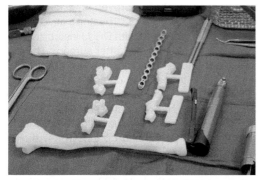

Fig. 6. Case 3: Intraoperative set-up with 3-dimensional–printed model of the radius malunion (bottom), patient-specific drill guides (middle-left), and patient-specific cutting guide (middle-right).

of fracture, and the bones that were osteotomized did not affect the improvement in motion. In a series of 9 patients, Price and colleagues[54] were able to achieve an average increase of 102° in forearm rotation after osteotomy for diaphyseal forearm malunions without radial head dislocation or DRUJ instability. All osteotomies were performed within 12 months of injury after a trial period of observation without immobilization. Nagy and colleagues looked at outcomes of osteotomy for symptomatic forearm malunion based on the patient's preoperative complaints, including loss of forearm rotation and DRUJ pain. They found that patients with a predominant loss of supination preoperatively had a greater improvement in range of motion after surgery than patients with a predominant loss of pronation. All patients that were operated on for a painful DRUJ had resolution of their pain with a stable joint after surgery.

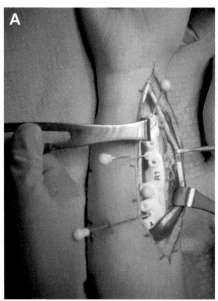
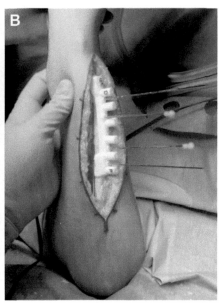

Fig. 7. Case 3: Drill guides secured to the radius (*A*) and ulna (*B*) with Kirschner wires.

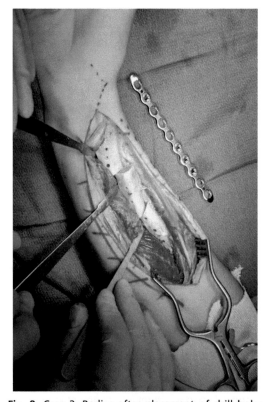

Fig. 8. Case 3: Radius after placement of drill holes and performing a double osteotomy of the diaphysis as directed by the preoperative plan and custom guides. A single osteotomy was also performed of the ulna (not pictured).

Use of computer-simulated surgical planning preoperatively and intraoperative use of custom 3-D–printed guides has gained popularity in recent years and is increasingly being used in orthopedic applications.[44] This has been shown to simplify the planning and execution of osteotomies for the correction of complex deformities and do so with more precision and good clinical outcomes.[60–63] Recent clinical studies have demonstrated the safety and efficacy of preoperative computer simulation and use of patient-specific surgical guides for the execution of corrective osteotomies for forearm malunions in children. Bauer and colleagues[44] reviewed the outcomes in 19 patients who underwent forearm osteotomies with preoperative surgical planning with simulation and patient-specific guides. All osteotomies went on to union and there were few minor complications. Forearm range motion improved on average from 101° preoperatively to 133° postoperatively. The 8 patients in their cohort with DRUJ instability preoperatively were corrected after surgery. The authors recommend the technique as a safe and effective way to perform complex and multiple osteotomies for forearm deformity correction in children. A newer prospective cohort study by Roth and colleagues[64] evaluated outcomes in 15 patients after 3-D–planned corrective osteotomy and use of patient-specific cutting guides. Average improvement of range of motion was from 67° preoperatively to 128° postoperatively, achieving 85% of motion of the contralateral forearm. Multivariate analysis showed that severe preoperative restriction in forearm pro-supination

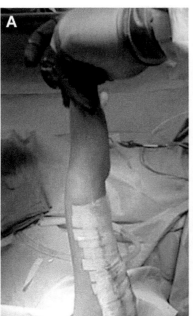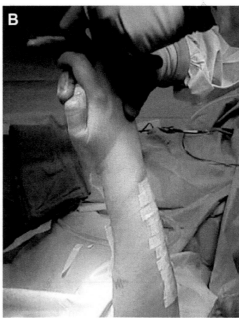

Fig. 9. Case 3: Intraoperative forearm rotation after corrective osteotomies and fixation. Full pronation and supination were observed without distal radioulnar joint dislocation or subluxation.

(<69°), a shorter interval until corrective osteotomy (<1 year), and greater angulation of the radius (>20°) were predictive of greater range of motion improvement after 3-D–guided osteotomy. Of interest, this study did not find a correlation between outcome and age at time of osteotomy.

A meta-analysis of individual participant data performed by Roth and colleagues analyzed 11 studies with a total of 71 children who underwent forearm osteotomies for malunion. The authors concluded that performance of osteotomy within 1 year of injury, an angular deformity of greater than 20°, and the use of 3-D computer-assisted techniques were predictive of superior functional outcome after corrective osteotomy for forearm malunions.

In a comparison between conventional and computer-assisted corrective osteotomy of the forearm, Bauer and colleagues[51] retrospectively compared 31 patients (mean age 31y, range 10–66y) who had conventional osteotomy versus 25 patients (mean age 28y, range 11–71y) who were treated with a computer-assisted method and patient-specific instrumentation. The mean operative time for the computer-assisted group was significantly shorter than in the conventional group (108 ± 26 min vs 140 ± 37 min), with similar clinical outcomes. There were 2 patients in the computer-assisted group who required revision for nonunion. The total direct cost for preoperative planning and instrumentation was 2415 USD per case. These results were corroborated by Benayoun and

colleagues in their study of 23 corrective osteotomies, 9 utilizing a patient-specific surgical guide and 14 without. Surgical times were shorter in the guide-use group by an average of 42 minutes, and there was also greater improvement in Patient-Rated Wrist Evaluation scores in the guide-use group. The mean total intraoperative radiation dose was lower in the group that did not use a patient-specific guide.

SUMMARY

Many pediatric forearm fractures can be treated nonoperatively if initial alignment or alignment after reduction falls within acceptable parameters for the patient's age and fracture type. If parameters are not met, the injury is missed, or reduction is lost, a malunion can occur. Malunited forearm fractures in the pediatric population may lead to limited forearm range of motion and functional limitations. The severity of the loss of motion and the specific functional limitations that the patient experience should be the surgeon's primary guide for making treatment decisions. In cases where range of motion limitations are minimal, well-tolerated, and not functionally limiting, nonoperative management is appropriate. In cases where there is substantial loss of forearm motion that impairs that patient's functional activities, operative intervention with corrective osteotomy should be considered and discussed with the patient and their caregivers. Corrective osteotomy can be safely and effectively performed with a variety of techniques. For simple uniplanar or biplanar angular deformity, osteotomies can often be planned based on preoperative radiographs and executed with the assistance of intraoperative fluoroscopy. For correction of multiplanar deformities, especially when there is a rotational (axial plane) component, advances in 3-D surgical planning and patient-specific cutting guides have made surgical correction of malunion in the forearm more precise and may decrease operative time. The cost to benefit ratio should be considered when using these technologies. For best functional results, osteotomy should be performed within 6 to 12 months of injury.

CLINICS CARE POINTS

- Most pediatric forearm fractures can be treated nonoperatively if initial alignment or alignment after reduction falls within acceptable parameters for the patient's age and fracture type. In general, more deformity can be accepted in patients under the age of 8, and distal deformity is better tolerated than proximal deformity.

- A malunion with angulation greater than 20° and/or malrotation more than 30° can cause noticeable difference in forearm rotation.

- The impact of limited forearm rotation varies between patients; however, 50° of pronation and supination are sufficient for most activities, with more pronation required for activities like typing and holding a cell phone.

- When forearm range of motion is limited or if the patient has DRUJ or radiocapitellar joint instability, surgical correction with osteotomy is indicated.

- Computer-simulated preoperative planning and use of patient-specific instrumentation is a safe, precise, and effective method for performing corrective osteotomy. The literature supports its use, and it may result in shorter operative times and has comparable clinical outcomes to conventional osteotomy.

DISCLOSURE

The authors have nothing to disclose.

SUPPLEMENTARY DATA

Supplementary data related to this article can be found online at https://doi.org/10.1016/j.hcl.2023.08.016.

REFERENCES

1. Noonan KJ, Price CT. Forearm and Distal Radius Fractures in Children. J Am Acad Orthop Surg 1998;6(3):146–56.
2. Truntzer J, Vopat ML, Kane PM, et al. Forearm diaphyseal fractures in the adolescent population: treatment and management. Eur J Orthop Surg Traumatol 2015;25(2):201–9.
3. Smith VA, Goodman HJ, Strongwater A, et al. Treatment of Pediatric Both-Bone Forearm Fractures. J Pediatr Orthop 2005;25(3):5.
4. Thomas EM, Tuson KW, Browne PS. Fractures of the radius and ulna in children. Injury 1975;7(2):120–4.
5. Fuller DJ, McCullough CJ. Malunited fractures of the forearm in children. J Bone Joint Surg Br 1982;64(3):364–7.
6. Schmittenbecher PP. State-of-the-art treatment of forearm shaft fractures. Injury 2005;36(1):S25–34.
7. Price CT, Scott DS, Kurzner ME, et al. Malunited forearm fractures in children. J Pediatr Orthop 1990;10(6):705–12.
8. Vittas D, Larsen E, Torp-Pedersen S. Angular Remodeling of Midshaft Forearm Fractures in Children. Clin Orthop Relat Res 1991;265:261–4.
9. Johari AN, Sinha M. Remodeling of forearm fractures in children. J Pediatr Orthop Part B 1999;8(2):84–7.
10. Naranje SM, Erali RA, Warner WC, et al. Epidemiology of Pediatric Fractures Presenting to Emergency Departments in the United States. J Pediatr Orthop 2016;36(4):e45–8.
11. Landin LA. Fracture patterns in children. Analysis of 8,682 fractures with special reference to incidence, etiology and secular changes in a Swedish urban population 1950-1979. Acta Orthop Scand Suppl 1983;202:1–109.
12. Ramirez R, Zlotolow D. Shoulder, Elbow, and Forearm Fractures and Dislocations. In: Textbook of hand and Upper Extremity surgery. Vol 2. 2nd ed. American Society for Surgery of the Hand; 2019.
13. Cheng JC, Ng BK, Ying SY, et al. A 10-year study of the changes in the pattern and treatment of 6,493 fractures. J Pediatr Orthop 1999;19(3):344–50.
14. Carey PJ, Alburger PD, Betz RR, et al. BOTH-BONE FOREARM FRACTURES IN CHILDREN. Orthopedics 1992;15(9):1015–9.
15. Zionts LE, Zalavras CG, Gerhardt MB. Closed Treatment of Displaced Diaphyseal Both-Bone Forearm Fractures in Older Children and Adolescents. J Pediatr Orthop 2005;25(4):507–12.
16. Ploegmakers JJW, Verheyen CCPM. Acceptance of angulation in the non-operative treatment of paediatric forearm fractures. J Pediatr Orthop B 2006;15:428–32.
17. Zlotolow DA. Pediatric Forearm Fractures: Spotting and Managing the Bad Actors. J Hand Surg 2012;37(2):363–6.

18. Price CT. Acceptable Alignment of Forearm Fractures in Children: Open Reduction Indications. J Pediatr Orthop 2010;30(Supplement 2):S82–4.
19. Daruwalla JS. A study of radioulnar movements following fractures of the forearm in children. Clin Orthop 1979;139:114–20.
20. Fuller DJ, Mccullough CJ. MALUNITED FRACTURES OF THE FOREARM IN CHILDREN.; 1982.
21. Miller BS, Taylor B, Widmann RF, et al. Cast immobilization versus percutaneous pin fixation of displaced distal radius fractures in children: a prospective, randomized study. J Pediatr Orthop 2005;25(4):490–4.
22. Kutsikovich JI, Hopkins CM, Gannon EW, et al. Factors that predict instability in pediatric diaphyseal both-bone forearm fractures. J Pediatr Orthop B 2018;27(4):304–8.
23. Franklin CC, Wren T, Ferkel E, et al. Predictors of conversion from conservative to operative treatment of pediatric forearm fractures. J Pediatr Orthop B 2014;23(2):150–4.
24. Bowman EN, Mehlman CT, Lindsell CJ, et al. Nonoperative treatment of both-bone forearm shaft fractures in children: Predictors of early radiographic failure. J Pediatr Orthop 2011;31(1):23–32.
25. Okoroafor UC, Cannada LK, McGinty JL. Obesity and Failure of Nonsurgical Management of Pediatric Both-Bone Forearm Fractures. J Hand Surg 2017;42(9):711–6.
26. Chia B, Kozin SH, Herman MJ, et al. Complications of Pediatric Distal Radius and Forearm Fractures. Inst Course Lect 2015;64:499–507.
27. Yang JJ, Chang JH, Lin KY, et al. Redisplacement of Diaphyseal Fractures of the Forearm After Closed Reduction in Children: A Retrospective Analysis of Risk Factors. J Orthop Trauma 2012;26(2):110–6.
28. Colaris JW, Allema JH, Reijman M, et al. Risk factors for the displacement of fractures of both bones of the forearm in children. Bone Jt J 2013;95-B(5):689–93.
29. Asadollahi S, Pourali M, Heidari K. Predictive factors for re-displacement in diaphyseal forearm fractures in children—role of radiographic indices. Acta Orthop 2017;88(1):101–8.
30. Pace JL. Pediatric and Adolescent Forearm Fractures: Current Controversies and Treatment Recommendations. J Am Acad Orthop Surg 2016;24(11):780–8.
31. Holdsworth BJ, Sloan JP. Proximal forearm fractures in children: residual disability. Injury 1982;14(2):174–9.
32. Blackburn N, Ziv I, Rang M. Correction of the malunited forearm fracture. Clin Orthop 1984;188:54–7.
33. Matthews LS, Kaufer H, Garver DF, et al. The effect on supination-pronation of angular malalignment of fractures of both bones of the forearm. J Bone Joint Surg Am 1982;64(1):14–7.
34. Trousdale RT, Linscheid RL. Operative treatment of malunited fractures of the forearm. J Bone Joint Surg Am 1995;77(6):894–902.
35. Nagy L, Jankauskas L, Dumont CE. Correction of Forearm Malunion Guided by the Preoperative Complaint. Clin Orthop 2008;466(6):1419–28.
36. Nilsson BE, Obrant K. The Range of Motion Following Fracture of the Shaft of the Forearm in Children. Acta Orthop Scand 1977;48(6):600–2.
37. Colaris JW, Oei S, Reijman M, et al. Three-dimensional imaging of children with severe limitation of pronation/supination after a both-bone forearm fracture. Arch Orthop Trauma Surg 2014;134(3):333–41.
38. Morrey BF, Askew LJ, Chao EY. A biomechanical study of normal functional elbow motion. J Bone Joint Surg Am 1981;63(6):872–7.
39. Valone LC, Waites C, Tartarilla AB, et al. Functional Elbow Range of Motion in Children and Adolescents. J Pediatr Orthop 2020;40(6):304–9.
40. Dumont CE, Thalmann R, Macy JC. The effect of rotational malunion of the radius and the ulna on supination and pronation: AN EXPERIMENTAL INVESTIGATION. J Bone Joint Surg Br 2002;84-B(7):1070–4.
41. Kasten P, Krefft M, Hesselbach J, et al. How Does Torsional Deformity of the Radial Shaft Influence the Rotation of the Forearm?: A Biomechanical Study. J Orthop Trauma 2003;17(1):57–60.
42. Tarr RR, Garfinkel AI, Sarmiento A. The effects of angular and rotational deformities of both bones of the forearm. An in vitro study. J Bone Joint Surg Am 1984;66(1):65–70.
43. Wongcharoenwatana J, Eamsobhana P, Chotigavanichaya C, et al. The effects of maximal radial bowing on forearm rotation in pediatric diaphyseal forearm fractures. Musculoskelet Surg 2021. https://doi.org/10.1007/s12306-021-00728-5.
44. Bauer AS, Storelli DAR, Sibbel SE, et al. Preoperative Computer Simulation and Patient-specific Guides are Safe and Effective to Correct Forearm Deformity in Children. J Pediatr Orthop 2017;37(7):504–10.
45. Sibbel SE. Pediatric Forearm Deformity: Use of 3D Modeling to Guide Deformity Correction. Tech Orthop 2019;34(1):2–5.
46. Weinberg DS, Park PJ, Boden KA, et al. Anatomic Investigation of Commonly Used Landmarks for Evaluating Rotation During Forearm Fracture Reduction. JBJS 2016;98(13):1103.
47. Evans EM. Rotational Deformity in the Treatment of Fractures of Both Bones of the Forearm. JBJS 1945;27(3). https://journals.lww.com/jbjsjournal/Fulltext/1945/27030/ROTATIONAL_DEFORMITY_IN_THE_TREATMENT_OF_FRACTURES.3.aspx.
48. Creasman C, Zaleske DJ, Ehrlich MG. Analyzing Forearm Fractures in Children. Clin Orthop Relat Res

1984;188. https://journals.lww.com/corr/Fulltext/1984/09000/Analyzing_Forearm_Fractures_in_Children_.6.aspx.

49. Sardelli M, Tashjian RZ, MacWilliams BA. Functional elbow range of motion for contemporary tasks. J Bone Joint Surg Am 2011;93(5):471–7.

50. van Geenen RCI, Besselaar PP. Outcome after corrective osteotomy for malunited fractures of the forearm sustained in childhood. J Bone Joint Surg Br 2007;89(2):236–9.

51. Bauer DE, Zimmermann S, Aichmair A, et al. Conventional Versus Computer-Assisted Corrective Osteotomy of the Forearm: a Retrospective Analysis of 56 Consecutive Cases. J Hand Surg 2017;42(6):447–55.

52. Roth KC, Walenkamp MMJ, van Geenen RCI, et al. Factors determining outcome of corrective osteotomy for malunited paediatric forearm fractures: a systematic review and meta-analysis. J Hand Surg Eur Vol 2017;42(8):810–6.

53. Paley D, Herzenberg JE, Tetsworth K, et al. Deformity planning for frontal and sagittal plane corrective osteotomies. Orthop Clin North Am 1994;25(3):425–65.

54. Price CT, Knapp DR. Osteotomy for Malunited Forearm Shaft Fractures in Children. J Pediatr Orthop 2006;26(2):4.

55. Jupiter JB, Ruder J, Roth DA. Computer-generated bone models in the planning of osteotomy of multidirectional distal radius malunions. J Hand Surg 1992;17(3):406–15.

56. Croitoru H, Ellis RE, Prihar R, et al. Fixation-based surgery: a new technique for distal radius osteotomy. Comput Aided Surg Off J Int Soc Comput Aided Surg 2001;6(3):160–9.

57. Kunz M, Ma B, Rudan JF, et al. Image-guided distal radius osteotomy using patient-specific instrument guides. J Hand Surg 2013;38(8):1618–24.

58. Miyake J, Murase T, Oka K, et al. Computer-Assisted Corrective Osteotomy for Malunited Diaphyseal Forearm Fractures. J Bone Jt Surg 2012;94(20):e150.

59. Miyake J, Murase T, Moritomo H, et al. Distal radius osteotomy with volar locking plates based on computer simulation. Clin Orthop 2011;469(6):1766–73.

60. Storelli DAR, Bauer AS, Lattanza LL, et al. The Use of Computer-aided Design and 3-Dimensional Models in the Treatment of Forearm Malunions in Children. Tech Hand Up Extrem Surg 2015;19(1):23–6.

61. Kataoka T, Oka K, Murase T. Rotational Corrective Osteotomy for Malunited Distal Diaphyseal Radius Fractures in Children and Adolescents. J Hand Surg 2018;43(3):286.e1–8.

62. Byrne AM, Impelmans B, Bertrand V, et al. Corrective Osteotomy for Malunited Diaphyseal Forearm Fractures Using Preoperative 3-Dimensional Planning and Patient-Specific Surgical Guides and Implants. J Hand Surg 2017;42(10):836.e1–12.

63. Saravi B, Lang G, Steger R, et al. Corrective Osteotomy of Upper Extremity Malunions Using Three-Dimensional Planning and Patient-Specific Surgical Guides: Recent Advances and Perspectives. Front Surg 2021;8:615026.

64. Roth KC, van Es EM, Kraan GA, et al. Outcomes of 3-D corrective osteotomies for paediatric malunited both-bone forearm fractures. J Hand Surg Eur Vol 2022;47(2):164–71.

Distal Radius Nonunions
A Rare Entity?

Sofia Bougioukli, MD, PhD, Kevin C. Chung, MD, MS*

KEYWORDS

- Distal radius fracture • Nonunion • Wrist arthrodesis
- Distal radius open reduction and internal fixation • Bone graft

KEY POINTS

- Distal radius nonunion is a rare complication following distal radius fracture.
- Pathogenesis of distal radius nonunion is multifactorial and includes injury, patient biology, and initial method of treatment.
- In established distal radius nonunions, definitive surgical treatment is necessary with open reduction and internal fixation of the distal radius with or without bone graft or conversion to a wrist arthrodesis.
- There is no consensus on the optimal surgical approach for managing distal radius nonunions.

INTRODUCTION

The majority of distal radius fractures heal uneventfully with either nonoperative treatment or open reduction and internal (ORIF) versus external fixation as indicated. However, in certain cases, nonunion can occur, leading to pain, instability, and disabling wrist and hand function. Distal radius nonunions are extremely uncommon. Most pertinent reports in the literature include only a small number of cases, making it challenging to definitively determine the incidence of distal radius fracture nonunions. In his classic report in 1942, Watson-Jones described one case of distal radius nonunion out of 3199 studied fractures,[1] whereas Cooney and colleagues did not find any nonunions in their series of 565 distal radius fractures.[2] In a study by Bacorn and Kurtzke, only 0.2% of 2100 distal radius fractures either failed to unite or demonstrated delayed healing.[3] Similarly, Segalman and Clark reported a total of 11 patients with 12 distal radius nonunions managed in their practice from 1973 to 1997.[4]

This low incidence of distal radius fracture nonunions seems to be multifactorial. It has been hypothesized that the fracture location in metaphyseal bone, common impaction and bony apposition of the fracture fragments, and generally minimal soft-tissue injury in low-energy injuries all contribute to creating a favorable environment for fracture healing in distal radius fractures.[5] Despite distal radius nonunion being a rare complication, and reports in the literature being few, it can be debilitating to the affected patients, compromising their wrist and hand function.

Distal radius nonunions require surgical treatment to relieve pain, provide stability, and improve function. Management of nonunions can be challenging, with multiple surgical treatment approaches having been described in the literature with varying success rates. To date, there is no consensus on the optimal approach for managing distal radius nonunions. Moreover, patients with distal radius nonunions often require multiple procedures to achieve union, which in turn leads to increased risk of complications, significant health care costs, disability, and prolonged time off work. The current review will address the pathogenesis, treatment options, and future hurdles in the management of distal radius fracture nonunions.

University of Michigan Medical School, Ann Arbor, MI, USA
* Corresponding author. University of Michigan Comprehensive Hand Center, Michigan Medicine, 1500 E. Medical Center Drive 2130 Taubman Center, SPC 5340, Ann Arbor, MI 48109-5340.
E-mail address: kecchung@med.umich.edu

Hand Clin 40 (2024) 49–61
https://doi.org/10.1016/j.hcl.2023.08.002
0749-0712/24/© 2023 Elsevier Inc. All rights reserved.

Table 1
Risk factors for nonunion of long bones[7-12]

Mechanical instability	Poor vascularity	Inadequate bone contact	Patient factors
Inadequate fixation	Open fracture	Soft tissue interposition	Age
Distraction of fracture fragments	Soft tissue injury	Malalignment	Infection
Bone loss	Arterial injury	Segmental bone defect	Medications (NSAIDs, anticoagulants, opiates etc.)
Poor bone quality	Periosteal stripping during ORIF	Distraction during fixation	Systemic medical conditions (DM, CKD, osteoporosis etc.)
			Smoking
			Alcohol abuse
			Radiation

Abbreviations: CKD, chronic kidney disease; DM, diabetes mellitus; NSAIDs, non-steroidal anti-inflammatory drugs; ORIF, open reduction and internal fixation.

RISK FACTORS ASSOCIATED WITH DISTAL RADIUS NONUNIONS

Bone healing requires a well-orchestrated sequence of biological events combined with mechanical stability to ensure successful fracture union.[6] In general, any alteration in the bone regeneration cascade as a result of poor local biology, infection, host inherent systemic factors, or biomechanical instability may lead to impaired healing (**Table 1**). A compromised regional biologic environment can be a result of inadequate local blood supply due to high-energy trauma with severe comminution, damage to nutrient vessels, or poor soft tissue envelope. It can also result from excessive periosteal stripping during surgical exposure and stabilization of the fracture.[7] Insufficient bone contact at the fracture site as a result of significant bone loss, soft tissue interposition, or excess distraction can also hinder bone healing.[8] Additionally, host factors such as age,[9] smoking,[10] metabolic bone disease, or concomitant systemic medical conditions and pertinent medications[11,12] also play a role in the pathogenesis of nonunions of long bones. Finally, mechanical instability from inadequate immobilization or fracture fixation also contributes to nonunion.[8] In the following paragraphs, the authors will review how these factors are implicated in distal radius nonunions.

Fracture comminution and open fractures with soft tissue stripping and bone loss are significant risk factors for nonunion.[13-16] Prommersberger and colleagues noted severe metaphyseal comminution of the initial distal radius injury in 18 out of the 23 studied patients with subsequent nonunions.[13] In their series of 758 distal radius fractures, Eglseder and colleagues identified 12 cases of nonunion. Seven out of 12 cases had an open fracture originally. The authors hypothesized that open distal radius fractures with associated soft tissue stripping had compromised local biology, leading to poor bone healing potential. In their series, they demonstrated that an open injury was associated with a 10 fold increase in nonunion rate (6.4% in open fractures vs 0.6% in closed injuries).[16] From a technical standpoint, insufficient immobilization,[14] inadequate stabilization across the fracture site with proximal and distal fixation, or over distraction at the radial fracture site all contribute to increased risk for fracture nonunion.[15] Several investigators have also suggested that the increase in distal radius fracture nonunions in recent years is a result of surgical interventions that attempt to restore radial length and inadvertently may create critical-sized osseous defects in the radius metaphysis.[4,13,15,17]

Concomitant distal ulna fracture or distal radioulnar joint dislocation may increase instability at the fracture site, with increased motion at the fracture site thus hindering union.[13,14] In their case series of 23 distal radius nonunions, Prommersberger and colleagues noticed that 9 of 23 patients had a concomitant fracture of the distal ulna, One patient had undergone a Darrach procedure and a second patient a resection of the radial head for a concomitant radial head fracture. The authors concluded that these procedures may have led to increased instability and thus may have compromised fracture healing of the distal radius.[13] In their report of 4 elderly female patients with distal radius nonunions, McKee et al. reported that 3 of the 4 nonunions had an associated distal ulna fracture.[5]

Patient factors including but not limited to tobacco use, alcohol, and medical comorbidities have also been studied for their potential association with radial fracture delayed healing. In his case series of distal radius nonunions using a free vascularized medial femoral condyle graft, Henry and colleagues described that all of the patients were smokers (6 of 6 patients).[18] Similarly, Smith and Wright reported that 100% (5 of 5) of their patients with distal radius nonunion were heavy smokers.[19] In the same cohort, 3 out of 5 patients had a history of alcohol abuse.[19] Segalman and Clark also noted alcohol abuse as a possible risk factor for radius nonunion.[4] Malnutrition, peripheral vascular disease, diabetes, and peripheral neuropathy have also been implicated in compromised distal radius fracture healing,[4,18] though clear correlation has not been proven.

EVALUATION AND DIAGNOSIS

As previously described, risk factors for distal radius fracture nonunion are multifactorial. As such, it is important to consider all pertinent risk factors when evaluating a patient with this condition, so as to understand the underlying pathophysiology and maximize the likelihood of success of subsequent interventions. History should focus on the initial fracture, including timing and mechanism of injury, open versus closed injury, as well as type and number of interventions undertaken. Past medical and social history should also be reviewed in detail, including but not limited to diabetes, renal failure, peripheral vascular disease, autoimmune disorders, osteoporosis, smoking, alcohol use, nutritional status, and vitamin D status. Medications used, such as nonsteroidal anti-inflammatory drugs, corticosteroids, anticoagulants, antiepileptics, and others should also be documented.[12] Finally, any postoperative complications including wound complications, infection, drainage, as well as use of antibiotics in the perioperative period should be analyzed.

Nonunion should be suspected in patients presenting with complains of persistent pain over the fracture site after range of motion (ROM) is initiated. Abnormal hand function with limited wrist and forearm ROM and grip strength can also be present. Another possible finding is worsening deformity of the wrist and often prominence of the distal ulna. As part of the physical examination, a thorough evaluation of the affected extremity should be undertaken. The treating physician should inspect the status of the soft tissue envelope as well as the position of the wrist. Tenderness to palpation over the fracture site, gross motion at the nonunion site, and wrist stability should also be assessed. Finally, a detailed neurovascular examination is needed to rule out any motor or sensory deficits.

The diagnosis of nonunion is confirmed with proper imaging. Plain radiographs are the initial imaging modality of choice (**Fig. 1**). The fracture site is evaluated for signs of cortical bridging and bone remodeling. Lateral flexion and extension views of the wrist can also be helpful in determining whether there is motion at the fracture site.[20] In general, in a healthy patient with a distal radius fracture, healing is expected within 3 months on plain radiographs. If a fracture fails to reach bony union by 4 to 6 months postinjury then it is considered a delayed union. A fracture that persists for a minimum of 9 months without signs of healing for at least 3 months constitutes a nonunion. If the status of the union is equivocal, then a computed tomographic scan should be obtained.

If adequate reduction and stabilization are observed in the setting of a distal radius nonunion, additional laboratory tests should be ordered to rule out undiagnosed metabolic or endocrine abnormalities that could compromise bone healing.[21] Vitamin D levels, calcium, magnesium, thyroid stimulating hormone, and free T4 are the most commonly ordered tests in such cases.[21] Finally, an underlying infectious process should always be suspected and ruled out in the setting of a nonunion. White blood cell count, erythrocyte sedimentation rate, and C reactive protein levels need to be evaluated if there are any concerns for a septic nonunion. Laboratory testing should be supplemented with a local bone biopsy from the nonunion site to definitively rule out an infection.

MANAGEMENT OF NONINFECTED NONUNIONS

Although the incidence and pathophysiology of distal radius fracture nonunions are somewhat unclear, the need for operative intervention for successful management of the nonunion is well documented in the literature. The treatment algorithm selected depends on the presence of infection, status of the radiocarpal and distal radioulnar joints, type of prior surgical interventions, and functional demands of the patient. Multiple surgical techniques exist for managing distal radius nonunions, including open reduction and internal fixation of the nonunion site with or without bone grafting or consideration of wrist arthrodesis (**Table 2**). No single technique has demonstrated clear superiority with regards to union rate and functional outcomes.

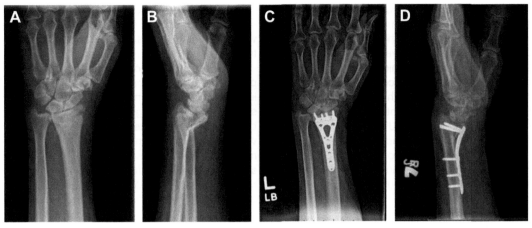

Fig. 1. 55 year old woman with past medical history of epilepsy and tobacco use presents with a left distal radius nonunion status post fall from motorhome 8 months ago. She was originally treated at an outside institution with ORIF (*A, B*), but subsequently developed significant wrist pain with limited wrist and hand ROM. Radiographic imaging demonstrated a nonunion of her distal radius (*C, D*).

For multiple years, the standard of care for distal radius nonunions was wrist arthrodesis.[4,5] The rationale was that attempts to fix a small, metaphyseal distal radius fracture were precarious at best and could not guarantee consistent results. In 1998, Segalman and Clark[4] treated a total of 9 patients with distal radius fracture nonunion. Open reduction and internal fixation with iliac crest bone graft (ICBG) was performed in 3 of 9 patients whereas the rest (6 of 9) were treated with wrist fusion. Both patient groups had a 100% union rate with minimal complications. The authors concluded that ORIF should be attempted when ≥5 mm subchondral bone is available distal to the nonunion site to increase the likelihood of successful union.[4] Otherwise, wrist arthrodesis was recommended (<5 mm subchondral bone). However, newer implants and improved surgical techniques for stabilizing small, periarticular fragments have made ORIF a reasonable option in the setting of distal radius nonunions regardless of distal fragment size.[13,23] In their study of 23 nonunions, Prommersberger and colleagues studied the effect of the size of the distal subchondral bone in clinical outcomes.[13] All of their patients were managed with ORIF with bone autograft from the iliac crest or femoral head, In their series, 10 of 23 patients had <5 mm of subchondral bone distal to the nonunion site and 13 of 23 with >5 mm. Only one patient did not achieve union in the large fragment group (>5 mm) and subsequently underwent wrist fusion. No differences with regards to wrist and forearm ROM, grip strength, and radiographic parameters were noted between the two cohorts.

Currently, for noninfected distal radius nonunions with adequate bone stock, the literature generally supports management of the nonunion with ORIF combined with bone grafting to attempt preservation of wrist motion. Surgical management in such cases includes aggressive debridement of the nonunion site to healthy looking, bleeding tissue, realignment of the fracture fragments, bone graft augmentation, good bony apposition, and stable fixation (**Fig. 2**). There is no consensus or specific recommendations with regards to optimal surgical approach. Volar, dorsal, or combined volar/dorsal approaches are all acceptable choices depending on the fracture nonunion pattern, direction of the deformity, previous approach, and surgical hardware, as well as the status of the soft tissue envelope.[13,23] With regards to fixation methods, various implants have been successfully used to stabilize the distal radius following nonunion debridement including volar and dorsal plating systems.[13,14,16,22–27] Ring recommended the use of 2 orthogonal plates to overcome the challenges stemming from the small distal fragment of the nonunited radius and provide superior biomechanical stability.[30] Fernandez and colleagues described their results in 10 patients with delayed union or nonunion of the distal radius addressed with debridement, bony alignment, plate fixation, and ICBG. Multiple different implants were used including volar plate fixation with a 3.5 mm or 2.7 mm T-shaped plate or dorsal fixation with a pi-plate, 3.5 mm dynamic compression plate or semitubular plate.[23] Union was noted in 10 of 10 cases at an average of 3 months postintervention, resulting in an average of 105° wrist flexion and extension, 145° forearm protonation/supination, and 73% grip strength as compared with the contralateral wrist. Similarly,

Table 2
Management of aseptic distal radius fracture nonunion

Authors (Year)	No of Nonunions	Management	Hardware Used	Union Rate (Time to Union)	Functional Outcomes	Complications
Harper et al,[22] 1990	2	ORIF + ICBG	Volar plate (not further specified)	2/2 (3–4 mo)	"Good" wrist and hand function	None reported
McKee et al,[5] 1997	3	ORIF + ICBG (1) OR arthrodesis (2)	Rush rod	2/3 (unclear)	Grip strength: 15 kg No pain with daily activities	Death (1)
Segalman et al[4] 1998	9	ORIF + ICBG (3) OR arthrodesis (6)	ORIF:Not reported Arthrodesis: • Single 3.5 mm dynamic compression plate (4) • Steinmann pin (1) • 3.5 mm recon plate	9/9 (3–12 mo)	Not reported	Complex regional pain syndrome (1) Postoperative infection (1)
Smith et al[19] 1999	5	ORIF + ICBG	Not reported	3/5 (Unknown)	Not reported	Persistent nonunion requiring wrist fusion in 2 of 5 pts
Fernandez et al,[23] 2001	10	ORIF + ICBG	Various implants (different volar/dorsal plates, K wires, compression screws)	10/10 (3 mo)	Grip strength: 73% vs contralateral wrist Flexion: 50° Extension: 55° Pronation: 75° Supination: 70°	Infection at ICBG harvest site (1) Hardware irritation (3)
Prommersberger et al,[13] 2002	23	ORIF ± ICBG (20) or femoral head graft (1)	Various implants (different volar/dorsal plates, K wires)	22/23 (unclear)	Large vs small fragment cohort respectively Grip strength: 29 ± 19 vs 23 ± 15 Extension: 32 ± 14° vs 19 ± 14° Flexion: 35 ± 19° vs 31 ±8° Pronation: 66 ± 22° vs 55 ± 37° Supination: 29 ± 27° vs 43 ± 35°	Persistent nonunion requiring wrist fusion (1) DRUJ arthrosis (1) Hardware irritation (3)

(continued on next page)

Table 2
(continued)

Authors (Year)	No of Nonunions	Management	Hardware Used	Union Rate (Time to Union)	Functional Outcomes	Complications
Crow et al,[24] 2004	1	ORIF with vascularized bone graft from 2nd metacarpal and cancellous bone allograft	Dual plating	1/1 (7.5 mo)	Grip strength: 18 kg Flexion: 60° Extension: 15° Full pronation/ supination DASH score: 24	None reported
Henry,[25] 2007	1	ORIF + genicular corticoperiosteal free flap	Dia-meta volar distal radius plate	1/1 (5 wk)	Grip strength: 90% vs contralateral wrist Flexion: 70° Extension: 70° Pronation: 80° Supination: 80°	None reported
Villamor et al,[26] 2008	1	Modified Sauvé–Kapandji	3.5 mm volar fixed angle plate	1/1 (4 mo)	Grip strength: 90% vs contralateral wrist "Full" wrist ROM	None reported
Karuppiah et al[27] 2010	1	Modified Sauvé–Kapandji	AO T-plate	1/1 (7 mo)	Grip strength: 51% vs contralateral wrist Flexion: 45° Extension: 30° Pronation: 30° Supination: 90° DASH: 15	None reported
Koo et al[14] 2011	1	ORIF + ulnar shortening osteotomy	3.5 mm locking compression plate	1/1 (4 mo)	Grip strength: 57% vs contralateral wrist Flexion: 40° Extension: 25° Pronation: 90° Supination: 30°	None reported
Mithani et al[28] 2014	8	ORIF	Dorsal spanning bridge plate ± volar locking plate	8/8	Flexion: 36 Extension: 40 Pronation: 80° Supination: 70° DASH: 28	DRUJ arthrosis requiring wrist fusion (1)

Saremi et al[29] 2016	10	Posterior interosseous bone flap with ORIF (6) OR arthrodesis (3)	ORIF: Locking T-plate Arthrodesis: recon plate	9/9 (3.8 mo)	Grip strength: 15.3 kg Flexion: 34° Extension: 43° Supination: 82° Pronation: 67°	None reported
Shinohara et al[17] 2017	1	ORIF	Volar locking plate	1/1 (3 mo)	No pain with daily activities	None reported
Henry[30] 2017	6	Free vascularized medial femoral condyle flap with ORIF OR arthrodesis	Unclear	6/6 (7 wk)	DASH: 18	Ulnocarpal impaction (1) Osteomyelitis (1)

Abbreviations: DASH, disabilities of the arm, Shoulder and Hand; ICBG, iliac crest bone graft; mo, months; No, Number; ORIF, open reduction and internal fixation; Pt, patient; Recon, reconstruction; ROM, range of motion; wks, weeks.

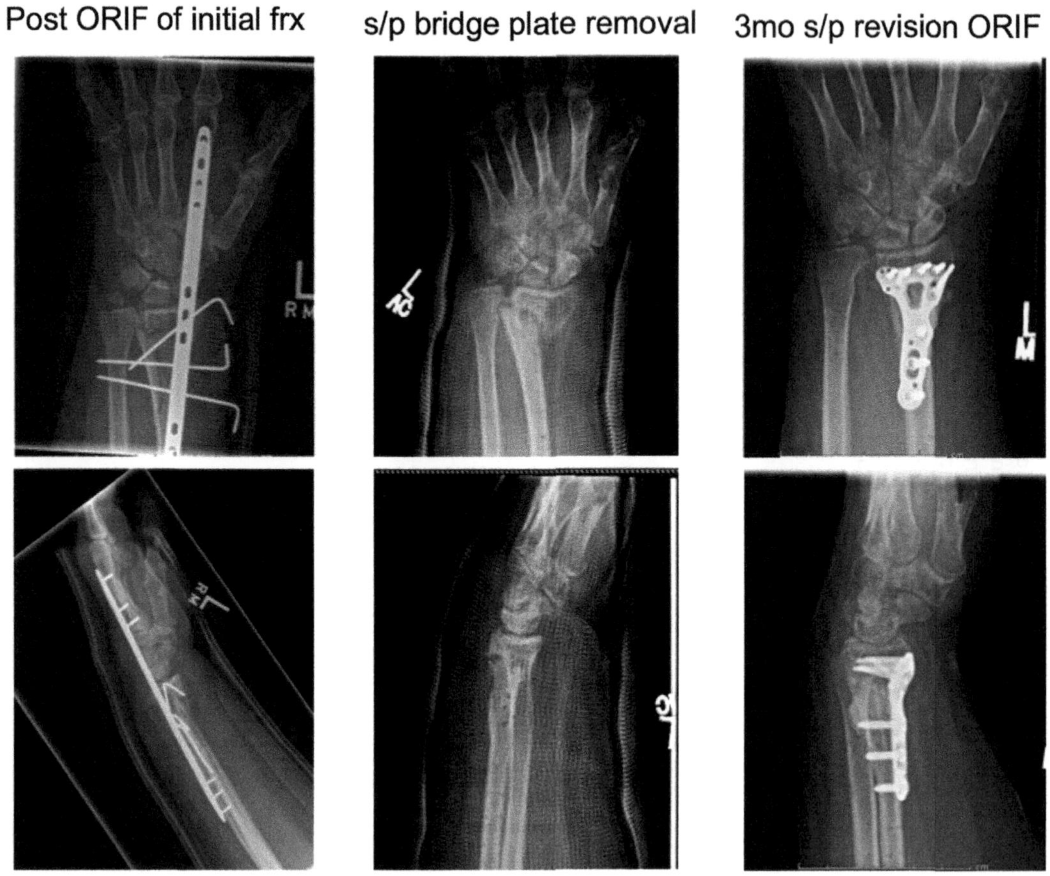

Post ORIF of initial frx   s/p bridge plate removal   3mo s/p revision ORIF

Fig. 2. A 60 year old woman with a past medical history of systemic lupus erythematosus presents for evaluation of left distal radius nonunion following an open distal radius fracture originally treated with irrigation and debridement, bridge plate fixation, and DRUJ CRPP. Loss of reduction was noted following hardware removal 3 months postoperatively. The patient was symptomatic with pain over the fracture site, wrist instability, and obvious wrist deformity. Her distal radius nonunion was treated 7 months after her initial fracture with repeat distal radius ORIF and cancellous bone allograft. Union was achieved at 3 months postoperatively. At her 6 month follow up she had painless wrist ROM (wrist extension: 40°, wrist flexion: 35°, forearm protonation/supination: 80/80°). ORIF; open reduction and internal fixation, s/p; status post, mo; months.

Eglseder and colleagues utilized volar or dorsal distal radius plates in their series of 10 distal radius nonunions with successful clinical and radiographic outcomes.[16] Mithani and colleagues[28] demonstrated the potential of dorsal spanning bridge plate fixation in 8 cases of distal radius nonunion. Union was achieved in all patients with significant improvements in ROM, grip strength, and DASH score. External fixation can also be used effectively in the definitive management of distal radius nonunions.[4,19]

In distal radius nonunions, bone graft is used to fill the defect along with ORIF to enhance bone healing. Bone autograft can be obtained from the iliac crest or resected distal ulna when a concomitant Darrach distal ulna resection procedure is performed. Allograft in the form of bone chips or structural bone graft (eg, fibula allograft) is an alternative option (**Figs. 3** and **4**). In patients with complex distal radius nonunions who have failed multiple surgical attempts at union and where there is a concern for a significant bone defect and compromised local biology, a free vascularized bone flap may be required to achieve union. In a consecutive case series of 9 patients, Saremi and colleagues[29] described the use of posterior interosseous bone flap to treat distal radius nonunions. Six patients were managed with ORIF and 3 with wrist arthrodesis due to severe distal radioulnar joint (DRUJ) arthrosis. The authors reported that all patients achieved union with improvements in their wrist and hand function without any donor-site morbidity.[29] Henry and colleagues demonstrated the successful use of a

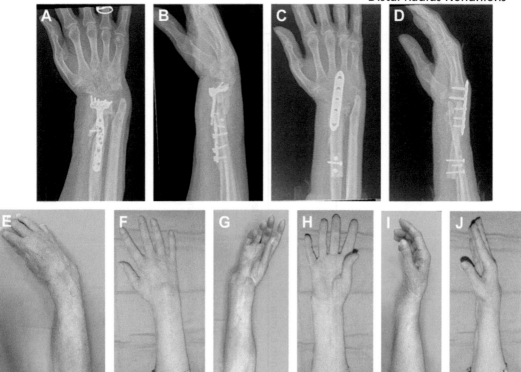

Fig. 3. This is a 60 year old woman with a right distal radius fracture following a ground level fall 8 years before presentation. She reportedly underwent 20 surgical procedures by 2 separate surgeons over the subsequent 8 years including but not limited to CRPP of her distal radius, ORIF, revision ORIF with ICBG, external fixator placement, bridge plate fixation, and finally fibula allograft with ORIF to achieve union. She underwent a Darrach procedure with the senior author for symptomatic ulna impaction syndrome and was recovering appropriately when she suddenly started noticing increasing radial sided wrist pain and deformity (*E, G, I*). Radiographic evaluation demonstrated hardware failure and fracture of the bone graft fracture in the radius (*A, B*). The patient was managed with hardware removal, irrigation and debridement, fibula allograft, and wrist fusion. Her plain radiographs 3 months postoperatively demonstrate a stable wrist status post fibular allograft placement with a dorsal plate and proximal lag screws, with no interval complications (*C, D*). Clinically the patient's dorsal incision is healing properly without signs of infection. She has no wrist pain and her wrist is in neutral position with correction of the deformity (*F, H, J*).

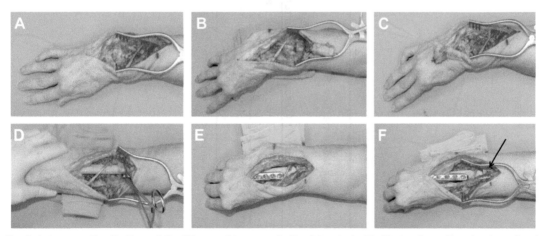

Fig. 4. Intraoperative findings of the 60 year old woman in **Fig. 3** treated with fibula allograft and wrist arthrodesis following a distal radius nonunion. Metallosis and devitalized scar tissue were noted in the wound (*A*). Excisional debridement of subcutaneous fat, fascia, muscle, and bone was carried out in this region to remove all devitalized tissue (*B, C*). The broken hardware was also removed (*C*). The total area of debridement was 8 cm × 3 cm. There were no signs of gross infection. Bleeding bone was noted at the proximal radius stump following debridement. A 10 cm fibular allograft was selected to bridge the resulting 8 cm radial defect and allow for overlapping at the proximal and distal sites (*D*). Distally, a 3.5 mm plate was selected for distal fixation (*E*). Proximally, three 2.7 mm lag screws were inserted to secure the allograft to the radius (*F; black arrow*). Bone graft harvested from the carpus earlier was used to fill the area around the distal fixation.

Table 3
Management of septic distal radius fracture nonunions

Authors Year	No of Nonunions	Management	Cultures	Antibiotics (Duration)	Definitive Fixation	Union
Ring et al,[31] 1999	2	Two stage approach	Not reported	Not specified	Wrist arthrodesis + Free vascularised fibula bone graft	2/2 (unknown)
Noaman et al,[32] 2020	15	Single stage approach	Not reported	Not specified (1 wk)	Distal radius resection + Free vascularised fibula bone graft + ORIF	13/15 (4 mo)

Abbreviaitons: No: Number; ORIF, open reduction and internal fixation; Recon, reconstruction; Pt, patient; ICBG, iliac crest bone graft; ROM, range of motion; mo, months; wk, week.

medial femoral condyle bone flap in a cohort of 6 patients with multiple comorbidities and failed prior procedures for their nonunion.[18] A 100% union rate was noted, resulting in improved DASH scores (18 vs 63 preoperatively). Finally, a case report presented a successful outcome of using vascularized bone graft from the second metacarpal with dual plating.[24]

Additional procedures at the ulnar side of the wrist may be required to preserve function, as DRUJ involvement is often present with deformity or posttraumatic arthritis. In the majority of cases, re-establishing the length of the radius will ensure restoration of DRUJ stability.[13] When severe, symptomatic arthrosis of the DRUJ is present, Darrach resection or DRUJ interposition arthroplasty can be considered to overcome persisting joint pain that is not alleviated despite having restored the radius length and alignment. In their case series, Fernandez and colleagues treated concomitant DRUJ pathology in 4 patients with either a hemiresection interposition (Bower's) arthroplasty or a Darrach procedure.[23]

Finally, failure to achieve union with multiple attempts at ORIF with bone grafting can be salvaged with wrist fusion. Wrist arthrodesis is also an acceptable choice in elderly patients with low functional demands. Wrist arthrodesis is performed using standard techniques. In brief, the nonunion site and the distal radius articular surface are debrided to bleeding cancellous bone followed by plate stabilization and bone grafting. Wrist arthrodesis has been associated with acceptable results in treatment of distal radius nonunions.[4,5,18,29] Bone autograft is usually harvested from the iliac crest but can also be obtained from the resected ulna if a Darrach procedure is performed at the same time.[30]

MANAGEMENT OF SEPTIC NONUNIONS

The literature on septic nonunions of the distal radius is very limited. Only 2 case series were identified in the English literature (**Table 3**). In general, there are 2 basic strategies in the management of infected nonunions of long bones; 1 versus 2 stage approaches. In the former, septic nonunion debridement and bone reconstruction are undertaken during the same procedure. In the 2 stage approach, the goal is to first eradicate the infection with meticulous irrigation and debridement, followed by prolonged antibiotic treatment and then additional surgical intervention for bone reconstruction.

Ring and colleagues reviewed the use of arthrodesis with a free fibula transfer for the management of 2 male patients with septic distal radius nonunion.[31] This was a 2 stage approach

with aggressive debridement and a course of antibiotics, followed by bone defect reconstruction once the infection was eradicated. The average length of fibula graft was 10 cm. Both patients achieved union at the proximal and distal host bone/fibula junction. No recurrence of the infection was reported, though the second patient had superficial wound dehiscence managed with local wound care.

In their patient cohort of 15 patients with septic nonunion of the distal radius, Noaman and colleagues described a single-stage approach with debridement of the nonunion and excision of the affected distal radius bone, and reconstruction of the resulting defect with a free proximal fibula vascularized bone graft.[32] The biceps femoris tendon slip that is attached to the harvested fibula graft is used to reinforce soft tissue reconstruction. Bone union was achieved in 13 of 15 patients at an average of 4 months with improved functional outcomes and no recurrence of the infection.

SUMMARY

Distal radius fracture nonunion is an uncommon complication. However, it can be debilitating to the affected patients, causing wrist pain, deformity, and limited ROM. Once the need for surgical intervention has been established, a number of different surgical approaches exist to treat a distal radius nonunion. ORIF using plate fixation and autologous bone graft has shown promising results as the first step in the management of distal radius nonunions, even in cases of small distal fragments. In complex cases of segmental bone defects and compromised local biology, free vascularized bone transfer can be used to enhance healing. Persistent nonunion despite multiple attempts at ORIF with bone grafting can be salvaged with wrist arthrodesis.

CLINICS CARE POINTS

- Distal radius nonunion is a rare complication following distal radius fracture.
- Distal radius nonunion has been associated with increased metaphyseal comminution, concomitant distal ulna fracture, inadequate immobilization and patient factors.
- Nonunion should be suspected in patients with persistent pain, limited range of motion and worsening wrist deformity after wrist remobilization.
- If adequate reduction and stabilization are observed in the setting of a distal radius

nonunion, additional laboratory tests should be ordered to rule out undiagnosed metabolic or endocrine abnormalities that could compromise bone healing.

- An underlying infectious process should always be ruled out in the setting of a nonunion with evaluation of white blood cell count, ESR, CRP and possibly a local bone biopsy.
- Treatment selection depends on the presence of infection, status of the radiocarpal and distal radioulnar joints, type of prior surgical interventions and functional demands of the patient.
- Currently, for non-infected distal radius nonunions with adequate bone stock, the literature generally supports management of the nonunion with ORIF combined with bone grafting to attempt preservation of wrist motion.
- Conversion to wrist arthrodesis is considered as a salvage procedure in cases of limited bone distally, failed nonunion repair or in elderly patients with low functional demands.

FUNDING

No funding was received for this study.

FINANCIAL DISCLOSURE

None of the authors has a financial interest in any of the drugs, products, or devices mentioned in this discussion or the manuscript being discussed.

REFERENCES

1. Watson-Jones R. Fractures and other bone and joint injuries. 2nd edition. Edinburgh: Livingstone; 1942.
2. Cooney WP 3rd, Dobyns JH, Linscheid RL. Complications of Colles' fractures. J Bone Joint Surg Am 1980;62:613–9.
3. Bacorn RW, Kurtzke JF. Colle's fracture: A study of two thousand cases from the New York State Workmen's Compensation Board. J Bone Joint Surg 1953;35A:643–58.
4. Segalman KA, Clark GL. Un-united fractures of the distal radius: a report of 12 cases. J Hand Surg Am 1998 Sep;23(5):914–9.
5. McKee MD, Waddell JP, Yoo D, et al. Nonunion of distal radial fractures associated with distal ulnar shaft fractures: a report of four cases. J Orthop Trauma 1997 Jan;11(1):49–53.
6. Giannoudis PV, Einhorn TA, Marsh D. Fracture healing: the diamond concept. Injury 2007;38(Suppl 4):S3–6.
7. Zura R, Mehta S, Della Rocca GJ, et al. Biological Risk Factors for Nonunion of Bone Fracture. JBJS Rev 2016;4(1):e5.
8. Nicholson JA, Makaram N, Simpson A, et al. Fracture nonunion in long bones: A literature review of risk factors and surgical management. Injury 2021; 52(Suppl 2):S3–11.
9. Zura R, Braid-Forbes MJ, Jeray K, et al. Bone fracture nonunion rate decreases with increasing age: A prospective inception cohort study. Bone 2017; 95:26–32.
10. Scolaro JA, Schenker ML, Yannascoli S, et al. Cigarette smoking increases complications following fracture: a systematic review. J Bone Joint Surg Am 2014;96(8):674–81.
11. Hernandez RK, Do TP, Critchlow CW, et al. Patient-related risk factors for fracture-healing complications in the United Kingdom General Practice Research Database. Acta Orthop 2012;83(6):653–60.
12. Zura R, Xiong Z, Einhorn T, et al. Epidemiology of Fracture Nonunion in 18 Human Bones. JAMA Surg 2016;151(11):e162775.
13. Prommersberger KJ, Fernandez DL, Ring D, et al. Open reduction and internal fixation of un-united fractures of the distal radius: does the size of the distal fragment affect the result? Chir Main 2002; 21:113–23.
14. Koo SC, Ho ST. Non-union of Fracture of Distal Radiusjournal of orthopaedics. trauma and rehabilitation 2011;15:21e24.
15. Weber SC, Szabo RM. Severely comminuted distal radial fractures as an unsolved problem: complications associated with external fixation and pins and plaster techniques. J Hand Surg 1986;11A:157–65.
16. Eglseder WA Jr, Elliott MJ. Nonunions of the distal radius. Am J Orthop (Belle Mead NJ) 2002;31(5):259–62.
17. Shinohara T, Hirata H. Distal radius nonunion after volar locking plate fixation of a distal radius fracture: a case report. Nagoya J Med Sci 2017;79(4):551–7.
18. Henry M. Vascularized medial femoral condyle bone graft for resistant nonunion of the distal radius. J Hand Surg Asian Pac 2017;22(1):23–8.
19. Smith VA, Wright TW. Nonunion of the distal radius. J Hand Surg Br 1999;24(5):601–3.
20. Harper WM, Jones JM. Non-union of Colles' fracture: report of two cases. J Hand Surg Br 1990;15(1):121–3.
21. Brinker MR, O'Connor DP, Monla YT, et al. Metabolic and endocrine abnormalities in patients with nonunions. J Orthop Trauma 2007;21(8):557–70.
22. Harper WM, Jones JM. Non-union of Colles' fracture: report of two cases. J Hand Surg 1990;15B:121–3.
23. Fernandez DL, Ring D, Jupiter JB. Surgical management of delayed union and nonunion of distal radius fractures. J Hand Surg 2001;26A:201–9.

24. Crow SA, Chen L, Lee JH, et al. Vascularized bone grafting from the base of the second metacarpal for persistent distal radius nonunion: a case report. J Orthop Trauma 2005;19(7):483–6.

25. Henry M. Genicular corticoperiosteal flap salvage of resistant atrophic non-union of the distal radius metaphysis. Hand Surg 2007;12(3):211–5.

26. Villamor A, Rios-Luna A, Villanueva-Martínez M, et al. Nonunion of distal radius fracture and distal radioulnar joint injury: a modified Sauvé-Kapandji procedure with a cubitus proradius transposition as autograft. Arch Orthop Trauma Surg 2008;128(12):1407–11.

27. Karuppiah SV, Johnstone AJ. Sauve-Kapandji as a salvage procedure to treat a nonunion of the distal radius. J Trauma 2010;68(5):E123–5.

28. Mithani SK, Srinivasan RC, Kamal R, et al. Salvage of distal radius nonunion with a dorsal spanning distraction plate. J Hand Surg [Am] 2014;39(5): 981–4.

29. Saremi H, Shahryar-Kamrani R, Ghane B, et al. Treatment of distal radius fracture nonunion with posterior interosseous bone flap. Iran Red Crescent Med J 2016;18(7):e38884.

30. Ring D. Nonunion of the distal radius. Hand Clin 2005;21(3):443–7.

31. Ring D, Jupiter JB, Toh S. Transarticular bony defects after trauma and sepsis: arthrodesis using vascularized fibular transfer. Plast Reconstr Surg 1999; 104(2):426–34.

32. Noaman H, Sorour Y, Marzouk A. Wrist arthroplasty for treatment of infected distal radius nonunion using free vascularised proximal fibular bone graft. Injury 2020;S0020-1383(20):30945–51.

Managing the Extra-Articular Distal Radius Malunion

Francisco Rodriguez-Fontan, MD[a], Alexander Lauder, MD[a,b],*

KEYWORDS

- Distal radius extra-articular fracture • Malunion • Osteotomy • Radial tilt • Radial inclination
- Radial height

KEY POINTS

- Malalignment of the distal radius alters the biomechanical relationships of the radiocarpal and distal radioulnar joints and may result in poor function.
- Malunion exists when radiographic malalignment correlates with clinical dysfunction, and the typical deformity involves dorsal angulation with shortening of the radius relative to the ulna leading to decreased wrist flexion, forearm rotation, and grip strength.
- Extra-articular malunions may be surgically corrected with opening wedge or closing wedge osteotomies with similar functional outcomes.
- Opening wedge osteotomies restore radial length and create an osseous void that may be treated with or without bone grafting, with similar union rates.
- Closing wedge osteotomies create increased stability with immediate cortical contact but accentuate the increased ulnar variance and often require ulnar-sided procedures, such as ulnar-shortening or ulnar head resection.

INTRODUCTION

Distal radius fractures (DRFs) are one of the most common upper-extremity injuries occurring in a bimodal distribution affecting children, young adults, and the elderly. DRFs account for more than 16% of adult fractures and may result from either low- or high-energy mechanisms.[1] Dorsally angulated extra-articular DRFs have adopted the eponym "Colles fractures" and are often encountered in the elderly after falling on outstretched hands.[2] Conversely, the DRF with volar angulation, or Smith fracture, accounts for only 5% of DRFs and typically results after falling on the hand in a flexed position or from a direct blow to the dorsum of the wrist.[1] Treatment paradigms historically involved manipulation and immobilization, which typically achieved osseous union and reasonable outcomes despite residual deformity. With a further understanding of wrist biomechanics and the widespread use of radiology, many fractures treated with closed reduction and casting lost reduction, yielding suboptimal outcomes when the deformity increased beyond certain radiologic parameters.[3–6]

DRFs can progress to malunion despite appropriate management with reduction and immobilization or surgical fixation.[7] Today, many fractures are treated surgically, and the advancement in implant design has decreased malunion rates.[8,9] DRF malunions account for approximately 11% and 23% of those treated operatively and nonoperatively, respectively.[4,9] As with other musculoskeletal injuries, malunion can lead to detrimental functional outcomes.[10] Defined radiographic parameters help monitor these injuries

a Department of Orthopedics, University of Colorado School of Medicine, 13001 East 17th Place, Aurora, CO 80045, USA; b Department of Orthopedics, Denver Health Medical Center, Denver, CO, USA
* Corresponding author. Department of Orthopedic Surgery, Denver Health Medical Center, 777 Bannock Street, Denver, CO 80207.
E-mail address: Lauder.Alexander@gmail.com

Hand Clin 40 (2024) 63–77
https://doi.org/10.1016/j.hcl.2023.06.002
0749-0712/24/Published by Elsevier Inc.

until the fracture heals within acceptable alignment.[11] When managing the malunited DRF, the treating physician must understand patient concerns and symptoms attributed to the malunion and also assess the anticipated functional impact of nonoperative management compared with pursuing surgical intervention in an attempt to restore preinjury anatomy and biomechanics. This article reviews the presentation, pathophysiology, radiologic evaluation, and treatment options and provides insight into the management of extra-articular DRFs.[1,12]

ANATOMY

The distal radius forms an anatomic pedestal supporting the biomechanics of the wrist and forearm.[13] The dorsal radius metaphyseal surface is grossly convex, converging to form the radial styloid. The contour forms the gliding surface of the 6 dorsal extensor compartments. The concave volar surface allows the attachment of the volar radiocarpal ligaments. The ulnar border articulates with the ulnar head via the sigmoid notch, providing rotatory and translatory motion of the radius around the ulna.[14] The distal radius can be divided into 3 columns: (1) the radial column, comprising the radial styloid and scaphoid facet; (2) the intermediate column, consisting of the sigmoid notch and lunate facet; and (3) the ulnar column, with the ulnar head/styloid and triangular fibrocartilage complex.[15]

The distal radius is composed of a subchondral bone plate, cancellous, and cortical bone.[16] The subchondral plate is arranged as a leaf-spring structure sustaining compression on the surface and tension on deeper layers. The trabeculae of the cancellous bone support the subchondral plate as a load-sharing construct distributing compressive forces.[16] These are arranged in columns and transmit loads toward the metaphysis and diaphysis. Although thin and flexible enough to transmit the loading, they coalesce through endosteal ridges at the cortex and form rods of thickened bone connecting the thinner metaphyseal cortex to the thicker diaphyseal cortex.[16,17] The brachioradialis inserts approximately 17 mm proximal to the radial styloid tip and is the primary deforming force in DRFs, accounting for resultant radial shortening and loss of radial inclination.[18] Normal wrist motion encompasses approximately 120° of flexion-extension, 50° of radial-ulnar deviation, and 150° of forearm pronosupination.[19] Approximately 80% of the axial force from the carpus is transmitted to the distal radius articular surface scaphoid and lunate facets in an ulnar-neutral wrist.[20]

The anatomic relationships between the radius and ulna are altered in the setting of extra-articular malunion.[21] The most common deformity occurs with loss of radial height and increased dorsal radial tilt, resulting in relative ulnar positive variance and increased load through the ulna.[22] The deformity typically limits forearm rotation and increases the risk of radiocarpal arthritic changes.[22] Compensatory adaptive nondissociative midcarpal instability may develop when there is a substantial deformity in DRF malunions (discussed later),[13] altering the contact pressures of the radiocarpal and capitolunate articulations.[21]

RADIOGRAPHIC ASSESSMENT AND WRIST BIOMECHANICS

Osseous alignment plays a critical role in the management of malunions. Four radiographic parameters are evaluated with standard posteroanterior and lateral wrist radiographs: radial height (normal range, 11–12 mm), radial inclination (22°–23°), ulnar variance (0 ± 1 mm), and volar tilt (11°–12°).[23] Extra-articular DRF malunion can be defined with the following parameters (**Fig. 1**)[9,24–28]:

- Greater than 10° dorsal tilt,
- Greater than 15° to 20° volar tilt,
- Less than 10° radial inclination,
- Greater than 3 mm radial height loss, and/or
- Positive ulnar variance greater than 1 mm.

Other parameters to consider include the following:

- Radial translation of the distal fragment and resultant effect on distal radioulnar joint (DRUJ) stability and lunate coverage,[29,30]
- Radiocarpal or midcarpal malalignment.[13,25]

These radiographic malunion parameters have been correlated to patient-reported outcomes as measured by the disabilities of the arm, shoulder, and hand (DASH) and Short Form-36 (SF-36) questionnaires.[24,31] A prospective study of 143 malunited DRFs analyzed the relationship between radiographic parameters and DASH scores at 2 years.[31] The study found that dorsal tilt greater than 10° and positive ulnar variance greater than 1 mm were associated with worse DASH scores. The DASH scores increased by at least 10 points if the malunion had one of these parameters, and more than 20 points if the malunion included both parameters.[31] DRF malunion was also associated with worse SF-36 scores and weaker grip strength.[24,31]

The progression of dorsal tilt increases the relative biomechanical load on the ulna, from baseline of 20% to as high as 60%[19,32] and may present with associated ulnar-sided wrist pain and ulnar

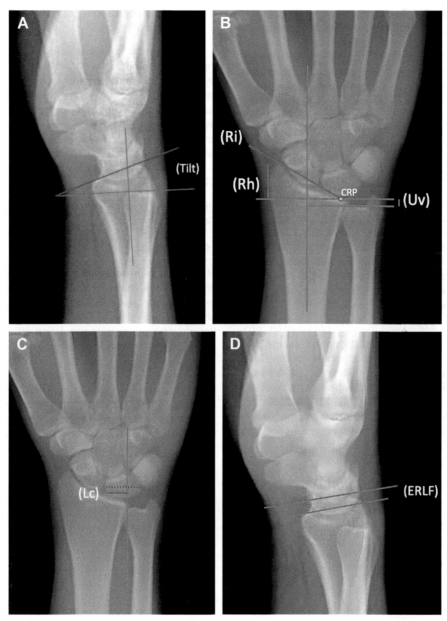

Fig. 1. Radiographic measurements in distal radius malunions. (*A*) Volar and dorsal tilt are measured on the 10° lateral radiograph as the angle between a perpendicular line to the longitudinal axis of the radius and the line connecting the apex of the volar and dorsal rim of the radius (tilt).[23] (*B*) Radial inclination (Ri) is measured as the angle between the long axis of the radial shaft and a line connecting the tip of the radial styloid with the ulnar central reference point (CRP), midway between the volar and dorsal ulnar corners. Ulnar variance (Uv) measures the difference in axial length between the CRP and the most distal extent of the ulnar head. Radial height (Rh) is measured from the tip of radial styloid to the CRP.[23] (*C*) Lunate coverage (Lc) percentage is measured with a line drawn through the ulnar edge of the lunate fossa parallel to the long axis of the radius. The distance from this line to the farthest radial point on lunate is measured (covered lunate, *solid line*). The covered lunate distance is divided by the full width of the lunate (*dotted line*) to provide the percentage of lunate coverage.[35] (*D*) The ERLF angle is measured by the angle comparing the longitudinal axis of the lunate with the lunate facet articular surface.[25]

abutment.[33] Dorsal angulation may lead to incongruency at the DRUJ and tightening of the interosseous membrane, leading to decreased forearm rotation and increased force requirements for pronosupination.[22,34] Conversely, increased coronal plane radial translation can lead to DRUJ instability[29,30] and should be suspected in the setting of DRUJ gapping, radial shaft convergence proximal to the fracture, and/or positive DRUJ stress testing.[30] Radiographic lunate coverage is another parameter that correlates to radial translation and DRUJ instability and has higher interobserver/intraobserver measurement reliability (see **Fig. 1**).[29] Normal lunate coverage is on average 45% (range, 25%–74%), and the contralateral uninjured side can be used for comparison in a clinical setting.[29,35]

Changes in distal radius articular angulation alter the load concentration of the carpus and shift the loading points of the radioscaphoid, radiolunate, and ulnocarpal articulations.[21,32] Compensatory adaptive nondissociative midcarpal instability can develop with alterations in the volar/dorsal tilt of the radius,[13] and assessment of carpal alignment on lateral radiographs should be performed routinely.[9,36] The Effective Radio-Lunate Flexion (ERLF) angle (**Fig. 2**)[25] describes carpal adaptation to the dorsally angulated distal radius malunion in 2 distinctive patterns.

- Type 1 ERLF, less than 25° of dorsal tilt, produces midcarpal malalignment where the lunate vertical axis is collinear to the distal radius axis and the midcarpal capitolunate articulation develops compensatory flexion;
- Type 2 ERLF, greater than 25° of dorsal tilt, yields radiolunate flexion with maintained midcarpal alignment that has associated

dorsal subluxation of the radiocarpal articulation.[9,25,37]

The former can progress to dorsal intercalated segment instability, which initially is well tolerated by patients whereby the latter tends to be immediately symptomatic.[25,37] Abnormal alignment may lead to progressive ligament attenuation, synovitis, ulnocarpal abutment, and posttraumatic arthritis owing to eccentric radiocarpal and midcarpal joint loading.[37]

CLASSIFICATION

DRF malunions can be classified according to **Table 1**.

PRESENTATION

Malunion can present with a myriad of complaints and symptoms: pain, instability, weakness, limited motion, and paresthesias. Commonly, dorsal angulation will restrict forearm pronation and wrist flexion, whereas a volar angulation will limit supination and extension.[9] Tendinopathy can present as weakened grip strength, tenosynovitis, and rarely, tendon ruptures.[38] Given the higher prevalence of dorsally angulated malunions, the flexor tendons (flexor pollicis longus most prevalent) are more commonly affected owing to bony prominence or vascular compromise.[39] Median nerve

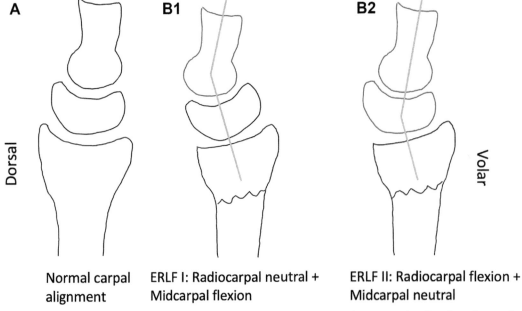

Fig. 2. Biomechanical adaptations to malunion. (*A*) Normal wrist position (10°–15° volar tilt, aligned carpus), (*B*) dorsally angulated distal radius malunion; (*B1*) ERLF type 1, less than 25° extension: radiocarpal alignment remains neutral resulting in midcarpal capitolunate flexion, (*B2*) ERLF type 2, greater than 25° extension: radiolunate flexion develops with dorsal radiocarpal subluxation, midcarpal alignment remains neutral.

Table 1
Classification of distal radius malunion

	Tilt	Malunion Characteristics
Intra-articular	*Variable*	*Discussed in subsequent article*
Extra-articular	Dorsal (most common)	Type I ERLF, <25° (leads to DISI) Type II ERLF, >25° (more symptomatic) ± Height and/or inclination loss Typical ulnar positive variance
	Volar (less common)	± Height and/or inclination loss Typical ulnar positive variance
	Neutral	± Height and/or inclination loss ± Coronal plane translation ± Change in ulnar variance
Combined	Intra-articular and extra-articular	*Discussed in subsequent article*

Abbreviation: DISI, dorsal intercalated segmental instability.

paresthesias secondary to a change in the carpal tunnel position, radioulnar joint synovitis, or osseous prominence may also develop in the setting of malunion.[9,40] Because of shortening of the radius relative to the ulna, ulnocarpal abutment or styloid impaction syndrome can lead to ulnar carpal arthropathy, manifesting as ulnar-sided wrist pain with loss of ulnar deviation, extension, pronation, and pain with loading.[9]

MANAGEMENT

Distal radius malunions are a frequent subject of malpractice claims owing to the resultant deformity[41–43] and associated disability.[31–33] Treatment considerations should incorporate the observed anatomic and radiographic deformity, functional status of the patient, and clinical presentation.[44,45] A true malunion exists when anatomic malalignment with associated functional impairment is attributed to the deformity.[46] Contraindications to surgical osteotomy include advanced joint degenerative changes and fixed carpal malalignment. In these instances, salvage procedures, such as partial or complete wrist arthrodesis, proximal row carpectomy, or hemiresection interposition arthroplasty, may be preferred.[47] Corrective osteotomy should be performed before advanced degenerative changes occur. Patients should be counseled that posttraumatic arthropathy may develop despite correction of the malalignment.[9]

OPERATIVE CONSIDERATIONS AND APPROACH

Preoperative planning of the corrective osteotomy should include orthogonal and contralateral wrist radiographs. Computed tomography (CT) of the injured wrist and/or contralateral wrist, and 3-

dimensional (3D) model reconstruction from CT may be useful adjuncts. The latter may aid the operative plan, anticipate, and predict the osteotomy location, direction, and correctional outcome.[48] The timing of surgery is based on many factors; early osteotomy is technically easier and decreases the duration of patient disability.[49] Correction within 12 weeks from injury has been shown to have favorable outcomes in correcting radiographic parameters and improving Mayo wrist scores.[50]

The goals of corrective osteotomy are to restore preinjury alignment, thereby improving function and pain. The deformity and surgeon's experience guide the modality implemented. Historically, corrective osteotomies for dorsally angulated malunions were performed using a dorsal approach with an opening wedge and plate fixation.[51] The advent of volar locking and fragment-specific plates has led to the use of a volar approach and plating (volar locking or orthogonal) with the advantage of less risk of extensor tendon irritation.[52–55] Both opening and closing wedge osteotomies can be performed volarly, through a Henry or transflexor carpi radialis approach, radially through first and second extensor compartments, dorsally between the second and fourth extensor compartments, or as a combination of these.[56] If an ulnar-sided procedure is needed, it can typically be approached from the flexor carpi ulnaris/extensor carpi ulnaris interval.

Advantages to the use of an opening wedge osteotomy include surgical restoration of height, inclination, tilt, and ulnar variance. The opening osteotomy may be incomplete or hinged—preserving one osseous cortex—or complete whereby no cortical contact is maintained. The use of graft augmentation may be beneficial in complete osteotomies.[57] Fernandez[58] suggested that up to

12 mm of radial length can be restored with a radial-sided opening wedge osteotomy, but some malunions need even more lengthening to restore native anatomy. In such cases, an adjunct ulnar-shortening osteotomy may be useful in patients with high functional demand,[58,59] or a Darrach ulnar head resection in older patients with lower functional demand.[59]

Closing wedge osteotomies have the advantage of providing direct cortical osseous contact, restoring inclination and tilt; however, this further shortens the radius and may require a secondary ulnar-sided procedure.[57] For distal radius malunions with acceptable sagittal deformity (ie, malunion <20° dorsal or 10° volar angulation) but significant ulnar positive variance, an isolated ulnar-sided procedure may be performed with favorable functional outcomes.[47,57,60–63]

Evaluating the center of rotation and angulation (CORA) preoperatively helps determine which osteotomy will be more suitable for deformity and length correction. Nagy's technique (**Fig. 3**, **Table 2**) involves tracing the deformity over the uninjured wrist radiographs.[64] By overlapping the contour of the malunited wrist radiographs to those of the uninjured side, lines are templated from the malunited volar and dorsal cortex toward the native volar and dorsal cortex, connecting the malunited and normal cortices. A perpendicular line is then made at the midpoint of both lines. The point where both perpendicular lines meet is the defined as the CORA. The CORA is marked on both posteroanterior and lateral radiographs and will help define the type of correction needed in the frontal and sagittal planes.[64] If the CORA lies at or close to the osseous margins, an incomplete opening wedge or closing osteotomy may provide sufficient correction. If the CORA lies away from the osseous margins, a complete opening wedge osteotomy may provide better correction.[47,64] Often, the CORA is outside the osseous margins in dorsally angulated malunion and at the bone margins in volarly angulated malunions.[47]

BONE GRAFTING AND OUTCOMES

Use of bone graft of any type is controversial in the management of distal radius malunions. Numerous structural (corticocancellous) and nonstructural (cancellous bone or substitute) grafts are available and may be considered depending on the type of osteotomy performed.[4] Closing wedge osteotomies allow for osseous apposition and compression, obviating adjunct grafting. Conversely, when performing an open wedge osteotomy, a bony void is created with radial lengthening that can be treated without grafting or augmented with autologous bone graft (ie, distal radius, olecranon, proximal tibia, iliac crest), allogeneic bone graft, or bone graft substitutes (ie, calcium phosphate, hydroxyapatite, bone morphogenic protein).[65] Historically, autologous structural corticocancellous iliac crest graft has been preferred, allowing a mechanical and biological advantage but with the cost of increased surgical time and associated donor site morbidity.[57] The advent of volar locked plating constructs has improved the implant stability, making cancellous grafts or bone substitutes suitable to fill in osseous defects with similar outcomes.[4,9,66] Interestingly, some studies demonstrated that the use of volar plates alone, without bone grafting, is sufficient to allow osseous healing without loss of correction.[54,67,68]

Incomplete, hinged osteotomies may improve union rates compared with complete osteotomies, as one cortex remains in contact. One study reported a significantly higher nonunion rate in complete osteotomies owing to the lack of contact between the distal radial fragment and the proximal shaft.[57] Ozer and colleagues[67] showed no healing time difference between allogeneic or no graft use in incomplete osteotomies.

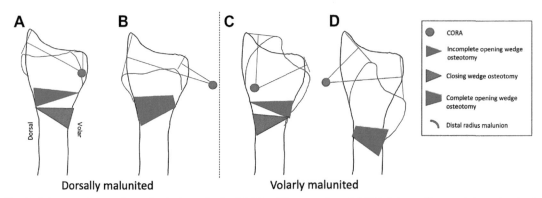

Fig. 3. Schemes of dorsally and volarly malunited DRFs with examples of CORA intersections points and osteotomy options. See **Table 2** for further description. (A&C) CORA close to cortex; (B&D) CORA away of cortex.

Table 2
Technical considerations of distal radius malunion correctional osteotomy

	Opening Wedge Osteotomy	Closing Wedge Osteotomy
Advantages	Restores height, inclination, and tilt	Restores inclination and tilt
Disadvantages	Creates osseous void	Accentuates ulnar positive variance
CORA	Away from osseous cortex	Close to osseous cortex
Volar approach	Volar opening wedge for volar malunion >15° (see **Fig. 3C, D**) • CORA close to cortex • Incomplete/hinged osteotomy ± bone graft (cancellous or corticocancellous triangular structural graft)	Volar closing wedge for dorsal malunion >20° (see **Fig. 3C**)
Dorsal approach	Dorsal opening wedge for dorsal malunion >20° (see **Fig. 3A, B**) • CORA away from cortex • Complete/under distraction osteotomy + bone graft (cancellous or corticocancellous trapezoidal structural graft)	Dorsal closing wedge for volar malunion >15° (see **Fig. 3A**) • + Ulnar-sided procedure
Ulnar-sided procedures	High-demand patient • Ulnar-shortening osteotomy Elderly, low-functioning patient[47,60] • Darrach: ulnar head resection • Ulnar head replacement • Sauvé-Kapandji: DRUJ arthrodesis and proximal ulna osteotomy • Hemiresection interposition arthroplasty Isolated ulnar-shortening osteotomy without radial osteotomy[47,57,60,61] • Indicated for malunions with acceptable sagittal plane alignment (<20° dorsal malunion or <10° volar malunion) with symptomatic positive ulnar variance	

Abbreviations: CORA, center of rotation and alignment; DRUJ, distal radioulnar joint.

Functional outcomes following distal radius osteotomies with the use of various grafting techniques for the treatment of malunion are summarized in **Table 3**. Overall, the published literature reports similar union rates, time to union, patient-reported outcomes, range of motion, and operative complications regardless of approach, fixation construct, or use of bone grafting.

SOFT TISSUE CONTRACTURES

Chronic DRF malunions may have associated soft tissue contractures owing to the altered anatomy of the wrist.[51,69,70] The brachioradialis often needs to be released to adequately restore radial height.[18] Following the correction of osseous alignment, loss of forearm rotation may result from DRUJ contracture, which may be managed with dorsal capsulectomy to restore pronation and/or volar capsulectomy to restore supination.[27]

COMPLICATIONS

Tendinopathy, tendon injury, delayed union, nonunion, and neuropathy are reported complications of surgical corrective osteotomy in distal radius malunions.[57] A retrospective cohort study of 60 patients undergoing correctional osteotomies of extra-articular malunion reported a complication rate of nearly 50% (25/60) with a reoperation rate of 22% (13/60).[57] Twenty-four patients in the cohort underwent complete opening distraction-type osteotomies with intercalary bone grafting, and 36 patients received opening wedge hinged osteotomies maintaining volar cortical contact. There were 7 nonunions (33%),

Table 3
Clinical outcomes following various bone grafting techniques in opening wedge osteotomies

Graft Type	Study	N	Age (mean years)	Follow-up (mean months)	Approach	Malunion Type	Type of Osteotomy (N)	Plating Technique	Union Rate	Time to Union (mean)	ROM Arc on Flexion-Extension (mean degrees)	DASH Score (preoperative and postoperative mean difference-MD/mean final score)	Complications (N)
No graft	Mahmoud et al,[79] 2012	22	31.8	18	Volar	Dorsal	Opening, Incomplete (19) Complete (3)	VLP	100%	10.4 wk	147.5	21.6 MD/12.9	• Intraoperative longitudinal split (1) • CRPS (1) • Median nerve neuritis (1) • Hardware irritation (1) • Ulnar-sided pain (2)
	Tarallo et al,[54] 2014	20	40	50	Volar	Dorsal	Opening (20)	VLP	100%	4 mo	130.6	28.5 MD/25.3	• Median nerve neuritis (2)
	Tiren et al,[80] 2014	11	52	8	Dorsal	Dorsal	Opening incomplete	Dorsal bicolumnar locking plates	100%	13 wk	138	10	• Symptomatic hardware (1)
	Scheer et al,[81] 2015	15	50.5	6	Volar	Dorsal	Opening, incomplete (9) Complete (6)	VLP	80%	NR	NR	NR	• Nonunion (3, complete osteotomies).
	Andreasson et al,[82] 2020	19	55	12	Volar and dorsal	Dorsal	Opening Incomplete	Carbon fiber volar plate	100%	NR	118	16 MD/20	• EPL rupture (1) • Hardware irritation (1) • Hardware failure (3)
	Ozer et al,[67] 2011	28	35	6	Volar	Dorsal	Opening incomplete	VLP	100%	11 wk	120	28 MD/10	
Structural graft	Ring et al,[66] 2002	10	43	30	Dorsal	Dorsal	Opening	Dorsal pi-shaped plate	100%	4 mo	98	NR	• Donor graft iliac site pain (1) • Hardware irritation (6)
	Yaradilmiş et al,[83] 2020	30 (15 smokers)	49.1	5.5	Volar	Dorsal	Opening complete	VLP	100%	14.1 wk; 16.6 wk (smokers)	118 (115 for smokers)	17.2 (17.5 for smokers)	• Superficial wound infection (2, smokers)
	Pecache et al,[84] 2020	13	NR	NR	Volar	Dorsal	Opening complete	VLP	100%	NR	NR	31.1 MD/25.5	• CRPS (1)

Nonstructural graft or substitute

Study	N											Complications
Ring et al,[66] 2002	10	45	7	Dorsal	Dorsal	Opening	Dorsal pi-shaped plate	100%	4 mo	132	NR	• Hardware irritation (6)
Andreasson et al,[82] 2020	19	59	12	Volar and dorsal	Dorsal	Opening incomplete	Carbon fiber volar plate	100%	NR	120	29 MD/16	• EPL rupture (1) • ECRL rupture (1) • CTS (1) • Hardware failure (1)
Abramo et al,[85] 2008	25	52	12	Radial and dorsal	Dorsal	Opening	Radial and dorsal plates	96%	NR	120	13 MD/23	• Persistent pain (2) • Hardware irritation (8) • Radial nerve paresthesia (6) • Nonunion and hardware failure (1)
Ozer et al,[67] 2011	28	37	6	Volar	Dorsal	Opening incomplete	VLP	100%	10 wk	123	32 MD/10	• EPL rupture (1)

Abbreviations: CTS, carpal tunnel syndrome; ECRL, extensor carpi radialis longus; EPL, extensor pollicis longus; N, number; NR, not recorded; VLP, volar locking plate.

3 cases of delayed healing, 1 iatrogenic extensor carpi radialis longus tendon laceration from an osteotome, and 3 delayed extensor pollicis longus tendon ruptures after surgery. Complete osteotomies whereby no cortical contact was maintained were associated with a greater risk of nonunion and delayed union.[57]

Volar plating can cause extensor tendon irritation from prominent dorsal screws, or flexor pollicis longus tendinopathy from plate prominence on the volar cortex.[57] Ulnar-shortening osteotomies have an inherent nonunion risk (10%–21%) owing to the ulna's distal watershed area.[71,72] When performed simultaneously with a radial osteotomy, there is a higher biological demand for both sites to heal. Hardware irritation is also common following ulnar-shortening osteotomy, often requiring a secondary procedure for plate removal.[73] Median nerve neuropathy is a reported complication following corrective osteotomy for DRF malunion that should be considered when performing osteotomies that result in radial lengthening,[40] leading some to recommend routine carpal tunnel release at the time of osteotomy.[74,75]

AUTHORS' PREFERRED TECHNIQUE

When there is significant extra-articular deformity and ulnar positive variance, the authors prefer an opening wedge osteotomy that is powerful enough to correct the deformity and restore the DRUJ kinematics. If a sliding or incomplete osteotomy achieves this goal, it is used. Otherwise, a complete osteotomy with iliac crest autologous structural bone graft is preferred. The site of osteotomy is chosen at the CORA (described above), and distraction is facilitated with the use of a brachioradialis tenotomy, dorsal periosteal release, traction via finger traps or addition of a lamina spreader in the osteotomy site when needed. Plate fixation is performed with a volar locking plate when there is sufficient bone stock distal to the CORA to accept the plate-screw construct. When the distal bone stock is minimal, or in the case of severe osteopenia or osteoporosis, a wrist-spanning bridge plate construct can be an alternative. The authors routinely perform a prophylactic carpal tunnel release with any lengthening to minimize the risk of secondary neuropraxia. The use of a radial closing wedge with ulnar-shortening osteotomy is avoided in an attempt to minimize multiple osseous healing sites. **Figs. 4–6** present 3 case examples of various osteotomies, reduction techniques, and bone grafting.

FUTURE DIRECTIONS

The use of CT 3D model reconstruction is an area of future research that may aid in preoperative

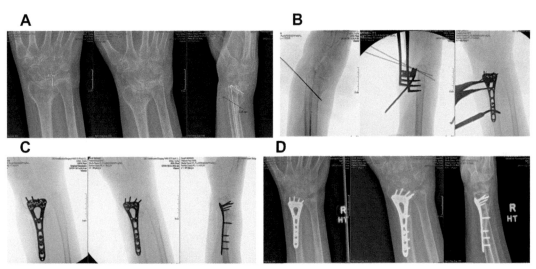

Fig. 4. Complete opening wedge osteotomy with cancellous bone allograft and volar locked plating in a 54-year-old woman with osteopenia. (*A*) Preoperative radiographs showed a 50° dorsally angulated malunion with 8 mm of ulnar positive variance. Red line indicates the planned osteotomy site. (*B*) Intraoperative fluoroscopy used a k-wire to identify the osteotomy site (*left*), placement of 2 k-wires parallel to the joint surface with the use of the volar locking plate as a reduction tool (*middle*), and a lamina spreader into the osteotomy site with a bone reduction clamp to assist reduction (*right*). (*C*) Intraoperative fluoroscopy after placement of allograft and final fixation. (*D*) Five-month postoperative imaging showed continued ongoing slow incorporation of the allograft with maintained alignment.

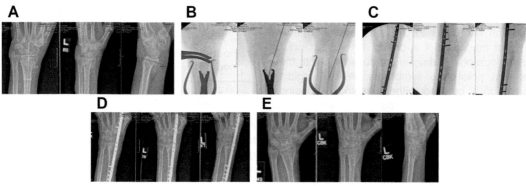

Fig. 5. Complete opening wedge osteotomy with iliac crest tricortical autograft and dorsal wrist spanning plate fixation in a 59-year-old woman with early malunion 8 weeks from injury. (*A*) Preoperative radiographs identified loss of radial inclination and impaction of the radial shaft to the subchondral articular surface (*line*). (*B*) A dorsal approach with restoration of alignment was assisted with a lamina spreader (*left*), provisional k-wire fixation (*middle*), and addition of tricortical iliac crest autograft (*right*). (*C*) Final intraoperative fixation. (*D*) Successive postoperative imaging at 2 days (*left*), 2 weeks (*middle*), and 3 months (*right*, note rapid healing with structural autograft). (*E*) Ten-month postoperative radiographs following removal of the wrist spanning plate.

planning.[48,76] 3D analysis and printing allow hands-on planning and may improve preoperative understanding of the deformity and surgical correction. A multicenter randomized control trial compared 12-month radiographic and patient-reported outcomes of standard 2D versus 3D preoperative planning for distal radius osteotomies in 40 adult patients.[77] The 3D group had significantly improved restoration of volar tilt and radial inclination but no significant differences in functional outcomes as measured with DASH scores, Patient-Rated Wrist Evaluation scores, pain and satisfaction scores, or grip strength.[77] 3D printing also allows for the production of case-specific cutting blocks, which may minimize measurement errors, improve precision of the osteotomy, and decrease surgical time[78]; however, further cost-benefit analyses are needed.

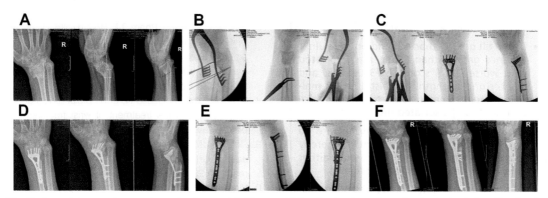

Fig. 6. Complete opening wedge osteotomy with iliac crest tricortical autograft and volar locked plate fixation in a 39-year-old man. (*A*) Preoperative radiographs identified 40° volar angulation and 1 cm of ulnar positive variance. Line indicates the planned osteotomy site. (*B*) Intraoperative fluoroscopy used k-wires to mark the osteotomy site (*left*) followed by the osteotomy (*middle, right*). (*C*) 4.5 kg of traction applied via finger traps allowed restoration of length. A lamina spreader was used to prevent the ulnar drift of the radial shaft to allow tricortical autograft placement (*left*) and final fixation (*middle, right*). (*D*) Three-week postoperative radiographs demonstrated loss of reduction and plastic deformity of the volar locking plate with volar translation of the graft after the patient reportedly fell. (*E*) Revision fixation using a stiffer plate was performed using the same distal locking holes. Intraoperative findings identified early incorporation of the distal portion of the graft, and the fixation was augmented with an orthogonal locked radial column plate. (*F*) Six-week postoperative radiographs demonstrated maintained alignment. This case highlights the significant forces through the osteotomy site and the importance of appropriate rigid fixation.

SUMMARY

Malunion can occur in DRFs treated nonoperatively or surgically. It is critical to understand if the radiographic malalignment correlates with the patient's presenting symptoms. When surgical correction is pursued, either opening or closing wedge osteotomies can be performed. Volar plates have led to more osteotomies performed through a volar exposure with fewer hardware-related complications and less need for structural bone grafting. Similar to other limb deformities, 3D analysis, printing, and planning can lead to more accurate osteotomies and fewer technical errors and is an area of future investigation.

CLINICS CARE POINTS

- Distal radius malunion may lead to ulnocarpal impaction, distal radioulnar joint instability, altered carpal alignment, and arthrosis. A true malunion exists when there is anatomic malalignment with associated functional impairment attributed to the deformity.
- The wrist is composed of 3 columns (radial, intermediate, and ulnar) with 3 notable articulations (radiocarpal, ulnocarpal, and distal radioulnar).[15] The most common deformity involves dorsal angulation and shortening of the radius relative to the ulna altering the native wrist biomechanics to either (1) adaptive midcarpal flexion or (2) radiocarpal flexion and dorsal subluxation.[13,25]
- Dorsal tilt greater than 10° and positive ulnar variance greater than 1 mm are associated with worse DASH scores, SF-36 scores, and weaker grip strength.[24,31] Distal radius malunions are a common subject of malpractice claims[41–43] and associated disability.[31–33]
- The goals of corrective osteotomy are to restore preinjury alignment, thereby improving function and pain, with either opening or closing wedge osteotomies.
- Opening wedge osteotomies restore radial length but create an osseous void that may be treated without bone grafting or augmented with either cortical or cancellous autograft or allograft. The use of bone grafting in opening wedge osteotomies is controversial but may improve union rates when performing complete osteotomies where no cortical contact remains.[57]
- Closing wedge osteotomies create immediate cortical contact but often require ulnar-sided procedures, such as ulnar shortening.

- Complications rates following extra-articular correctional osteotomies for distal radius malunions approach 50% and include tendinopathy, tendon injury, delayed union, nonunion, and neuropathy.[57]

DISCLOSURE

All authors have no conflicts of interest in relation to this article. This article received no specific grant from any funding agency in the public, commercial, or not-for-profit sectors.

REFERENCES

1. Shehovych A, Salar O, Meyer C, et al. Adult distal radius fractures classification systems: essential clinical knowledge or abstract memory testing? Ann R Coll Surg Engl 2016;98(8):525–31.
2. Thurston AJ. 'Ao' or eponyms: the classification of wrist fractures. ANZ J Surg 2005;75(5):347–55.
3. Altissimi M, Antenucci R, Fiacca C, et al. Long-term Results of Conservative Treatment of Fractures of the Distal Radius. Clin Orthop Relat Res 1986;206: 202–10.
4. Chung K. Hand surgery Update V. 5th edition. Chicago, IL: American Society for Surgery of the Hand; 2011.
5. Gartland JJ Jr, Werley CW. Evaluation of healed Colles' fractures. J Bone Jt Surg Am Vol 1951;33-a(4):895–907.
6. McQueen M, Caspers J. Colles fracture: does the anatomical result affect the final function? J Bone Jt Surg Br Vol 1988;70(4):649–51.
7. Delclaux S, Trang Pham TT, Bonnevialle N, et al. Distal radius fracture malunion: Importance of managing injuries of the distal radio-ulnar joint. Orthopaedics & traumatology, surgery & research 2016; 102(3):327–32.
8. Obert L, Loisel F, Gasse N, et al. Distal radius anatomy applied to the treatment of wrist fractures by plate: a review of recent literature. Sicot-J. 2015;1:14.
9. Cognet JM, Mares O. Distal radius malunion in adults. Orthopaedics & traumatology, surgery & research 2021;107(1S):102755.
10. Singaram S, Naidoo M. The physical, psychological and social impact of long bone fractures on adults: A review. Afr J Prim Health Care Fam Med 2019; 11(1):e1–9.
11. Kamal RN, Shapiro LM. American Academy of Orthopaedic Surgeons/American Society for Surgery of the Hand Clinical Practice Guideline Summary Management of Distal Radius Fractures. J Am Acad Orthop Surg 2022;30(4):e480–6.
12. Meinberg EG, Agel J, Roberts CS, et al. Fracture and Dislocation Classification Compendium-2018. J Orthop Trauma 2018;32(Suppl 1):S1–s170.

13. Bushnell BD, Bynum DK. Malunion of the distal radius. J Am Acad Orthop Surg 2007;15(1):27–40.
14. Kleinman WB. Stability of the distal radioulna joint: biomechanics, pathophysiology, physical diagnosis, and restoration of function what we have learned in 25 years. J Hand Surg 2007;32(7):1086–106.
15. Rhee PC, Medoff RJ, Shin AY. Complex Distal Radius Fractures: An Anatomic Algorithm for Surgical Management. J Am Acad Orthop Surg 2017;25(2):77–88.
16. Bain GI, MacLean SBM, McNaughton T, et al. Microstructure of the Distal Radius and Its Relevance to Distal Radius Fractures. J Wrist Surg 2017;6(4):307–15.
17. Meena S, Sharma P, Sambharia AK, et al. Fractures of distal radius: an overview. J Fam Med Prim Care 2014;3(4):325–32.
18. Koh S, Andersen CR, Buford WL Jr, et al. Anatomy of the distal brachioradialis and its potential relationship to distal radius fracture. J Hand Surg 2006;31(1):2–8.
19. Werner FW, Glisson RR, Murphy DJ, et al. Force transmission through the distal radioulnar carpal joint: effect of ulnar lengthening and shortening. Handchir Mikrochir Plast Chir 1986;18(5):304–8.
20. Palmer AK, Werner FW. Biomechanics of the distal radioulnar joint. Clin Orthop Relat Res 1984;187:26–35.
21. Pogue DJ, Viegas SF, Patterson RM, et al. Effects of distal radius fracture malunion on wrist joint mechanics. J Hand Surg Am 1990;15(5):721–7.
22. Kihara H, Palmer AK, Werner FW, et al. The effect of dorsally angulated distal radius fractures on distal radioulnar joint congruency and forearm rotation. J Hand Surg 1996;21(1):40–7.
23. Medoff RJ. Essential radiographic evaluation for distal radius fractures. Hand Clin 2005;21(3):279–88.
24. Brogren E, Hofer M, Petranek M, et al. Relationship between distal radius fracture malunion and arm-related disability: a prospective population-based cohort study with 1-year follow-up. BMC Muscoskel Disord 2011;12:9.
25. Batra S, Debnath U, Kanvinde R. Can carpal malalignment predict early and late instability in nonoperatively managed distal radius fractures? Int Orthop 2008;32(5):685–91.
26. Evans BT, Jupiter JB. Best Approaches in Distal Radius Fracture Malunions. Curr Rev Musculoskelet Med 2019;12(2):198–203.
27. Graham TJ. Surgical Correction of Malunited Fractures of the Distal Radius. J Am Acad Orthop Surg 1997;5(5):270–81.
28. Ring D, Prommersberger KJ, Gonzalez del Pino J, et al. Corrective osteotomy for intra-articular malunion of the distal part of the radius. J Bone Jt Surg Am Vol 2005;87(7):1503–9.
29. Ross M, Di Mascio L, Peters S, et al. Defining residual radial translation of distal radius fractures: a potential cause of distal radioulnar joint instability. J Wrist Surg 2014;3(1):22–9.
30. Fujitani R, Omokawa S, Akahane M, et al. Predictors of distal radioulnar joint instability in distal radius fractures. J Hand Surg 2011;36(12):1919–25.
31. Brogren E, Wagner P, Petranek M, et al. Distal radius malunion increases risk of persistent disability 2 years after fracture: a prospective cohort study. Clin Orthop Relat Res 2013;471(5):1691–7.
32. Short WH, Palmer AK, Werner FW, et al. A biomechanical study of distal radial fractures. J Hand Surg 1987;12(4):529–34.
33. Taleisnik J, Watson HK. Midcarpal instability caused by malunited fractures of the distal radius. J Hand Surg 1984;9(3):350–7.
34. Hirahara H, Neale PG, Lin YT, et al. Kinematic and torque-related effects of dorsally angulated distal radius fractures and the distal radial ulnar joint. J Hand Surg 2003;28(4):614–21.
35. Gilula LA, Weeks PM. Post-traumatic ligamentous instabilities of the wrist. Radiology 1978;129(3):641–51.
36. McQueen MM, Hajducka C, Court-Brown CM. Redisplaced unstable fractures of the distal radius. J Bone Jt Surg Br Vol 1996;78-B(3):404–9.
37. Park MJ, Cooney WP 3rd, Hahn ME, et al. The effects of dorsally angulated distal radius fractures on carpal kinematics. J Hand Surg 2002;27(2):223–32.
38. Komura S, Hirakawa A, Yamamoto K, et al. Delayed rupture of the flexor tendons as a complication of malunited distal radius fracture after nonoperative management: A report of two cases. Trauma Case Rep 2019;21:100198.
39. Proubasta IR, Lamas CG, Natera L, et al. Delayed rupture of all finger flexor tendons (excluding thumb) following nonoperative treatment of Colles' fracture: A case report and literature review. J Orthop 2015;12(Suppl 1):S65–8.
40. Gary C, Shah A, Kanouzi J, et al. Carpal Tunnel Syndrome Following Corrective Osteotomy for Distal Radius Malunion: A Rare Case Report and Review of the Literature. Hand 2017;12(5):Np157–np161.
41. DeNoble PH, Marshall AC, Barron OA, et al. Malpractice in distal radius fracture management: an analysis of closed claims. J Hand Surg 2014;39(8):1480–8.
42. Khan IH, Giddins G. Analysis of NHSLA claims in hand and wrist surgery. J Hand Surg 2010;35(1):61–4.
43. Matsen FA 3rd, Stephens L, Jette JL, et al. The quality of upper extremity orthopedic care in liability claims filed and claims paid. J Hand Surg 2014;39(1):91–9.
44. Arora R, Gabl M, Gschwentner M, et al. A Comparative Study of Clinical and Radiologic Outcomes of Unstable Colles Type Distal Radius

Fractures in Patients Older Than 70 Years: Nonoperative Treatment Versus Volar Locking Plating. J Orthop Trauma 2009;23(4):237–42.

45. Chung KC, Kim HM, Malay S, et al. Comparison of 24-Month Outcomes After Treatment for Distal Radius Fracture: The WRIST Randomized Clinical Trial. JAMA Netw Open 2021;4(6):e2112710.

46. Mulders MA, d'Ailly PN, Cleffken BI, et al. Corrective osteotomy is an effective method of treating distal radius malunions with good long-term functional results. Injury 2017;48(3):731–7.

47. Prommersberger KJ, Pillukat T, Mühldorfer M, et al. Malunion of the distal radius. Arch Orthop Trauma Surg 2012;132(5):693–702.

48. Belloti JC, Alves BVP, Faloppa F, et al. The malunion of distal radius fracture: Corrective osteotomy through planning with prototyping in 3D printing. Injury 2021;52(Suppl 3):S44–s48.

49. Jupiter JB, Ring D. A comparison of early and late reconstruction of malunited fractures of the distal end of the radius. J Bone Jt Surg Am Vol 1996; 78(5):739–48.

50. Bilgin SS, Armangil M. Correction of nascent malunion of distal radius fractures. Acta Orthop Traumatol Turcica 2012;46(1):30–4.

51. Fernandez DL. Correction of post-traumatic wrist deformity in adults by osteotomy, bone-grafting, and internal fixation. J Bone Jt Surg Am Vol 1982; 64(8):1164–78.

52. Malone KJ, Magnell TD, Freeman DC, et al. Surgical correction of dorsally angulated distal radius malunions with fixed angle volar plating: a case series. J Hand Surg 2006;31(3):366–72.

53. Gaspar MP, Kho JY, Kane PM, et al. Orthogonal Plate Fixation With Corrective Osteotomy for Treatment of Distal Radius Fracture Malunion. J Hand Surg 2017;42(1):e1–10.

54. Tarallo L, Mugnai R, Adani R, et al. Malunited extra-articular distal radius fractures: corrective osteotomies using volar locking plate. J Orthop Traumatol 2014;15(4):285–90.

55. Del Piñal FG-BF, Studer A, Regalado J, et al. Sagittal Rotational Malunions of the Distal Radius: The Role of Pure Derotational Osteotomy. J Hand Surg 2009; 34E(2):160–5.

56. Hozack BA, Tosti RJ. Fragment-Specific Fixation in Distal Radius Fractures. Curr Rev Musculoskelet Med 2019;12(2):190–7.

57. Haghverdian JC, Hsu JY, Harness NG. Complications of Corrective Osteotomies for Extra-Articular Distal Radius Malunion. J Hand Surg 2019;44(11): 987 e1–e987 e9.

58. Fernandez DL. Reconstructive procedures for malunion and traumatic arthritis. Orthop Clin N Am 1993;24(2):341–63.

59. Marcuzzi A, Lana D, Laselva O, et al. Combined radius addition osteotomy and ulnar shortening to correct extra-articular distal radius fracture malunion with severe radial deviation and ulnar plus. Acta Biomed 2019;90(12-S):167–73.

60. Kamal RN, Leversedge FJ. Ulnar shortening osteotomy for distal radius malunion. J Wrist Surg 2014; 3(3):181–6.

61. Hassan S, Shafafy R, Mohan A, et al. Solitary ulnar shortening osteotomy for malunion of distal radius fractures: experience of a centre in the UK and review of the literature. Ann R Coll Surg Engl 2019; 101(3):203–7.

62. Löw S, Mühldorfer-Fodor M, Pillukat T, et al. Ulnar shortening osteotomy for malunited distal radius fractures: results of a 7-year follow-up with special regard to the grade of radial displacement and post-operative ulnar variance. Arch Orthop Trauma Surg 2014;134(1):131–7.

63. Srinivasan RC, Jain D, Richard MJ, et al. Isolated ulnar shortening osteotomy for the treatment of extra-articular distal radius malunion. J Hand Surg 2013; 38(6):1106–10.

64. Jupiter JB, Ring DC. AO manual of fracture management—hand and wrist. 1st edition. Switzerland: Thieme AO Publishing; 2005.

65. Rodriguez-Fontan F. Fracture healing, the diamond concept under the scope: hydroxyapatite and the hexagon. Medicina (B Aires) 2022;82(5):764–9. Consolidación de fractura, una mirada al concepto diamante: hidroxiapatita y el hexágono.

66. Ring D, Roberge C, Morgan T, et al. Osteotomy for malunited fractures of the distal radius: a comparison of structural and nonstructural autogenous bone grafts. J Hand Surg 2002;27(2):216–22.

67. Ozer K, Kiliç A, Sabel A, et al. The role of bone allografts in the treatment of angular malunions of the distal radius. J Hand Surg Am 2011;36(11):1804–9.

68. Disseldorp DJ, Poeze M, Hannemann PF, et al. Is Bone Grafting Necessary in the Treatment of Malunited Distal Radius Fractures? J Wrist Surg 2015; 4(3):207–13.

69. Prommersberger KJ, Froehner SC, Schmitt RR, et al. Rotational deformity in malunited fractures of the distal radius. J Hand Surg 2004;29(1):110–5.

70. Adams BD. Effects of radial deformity on distal radioulnar joint mechanics. J Hand Surg 1993;18(3): 492–8.

71. Teunissen JS, Wouters RM, Al Shaer S, et al. Outcomes of ulna shortening osteotomy: a cohort analysis of 106 patients. J Orthop Traumatol 2022; 23(1):1.

72. Barbaric K, Rujevcan G, Labas M, et al. Ulnar Shortening Osteotomy After Distal Radius Fracture Malunion: Review of Literature. Open Orthop J 2015;9: 98–106.

73. Chan SK, Singh T, Pinder R, et al. Ulnar Shortening Osteotomy: Are Complications Under Reported? J Hand Microsurg 2015;7(2):276–82.

74. Hove LM, Nilsen PT, Furnes O, et al. Open reduction and internal fixation of displaced intraarticular fractures of the distal radius. 31 patients followed for 3-7 years. Acta Orthop Scand 1997;68(1):59–63.

75. Ruch DS, Wray WH 3rd, Papadonikolakis A, et al. Corrective osteotomy for isolated malunion of the palmar lunate facet in distal radius fractures. J Hand Surg 2010;35(11):1779–86.

76. Yoshii Y, Ogawa T, Hara Y, et al. An image fusion system for corrective osteotomy of distal radius malunion. Biomed Eng Online 2021;20(1):66.

77. Buijze GA, Leong NL, Stockmans F, et al. Three-Dimensional Compared with Two-Dimensional Preoperative Planning of Corrective Osteotomy for Extra-Articular Distal Radial Malunion: A Multicenter Randomized Controlled Trial. J Bone Jt Surg Am Vol 2018;100(14):1191–202.

78. Assink N, Meesters AML, Ten Duis K, et al. A Two-Step Approach for 3D-Guided Patient-Specific Corrective Limb Osteotomies. J Pers Med 2022; 12(9). https://doi.org/10.3390/jpm12091458.

79. Mahmoud M, El Shafie S, Kamal M. Correction of dorsally-malunited extra-articular distal radial fractures using volar locked plates without bone grafting. J Bone Jt Surg Br Vol 2012;94(8):1090–6.

80. Tiren D, Vos DI. Correction osteotomy of distal radius malunion stabilised with dorsal locking plates without grafting. Strategies in trauma and limb reconstruction 2014;9(1):53–8.

81. Scheer JH, Adolfsson LE. Non-union in 3 of 15 osteotomies of the distal radius without bone graft. Acta Orthop 2015;86(3):316–20.

82. Andreasson I, Kjellby-Wendt G, Fagevik Olsén M, et al. Functional outcome after corrective osteotomy for malunion of the distal radius: a randomised, controlled, double-blind trial. Int Orthop 2020; 44(7):1353–65.

83. Yaradılmış YU, Tecirli A, Örs Ç. Distal radius correction osteotomy with tricortical bone graft is a successful method in heavy smokers. J Orthop 2020; 18:150–4.

84. Pecache MB, Calleja HM. Corrective Osteotomy of Distal Radius Malunion Using a Rectangular-shaped Iliac Bone Graft and Volar Plating. Tech Hand Up Extrem Surg 2020;25(3):130–5.

85. Abramo A, Tägil M, Geijer M, et al. Osteotomy of dorsally displaced malunited fractures of the distal radius: No loss of radiographic correction during healing with a minimally invasive fixation technique and an injectable bone substitute. Acta Orthop 2008;79(2):262–8.

Managing the Intra-articular Distal Radius Malunion

Chelsea C. Boe, MD*, Stephen A. Kennedy, MD, FRCSC

KEYWORDS

• Intra-articular distal radius malunion • Corrective osteotomy • Arthroscopically assisted correction
• 3-D planning for malunion • Patient-specific instrumentation

KEY POINTS

• Not all articular malunions require correction.
• Young, active patients with symptomatic intra-articular malunions with significant radiologic derangement will likely have improved wrist function following corrective osteotomy.
• Normal wrist function should not be expected after intra-articular malunion correction.
• Long-term post-traumatic arthritis is to be expected regardless of intervention.

INTRODUCTION

Distal radius malunion is a well-known complication of distal radius fractures,[1–3] most commonly from re-displacement following closed reduction or lack of timely treatment.[4] Based on review of the literature and consensus expert opinion regarding acceptable healing parameters, the authors define malunion as follows:

• Radial inclination less than 10°
• Volar tilt greater than 20°
• Dorsal tilt greater than 20°
• Radial height less than 10 mm
• Articular step off greater than 2 mm[5]
• Significant radiocarpal translation

Volar and dorsal translation of the radiocarpal joint should be considered in evaluation of distal radius malunion as a hallmark of instability and potential source of pain. This is best evaluated by a longitudinal line extending from the center of axis of rotation of the capitate, which should normally intersect with the long axis of the radius. Radiocarpal subluxation is among the variables most significantly associated with impaired long-term function.[6]

In defining malunion, it is important to distinguish the type of malunion, namely intra-articular, extra-articular, or combined.[7,8] Extra-articular malunions will be discussed separately in a different chapter and we will focus specifically on the approach and consideration of intra-articular malunions.

Biomechanical data have demonstrated that altered alignment of the distal radial surface has direct and predictable impacts on contact pressures and transmission of force through the carpus and forearm. Dorsal angulation greater than 20° results in dorsal loading across the carpus and relative off-loading of the volar lunate facet.[9] This degree of angulation (20° dorsal relative to the normal position) additionally translates the radiocarpal articulation dorsal relative to the ulnar head, causing incongruency in distal radioulnar joint contact, tightening of the interosseous membrane, and reduced protonation and supination.[10] In vivo studies have further suggested that extreme ulnar positive variance (significant radial shortening) can block the dorsal translation of the distal radius relative to the ulnar head effecting a block to supination specifically.[11] Increasing dorsal angulation additionally results in increased

Department of Orthopaedics and Sports Medicine, University of Washington, Box 359798, 325 9th Avenue, Seattle, WA 98104, USA
* Corresponding author.
E-mail address: cboe@uw.edu

Hand Clin 40 (2024) 79–87
https://doi.org/10.1016/j.hcl.2023.08.015

force transmission through the ulna and the ulno-carpal joint, with significant change detectable at 20° dorsal angulation relative to the normal position.[9]

Similar to extreme alterations of dorsal tilt, increased palmar tilt can cause alterations of the distal radioulnar joint articulation, abnormal tensioning of the triangular fibrocartilage complex, and reduced forearm rotation.[12] Supination deficit is reported in volar malunions, though protonation deficit appears to be more common with significant increase of palmar tilt.[13]

The clinical impact of radiographic malunion is well established in the case of distal radius fractures. Loss of normal volar tilt results in decrease in functional outcome, manifested as higher Disabilities of the Shoulder and Hand (DASH) scores and higher Visual Analog Scalescores.[14] Loss of radial height can result in ulnar wrist pain, loss of grip strength, and reduction forearm range of motion secondary to distal radioulnar joint impingement.[15,16]

Cadaveric studies have shown increased contact pressures with articular incongruity as little as 1 mm,[17,18] and 2 mm of incongruity in clinical studies has been associated with universal development of radiographic arthritis.[19] Radiographic arthrosis develops in many cases within 1 year of injury,[2] often translates to clinical symptoms, and is consistently reported as a predictor of worse functional outcome.[15,19–22] Articular step off broadly has been associated with loss of wrist flexion[23] and specific displacement of the volar lunate facet associated with substantial loss of supination as well as loss of both flexion and extension.[24] In a series of 13 patients with volar lunate facet malunion, Ruch and colleagues noted an average supination of 38°, which was corrected to 87° upon correction of the malunion.[24]

While malunions are tolerated quite well in the elderly and patients with low functional demands despite significant anatomic derangement, this is not true for all patients.[25] The physiologically younger and high-demand patient population with articular derangement after distal radius fracture represents a group at highest risk for prolonged disability, and thus a potential target group for intervention to restore anatomic alignment and potentially change the natural history of these injuries. There is a strong association between loss of normal anatomic relationships of the distal radius and loss of congruence of the articular surface with diminished functional outcome and ongoing pain following distal radius fracture.[26,27]

Previous aversion to intervention for these malunions included difficulty in accessing the articular

surface, risk for increased articular damage in recreating a fracture through the articular surface, devascularization of small articular fragments, and concern regarding secure fixation of these fragments.[8,28] Advancements in distal radius plating, specifically smaller implants and fragment-specific instrumentation, has led to increasing belief in the feasibility of stable fixation for small articular fragments in AO type B and C fracture malunions. Advanced imaging availability including 3D modeling and patient-specific instrumentation have further piqued interest in the possibility of recreating complex fracture patterns and restoring or significantly improving articular congruity in this setting. Techniques such as dry arthroscopy and arthroscopically assisted fracture fixation have led to additional options for visualizing the joint without open arthrotomy and have the potential to become inside-out type techniques to recreate precise osteotomies through initial fracture lines.[28–30]

INDICATIONS

The indications for intervention in the setting of articular malunion remain incompletely defined. Most authors agree that not all fractures that can be defined as radiographic malunions are appropriate for intra-articular osteotomies.[31,32] Relative contraindications include patients with low functional demands, elderly patients with satisfactory wrist function despite malunion, patients who are poor surgical candidates due to medical comorbidities, inability to comply with postoperative recommendations, or poor tolerance for complications (which are not infrequent[32,33]).

Corrective osteotomy is not recommended in the setting of established post-traumatic arthrosis.[31] Depending on the treatment plan, a diagnostic arthroscopy may be considered to evaluate the state of the cartilage and confirm absence of arthrosis prior to performing osteotomy.[28,29] MRI can be utilized to evaluate the cartilage surface, though diagnostic arthroscopy is considered the gold standard. In the setting of established arthrosis, consideration should be given to salvage procedures such as limited wrist arthrodesis (**Figs. 1** and **2**).

Some authors recommend osteotomy only in the setting of symptomatic malunion. However, given the rapid rate of arthrosis in the setting of significant articular incongruity, this "wait and see" approach may result in delayed treatment to deleterious effect.[19,34] Others suggest early intervention in the setting of a high-demand or young patient in whom articular malalignment would reasonably be expected to translate to symptoms

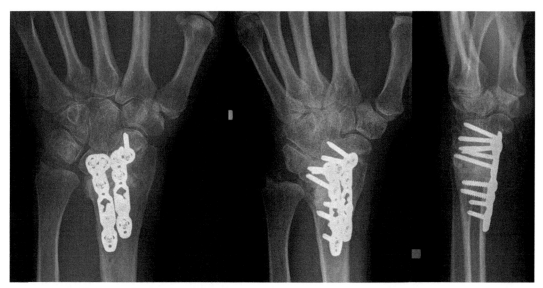

Fig. 1. Radioscapholunate fusion for arthrosis following intra-articular distal radius malunion. (Image courtesy of Douglas Hanel, MD.)

in the future.[32] The majority of authors agree that intervention should be considered in the setting of a physiologically young, active patient with radiocarpal subluxation, articular step off of 2 mm or more without arthrosis, and/or malunion of the volar lunate facet independent of symptoms.[31]

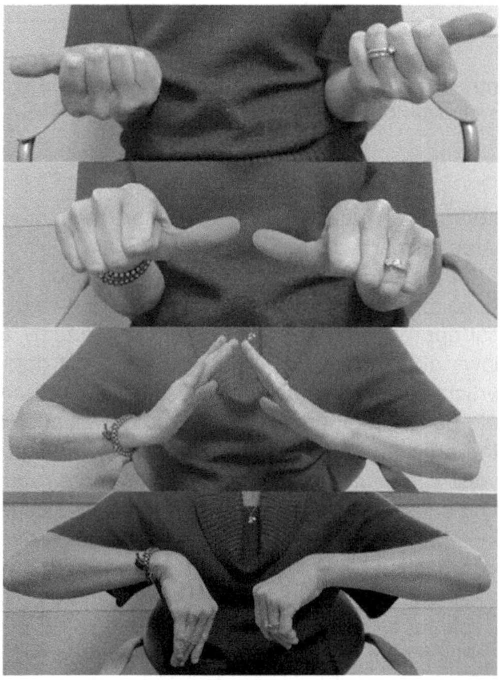

TIMING

The timing of surgical intervention continues to be debated. When recognized early, fracture callus can be more clearly identified and the fracture planes recreated with relative ease.[8,28] Additionally, treating nascent malunions avoids the potential complications of soft tissue contracture which may limit ultimate correction when intervention is significantly delayed. Jupiter and Ring demonstrated that early malunion correction (within 8 weeks) is technically easier and results in a shorter period of disability for the patient when compared to delayed intervention.[7] While the malunions in this series were largely extra-articular, it would stand to reason that the conclusions would be equally, if not more applicable, in the setting of more complex fracture deformities involving the articular surface.

In treatment of articular malunions involving the lunate facet, superior results were obtained with correction of the palmar lunate facet at an average of 5.4 months[24] compared to similar malunions treated at an average of 24 months.[15] Furthermore, del Pinal and colleagues demonstrated that malunions treated late appear to be more at risk for creation of articular gaps which cannot be fully corrected.[29] These results call into question the theory that allowing full bone healing and correction of osteopenia will improve fixation at

Fig. 2. Range of motion (ROM) following radioscapholunate fusion. Wrist ROM 75-degree arc on the left (extension 45°, flexion 30°). Contralateral wrist ROM was 125-degree arc (extension 65°, flexion 60°). Ulnar deviation is 30° on the right compared to 50° on the left. Radial deviation is 10° on the right and 25° on the left. (Images courtesy of Douglas Hanel, MD.)

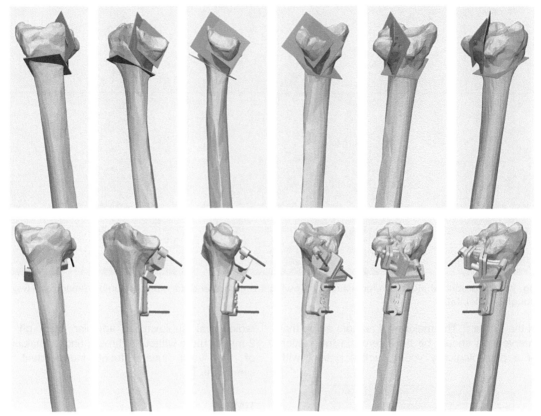

Fig. 3. 3D models demonstrating preoperative plan for intra-articular distal radius malunion correction with custom cutting guides and patient-specific instrumentation. (Images courtesy of Brian Pridgen, MD.)

the time of corrective osteotomy in the setting of intra-articular displacement.

APPROACH

In discussing the approach to intra-articular malunions, it is important to recognize that these deformities are 3-dimensional (3D) which may require correction in multiple planes.[7] There are specific fractures, namely volar shear fractures or malunions involving the volar lunate facet, in which the malunion can be approached from a single volar approach through the original fracture line and satisfactory correction can be achieved.[8,31,32,35] Ruch and colleagues presented 13 patients with malunited palmar lunate facet fractures approached volarly and demonstrated that the articular step off could be corrected to an average of less than 1 mm of displacement.[24] This approach provides excellent correction for an isolated volar fragment, maintaining attachment of the palmar radioulnar ligament.[36,37] However, there is dispute about whether articular congruity and anatomic alignment can be fully corrected from a volar-only

approach in malunions involving more than an isolated palmar facet fragment.[38]

Intra-articular evaluation and correction has been reported to be more effective through a dorsal approach,[39] where a dorsal capsulotomy allows direct observation and correction of dorsal articular fragments as well as centrally depressed die-punch fragments.[40,41] The same evaluation of the articular surface is less advisable through a volar capsulotomy secondary to the more robust and critical palmar capsular ligaments,[36,37] allowing only indirect evaluation of the articular surface approached through the fracture planes. Thus, in more complex articular deformities, there may be a role for a combined.[32]

Placement of fixation is typically dictated by the unique malunion being treated. Volar locking plate fixation is generally preferred with lower complication rates compared to dorsal fixation, as excellent results can be achieved with volar fixation in the majority of articular malunion cases.[42] However, in the setting of complex deformity and the need for independent fixation of dorsal fragments, both dorsal and volar fixation may be required.[38]

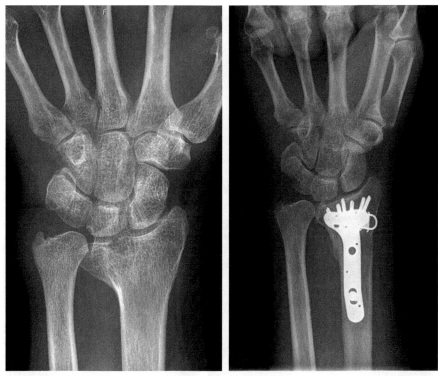

Fig. 4. Preoperative and 3 months postoperative posteroanterior (PA) radiographs of intra-articular distal radius malunion, corrected with custom guides as shown in **Fig. 3**. (Images courtesy of Brian Pridgen, MD.)

It is important to note that procedures with combined fixation are associated with a high rate of implant removal, independent of location of fixation.[32,33]

ARTHROSCOPY

Arthroscopy has been advocated as an alternative to an open arthrotomy for improved visualization of the articular surface to address articular malunions.[43] As described by del Pinal and colleagues in a case series of 4 patients, this approach had the advantage of avoiding detachment of fragments from surrounding supporting ligaments by performing osteotomies through arthroscopy portals, with effective recreation and correction of even irregularly shaped fragments.[28] Del Pinal, and colleagues further reported a series of 11 fractures treated with inside-out arthroscopic-assisted osteotomy with complete correction of articular step off in up to 3 articular fragments with outcomes comparable to those reported with open techniques.[29] Of note, interventions occurred an average of 9 weeks after fracture, when fracture lines were easily identifiable by direct arthroscopic inspection which may have contributed to the high success of the procedure. However, it is important

to recognize that these procedures required 2 surgeons skilled in arthroscopy and comfortable with dry technique.[29,30]

PATIENT-SPECIFIC INSTRUMENTATION

For complex, multiplanar deformities, advanced imaging in the form of a computed tomography (CT) scan, with or without 3-D renderings, is imperative for preoperative planning.[24,32] This is especially significant for rotational deformities that are easily underappreciated on plain radiographs.[44,45]

Modern technology allows for use of such 3-D modeling to generate patient-specific drill guides to facilitate precise re-creation of intra-articular fragments without the need for arthrotomy, thus, preserving ligamentous and capsular attachments.[46–48] Oka and colleagues described the use of patient-specific guides for intra-articular distal radius osteotomy[49] and further studies have validated the feasibility and success even in the setting of multiple articular fragments.[46,50,51] A meta-analysis published in 2017 reviewing 68 patients from 15 different studies with intra-articular malunions treated by 3D-planned corrective osteotomy demonstrated

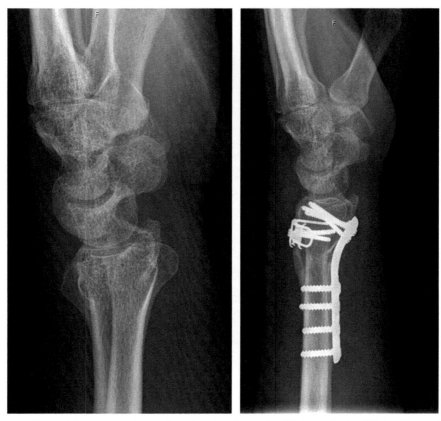

Fig. 5. Preoperative and 3-month postoperative lateral radiographs of intra-articular distal radius malunion, corrected with custom guides as shown in **Fig. 3**. (Images courtesy of Brian Pridgen, MD.)

statistically significant improvement in all radiographic parameters, nearly all to within 5° of normal.[52]

There are numerous advantages of patient-specific guides for intra-articular osteotomy, including the ability to custom design and de-rotate quite complex deformities in a predictable and reliable fashion (**Figs. 3** and **4**). However, there is substantial expense, required planning and manufacturing time, as well as the need for additional radiation from CT scans of bilateral wrists for the surgical planning.[46] A randomized, controlled trial comparing 3D planning versus conventional planning for distal radial osteotomies failed to find a significant difference in mean postoperative DASH scores or patient-related wrist evaluation scores with the use of 3D guides.[43] However, this study evaluated extra-articular osteotomies and thus may not translate to the more complex correction in the setting of intra-articular malunion.[53] To our knowledge, that study has not been replicated in intra-articular malunions, especially in C-type fractures, where increased nuance of the joint

surface may mean significant differences in surgical correction could be detected.

OUTCOMES

Despite the universally acknowledged technically challenging nature of these operations, functional and radiographic outcomes can be significantly improved with careful planning.[8,38,46,54] Significant improvement in articular step off has been demonstrated across multiple studies, with correction to <1 mm regardless of surgical approach, use of arthroscopy, 3D planning, or custom cutting guides.[8,24,28,29,38,46,51] Ring and colleagues reported a series of 23 patients treated for articular malunion with significant improvement in flexion, extension, protonation, supination, ulnar variance, and articular congruity compared with preoperative motion.[8] Similar results were achieved by Zhang at al., who noted significant correction of radial length, radial inclination, volar tilt, and ulnar variance with improvement in range of motion and grip strength.[38] These functional results were comparable to treatment of extra-articular osteotomy and have been validated by other authors[51] Patients can expect to have motion corrected to 70% to 89% of the contralateral side[26,32] (**Fig. 5**), and grip strength to 71% to 85% of the contralateral side.[8,24,26,29,31,32] Accordingly, patient-reported outcome measures and satisfaction are also consistent significantly improved following corrective osteotomy.[32,38,46,51] DASH scores are reported between 7.6 and 16.[24,26,29,32] Osteonecrosis has not been reported, despite fears related to osteotomy of small articular fragments.[8,32]

Improvement in functional outcomes appears to be durable over time. Zhang and colleagues demonstrated grip strength, DASH, Modified Mayo Wrist Score, and range of motion were maintained with no significant change between 3 and 18 months, though they did note that several patients with AO C-type fractures developed arthritis within 6 months.[38] Similar durability was reported at an average follow-up of 78 months with no significant association between functional outcome and length of follow-up.[32] Lozano-Calderon et al. evaluated long-term outcomes in 23 wrists which underwent correction of distal radial malunion at an average of 9 months post injury and found no significant difference in immediate compared with long-term (average 13 year) radiographic parameters.[15] However, this study noted that all patients who had intra-articular malunion had severe post-traumatic arthritis at long-term follow-up despite maintained surgical correction.[26] This is similar to other authors, who noted that normal wrist function is rarely ever achieved.[8,38,51]

SUMMARY

Intra-articular distal radius malunions are technically challenging surgical procedures which require meticulous technique and preoperative planning for multiplanar corrections often requiring numerous osteotomies including small, articular fragments. When performed well technically, significant improvement in radiographic alignment as well as functional outcomes can be expected. Based on currently available data, corrective osteotomy for articular malunion is indicated in symptomatic patients with significant alterations in their joint surface without evidence of arthrosis. Surgery is also indicated in young, active patients with early radiographic evidence of malunion which is likely to translate to symptomatic malunion or accelerated arthrosis. Preoperative planning should include advanced imaging to define articular fragments and facilitate planning of osteotomies, with consideration given to custom cutting guides and patient-specific instrumentation, especially in the setting of complex multiplanar malunions. For the experienced arthroscopist, arthroscopy may be helpful to visualize the joint during the procedure and confirm adequate correction of articular step offs, obviating the need for dorsal arthrotomy. It is important to recognize that restoration of the articular congruity and anatomic parameters do not always lead to restoration of normal wrist function. Moreover, the natural history of these significant articular injuries and predisposition to development of arthritis may not be significantly altered despite the improvement in anatomic alignment.

CLINICS CARE POINTS

- Functional deficits are anticipated with articular step off exceeding 2 mm, radial height less than 10 mm, radial inclination less than 10°, volar tilt exceeding 20°, dorsal tilt exceeding 20°, or significant radiocarpal translation.

- Nascent malunions should be treated early when long-term function is anticipated to be significantly impacted by the degree of deformity, especially in high-demand patients.

- Arthroscopic-assisted procedures allow direct visualization of the articular surface, though may be technically challenging.

- Custom molded 3D computer-assisted cutting guides may reduce operative time and allow predictable correction of deformity.

- Radiographic correction of articular malunion may not completely resolve functional limitations.

REFERENCES

1. Amadio PC, Botte MJ. Treatment of malunion of the distal radius. Hand Clin 1987;3(4):541–61.
2. Fernandez DL. Reconstructive procedures for malunion and traumatic arthritis. Orthop Clin North Am 1993;24(2):341–63.
3. Jenkins NH, Mintowt-Czyz WJ. Mal-union and dysfunction in Colles' fracture. J Hand Surg Br 1988;13(3):291–3.
4. Walenkamp MM, Aydin S, Mulders MA, et al. Predictors of unstable distal radius fractures: a systematic review and meta-analysis. J Hand Surg Eur 2016; 41(5):501–15.
5. Haase SC, Chung KC. Management of malunions of the distal radius. Hand Clin 2012;28(2):207–16.

6. McQueen MM, Hajducka C, Court-Brown CM. Re-displaced unstable fractures of the distal radius: a prospective randomised comparison of four methods of treatment. J Bone Joint Surg Br 1996; 78(3):404–9.

7. Jupiter JB, Ring D. A comparison of early and late reconstruction of malunited fractures of the distal end of the radius. J Bone Joint Surg Am 1996; 78(5):739–48.

8. Ring D, Prommersberger KJ, Gonzalez del Pino J, et al. Corrective osteotomy for intra-articular mal-union of the distal part of the radius. J Bone Joint Surg Am 2005;87(7):1503–9.

9. Short WH, Palmer AK, Werner FW, et al. A biomechanical study of distal radial fractures. J Hand Surg Am 1987;12(4):529–34.

10. Kihara H, Palmer AK, Werner FW, et al. The effect of dorsally angulated distal radius fractures on distal radioulnar joint congruency and forearm rotation. J Hand Surg Am 1996;21(1):40–7.

11. Ishikawa J, Iwasaki N, Minami A. Influence of distal radioulnar joint subluxation on restricted forearm rotation after distal radius fracture. J Hand Surg Am 2005;30(6):1178–84.

12. Bessho Y, Nakamura T, Nagura T, et al. Effect of volar angulation of extra-articular distal radius frac-tures on distal radioulnar joint stability: a biomechan-ical study. J Hand Surg Eur 2015;40(8):775–82.

13. Prommersberger KJ, Froehner SC, Schmitt RR, et al. Rotational deformity in malunited fractures of the distal radius. J Hand Surg Am 2004;29(1):110–5.

14. Batra S, Gupta A. The effect of fracture-related fac-tors on the functional outcome at 1 year in distal radius fractures. Injury 2002;33(6):499–502.

15. Harness NG, Jupiter JB, Orbay JL, et al. Loss of fix-ation of the volar lunate facet fragment in fractures of the distal part of the radius. J Bone Joint Surg Am 2004;86(9):1900–8.

16. McQueen M, Caspers J. Colles fracture: does the anatomical result affect the final function? J Bone Joint Surg Br 1988;70(4):649–51.

17. Wagner WF Jr, Tencer AF, Kiser P, et al. Effects of intra-articular distal radius depression on wrist joint contact characteristics. J Hand Surg Am 1996; 21(4):554–60.

18. Baratz ME, Des Jardins J, Anderson DD, et al. Dis-placed intra-articular fractures of the distal radius: the effect of fracture displacement on contact stresses in a cadaver model. J Hand Surg Am 1996;21(2):183–8.

19. Knirk JL, Jupiter JB. Intra-articular fractures of the distal end of the radius in young adults. J Bone Joint Surg Am 1986;68(5):647–59.

20. Bradway JK, Amadio PC, Cooney WP. Open reduc-tion and internal fixation of displaced, comminuted intra-articular fractures of the distal end of the radius. J Bone Joint Surg Am 1989;71(6):839–47.

21. Catalano LW 3rd, Cole RJ, Gelberman RH, et al. Dis-placed intra-articular fractures of the distal aspect of the radius. Long-term results in young adults after open reduction and internal fixation. J Bone Joint Surg Am 1997;79(9):1290–302.

22. Trumble TE, Schmitt SR, Vedder NB. Factors affecting functional outcome of displaced intra-articular distal radius fractures. J Hand Surg Am 1994;19(2):325–40.

23. Forward DP, Davis TR, Sithole JS. Do young patients with malunited fractures of the distal radius inevi-tably develop symptomatic post-traumatic osteoar-thritis? J Bone Joint Surg Br 2008;90(5):629–37.

24. Ruch DS, Wray WH 3rd, Papadonikolakis A, et al. Corrective osteotomy for isolated malunion of the palmar lunate facet in distal radius fractures. J Hand Surg Am 2010;35(11):1779–86.

25. Slagel BE, Luenam S, Pichora DR. Management of post-traumatic malunion of fractures of the distal radius. Orthop Clin North Am 2007;38(2):203–16, vi.

26. Cooney WP 3rd, Dobyns JH, Linscheid RL. Compli-cations of Colles' fractures. J Bone Joint Surg Am 1980;62(4):613–9.

27. Lozano-Calderon SA, Brouwer KM, Doornberg JN, et al. Long-term outcomes of corrective osteotomy for the treatment of distal radius malunion. J Hand Surg Eur 2010;35(5):370–80.

28. del Pinal F, Garcia-Bernal FJ, Delgado J, et al. Correction of malunited intra-articular distal radius fractures with an inside-out osteotomy technique. J Hand Surg Am 2006;31(6):1029–34.

29. del Pinal F, Cagigal L, Garcia-Bernal FJ, et al. Arthro-scopically guided osteotomy for management of intra-articular distal radius malunions. J Hand Surg Am 2010;35(3):392–7.

30. del Pinal F, Garcia-Bernal FJ, Pisani D, et al. Dry arthroscopy of the wrist: surgical technique. J Hand Surg Am 2007;32(1):119–23.

31. Prommersberger KJ, Ring D, Gonzalez del Pino J, et al. Corrective osteotomy for intra-articular mal-union of the distal part of the radius. Surgical tech-nique. J Bone Joint Surg Am 2006;88(Suppl 1 Pt 2):202–11.

32. Buijze GA, Prommersberger KJ, Gonzalez Del Pino J, et al. Corrective osteotomy for combined intra- and extra-articular distal radius malunion. J Hand Surg Am 2012;37(10):2041–9.

33. Haghverdian JC, Hsu JY, Harness NG. Complica-tions of Corrective Osteotomies for Extra-Articular Distal Radius Malunion. J Hand Surg Am 2019; 44(11):987 e981–e987 e989.

34. Axelrod T, Paley D, Green J, et al. Limited open reduction of the lunate facet in comminuted intra-articular fractures of the distal radius. J Hand Surg Am 1988;13(3):372–7.

35. Thivaios GC, McKee MD. Sliding osteotomy for deformity correction following malunion of volarly

displaced distal radial fractures. J Orthop Trauma 2003;17(5):326–33.

36. Nakamura T, Makita A. The proximal ligamentous component of the triangular fibrocartilage complex. J Hand Surg Br 2000;25(5):479–86.

37. Palmer AK, Werner FW. The triangular fibrocartilage complex of the wrist–anatomy and function. J Hand Surg Am 1981;6(2):153–62.

38. Zhang H, Zhu Y, Fu F, et al. Corrective Osteotomy with Volar and Dorsal Fixation for Malunion of Intra-Articular Fracture of the Distal Radius: A Retrospective Study. Orthop Surg 2022;14(8):1751–8.

39. Krimmer H, Schandl R, Wolters R. Corrective osteotomy after malunited distal radius fractures. Arch Orthop Trauma Surg 2020;140(5):675–80.

40. Ipaktchi K, Livermore M, Lyons C, et al. Current concepts in the treatment of distal radial fractures. Orthopedics 2013;36(10):778–84.

41. Ring D, Jupiter JB, Brennwald J, et al. Prospective multicenter trial of a plate for dorsal fixation of distal radius fractures. J Hand Surg Am 1997;22(5):777–84.

42. Tarallo L, Mugnai R, Adani R, et al. Malunited extra-articular distal radius fractures: corrective osteotomies using volar locking plate. J Orthop Traumatol 2014;15(4):285–90.

43. Gobel F, Vardakas DG, Riano F, et al. Arthroscopically assisted intra-articular corrective osteotomy of a malunion of the distal radius. Am J Orthop (Belle Mead NJ) 2004;33(6):275–7.

44. Prommersberger KJ, Pillukat T, Muhldorfer M, et al. Malunion of the distal radius. Arch Orthop Trauma Surg 2012;132(5):693–702.

45. Vroemen JC, Dobbe JG, Sierevelt IN, et al. Accuracy of distal radius positioning using an anatomical plate. Orthopedics 2013;36(4):e457–62.

46. Schweizer A, Furnstahl P, Nagy L. Three-dimensional correction of distal radius intra-articular malunions using patient-specific drill guides. J Hand Surg Am 2013;38(12):2339–47.

47. Stockmans F, Dezillie M, Vanhaecke J. Accuracy of 3D Virtual Planning of Corrective Osteotomies of the Distal Radius. J Wrist Surg 2013;2(4):306–14.

48. Pillukat T, Osorio M, Prommersberger KJ. [Correction of Intraarticular Malunion of the Distal Radius Based on a Computer-Assisted Virtual Planning]. Handchir Mikrochir Plast Chir 2018;50(5):310–8.

49. Oka K, Moritomo H, Goto A, et al. Corrective osteotomy for malunited intra-articular fracture of the distal radius using a custom-made surgical guide based on three-dimensional computer simulation: case report. J Hand Surg Am 2008;33(6):835–40.

50. Murase T, Oka K, Moritomo H, et al. Three-dimensional corrective osteotomy of malunited fractures of the upper extremity with use of a computer simulation system. J Bone Joint Surg Am 2008;90(11):2375–89.

51. Roner S, Schweizer A, Da Silva Y, et al. Accuracy and Early Clinical Outcome After 3-Dimensional Correction of Distal Radius Intra-Articular Malunions Using Patient-Specific Instruments. J Hand Surg Am 2020;45(10):918–23.

52. de Muinck Keizer RJO, Lechner KM, Mulders MAM, et al. Three-dimensional virtual planning of corrective osteotomies of distal radius malunions: a systematic review and meta-analysis. Strategies Trauma Limb Reconstr 2017;12(2):77–89.

53. Buijze GA, Leong NL, Stockmans F, et al. Three-Dimensional Compared with Two-Dimensional Preoperative Planning of Corrective Osteotomy for Extra-Articular Distal Radial Malunion: A Multicenter Randomized Controlled Trial. J Bone Joint Surg Am 2018;100(14):1191–202.

54. Marx RG, Axelrod TS. Intraarticular osteotomy of distal radial malunions. Clin Orthop Relat Res 1996;327:152–7.

Role of Three-Dimensional Guides in Management of Forearm and Wrist Malunions

Geert Alexander Buijze, MD, PhD, FEBHS[a,b,c],*, Andreas Verstreken, MD[d],
Frederik Verstreken, MD, FEBHS[d,e]

KEYWORDS

- Malunion • Three-dimensional (3D) guides • Printed bone models • Distal radius • Wrist • Forearm

KEY POINTS

- Malunion is the most common complication following a distal radius fracture.
- Restoring anatomy of the forearm and wrist in malunions is an essential but technically demanding procedure aiming for an optimal functional outcome.
- Three-dimensional (3D) visualization and printed bone models are valuable tools to improve understanding of the malunion pattern.
- 3D computer planning and patient-specific intraoperative guides allow for more accurate and reproducible correction, especially in complex malunion patterns.
- The major disadvantage to date for 3D guides is costs related to outsourced 3D planning and guide production.

 Video content accompanies this article at http://www.hand.theclinics.com.

INTRODUCTION

Malunion of the distal radius is a common complication, with a reported incidence of up to 23% of nonsurgically treated distal radius fractures.[1,2] Malunion can result in persistent wrist pain and functional impairment. In addition, secondary carpal malalignment and intra-articular deformities can lead to early degenerative changes.[3–5]

When surgical treatment is deemed necessary, a corrective osteotomy is the procedure of choice, and clinical studies have shown a significant correlation between the precise restoration of normal anatomy and the improvement in clinical outcome.[6–8] Planning and performing a corrective osteotomy can be technically challenging.

Conventional two-dimensional (2D) radiographs are limited in the visualization of complex intra-articular and/or rotational deformities of the malunited wrist.[9] In a clinical series of 15 patients, restoration of bony alignment to within 5° of angular deformity and 2-mm ulnar variance was obtained in only 40% (6/15) of patients, despite careful preoperative planning.[10] In another case series of 60 patients with corrective osteotomy of extra-articular distal radius fractures, a complication rate of 42% was reported, with tendon injuries and delayed or nonunion being the most commonly reported problems.[11]

Three-dimensional (3D) technology might address some of these challenges and improve outcomes following corrective surgery. In the

---

[a] Hand, Upper Limb, Peripheral Nerve, Brachial Plexus and Microsurgery Unit, Clinique Générale Annecy, France; [b] Hand and Upper Extremity Surgery Unit, CHU Lapeyronie, University of Montpellier, Montpellier, France; [c] Department of Orthopaedic Surgery, Amsterdam UMC, University of Amsterdam, Amsterdam, Netherlands; [d] Orthopedic Department, Antwerp University Hospital, Drie Eikenstraat 655, Edegem 2650, Belgium; [e] Orthopedic Department, AZ Monica Hospital, F. Pauwelslei 1, Antwerp 2100, Belgium
* Corresponding author.
E-mail address: gabuijze@hotmail.com

Hand Clin 40 (2024) 89–95
https://doi.org/10.1016/j.hcl.2023.09.002
0749-0712/24/© 2023 Elsevier Inc. All rights reserved.

current review, the authors discuss the added value of 3D planning and surgical guidance compared with more conventional techniques in the correction of malunions of the wrist and forearm.

CURRENT EVIDENCE

In the early 1990s, Jupiter and colleagues[12] reported on the use of computer-assisted design and manufacturing technology to create solid models of 5 unusually complex, multiplanar malunited distal radius fractures. In their experience, preoperative planning was dramatically enhanced by the ability to perform the surgical procedure on these models in advance, with a model of the uninjured limb used for comparison. Since the early development of 3D computer-assisted planning and surgical guidance, an exponential number of studies have been performed.

There has only been one prospective randomized study comparing 2D planning with 3D computer-assisted planning. Unfortunately, for feasibility reasons, the study excluded the more complex deformities. Buijze and colleagues[13] randomized 40 patients undergoing corrective osteotomies for extra-articular distal radius malunion to a conventional 2D planning group and a 3D computer-assisted planning group. Surgical procedures were performed by highly experienced surgeons in both groups. They found no significant difference in patient-based functional outcomes. However, the notable trend toward a minimal clinically important difference for both the DASH (Disabilities of the Arm, Shoulder and Hand) scores (>10 points) and the Patient-Rated Wrist Evaluation (PRWE) scores (>6 points) in favor of 3D planned surgical guidance raised doubt about the likelihood of a type II error (ie, incorrectly retaining a false null hypothesis). Post hoc analysis confirmed that the study was underpowered. There were also no significant differences in pain, satisfaction, range of motion, and grip strength. They did, however, find significantly ($P<.05$) less residual deformity based on radiographic parameters (radial inclination and volar angulation but not ulnar variance) in the 3D-guided group. One notable secondary finding was significantly less extensor tendon pathologic condition in the 3D planning group. This was hypothesized to be a result of the preoperative quantification of bone geometry with predefined screw lengths, reducing the risk of dorsally protruding screws. The investigators postulated that the high degree of experience and skill of participating surgeons may have led to underestimation of the true benefit of 3D guidance in achieving

accurate anatomic reconstruction and improving patient outcomes.

All other studies looking at the value of 3D computer planning were retrospective case series or systematic reviews. de Muinck Keizer and colleagues[9] performed a systematic review including 15 studies and 68 patients treated with 3D virtual planning for both extra-articular and intra-articular malunions. They demonstrated radiographic parameters to within 5° (angulation) or 2 mm (ulnar variance) of their normal values in 96% of patients. This was superior to the 40% achieved with 2D preoperative planning in a different clinical series, using the same criteria for restoration of anatomy.[10] Moreover, the investigators demonstrated a significant ($P<.05$) improvement of wrist range of motion and grip strength. The investigators reported an overall complication rate of 16% in comparison with a case series of 60 patients with conventional 2D planning with a complication in 42% (25/60) of patients.[9,11] More recent case series on 3D corrective osteotomies of the distal radius showed comparable results, reinforcing the growing evidence in support of 3D technology.[14,15]

The use of 3D technology and patient-specific guides seems to be of most benefit for complex deformities in forearm and wrist malunions,[9,16] as it allows precise reconstruction of intra-articular step-offs and gaps.[16,17] Further findings in favor of 3D technology are its reproducibility and correction safety for forearm and wrist malunions as well as its potential reduction in operation time, blood loss, and radiation exposure during surgery.[5,13]

Case 1: Three-Dimensional–Assisted Correction of Distal Radius Deformity, Following Fracture and Growth Arrest

A 13-year-old boy presents left wrist pain, deformity, and limited range of motion (**Fig. 1**A). He sustained a fracture of the left distal radius 6 years earlier, treated by closed reduction and immobilization. Radiographs of both forearms confirmed gross deformity of the distal radius, with shortening and angulation deformity (**Fig. 1**B). Based on computed tomographic (CT) scans, 3D stereolithography (STL) files of the bones of both forearms were generated, and the deformity was compared with the mirror image of the contralateral radius. A virtual surgical reconstruction to restore anatomy was planned, and patient-specific instruments were designed (**Fig. 1**C). Harvesting of a precise matching corticocancellous graft was possible with cutting guides for the iliac crest (**Fig. 1**D). The surgery was performed with 3D printed models and patient-specific instruments (**Fig. 1**E). Radiographs

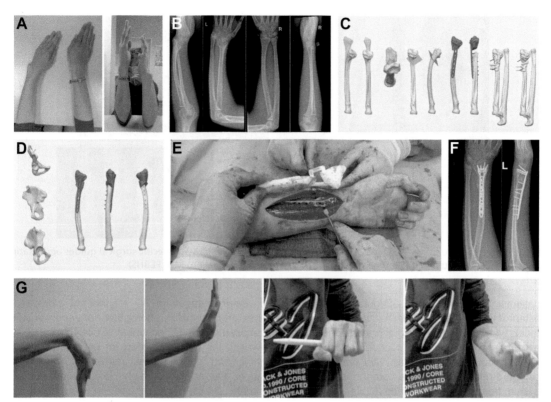

Fig. 1. Distal radius malunion and growth arrest (*A*), radiographs (*B*), 3D planning of surgical correction (*C*), 3D planning of iliac crest bone graft harvesting (*D*), 3D printed models and patient-specific instruments (*E*), postoperative radiographs (*F*), clinical outcome (*G*). (*Images copyright of* Frederik Verstreken, MD, FEBHS)

precisely matched the preoperative 3D plan, and bone healing was confirmed at 4 months (**Fig. 1**F). The patient had an excellent clinical outcome and function at 4 months postoperatively (**Fig. 1**G).

Case 2: Both Bone Forearm Malunion Following Diaphyseal Fracture

A 7-year-old boy was treated with closed reduction and casting for both bone forearm factures of the left arm (Video 1). He presented 11 months following treatment with symptomatic malunion of both the radius and the ulna, causing pain and functional disability (**Fig. 2**A). Based on bilateral CT scans of the forearm, 3D planning of surgical correction was performed (**Fig. 2**B). Patient-specific surgical guides and fixation plates were designed and 3D printed (**Fig. 2**C). The clinical outcome was excellent with restoration of normal alignment and return to pain-free full functioning (**Fig. 2**D).

Case 3: Intra-articular Distal Radius Malunion Following Prior Failed Surgery

The patient presented to clinic with pain and deformity of the right wrist. The patient had an intra-articular distal radius fracture that was initially treated with closed reduction percutaneous pinning with subsequent malunion with shortening and articular incongruity (**Fig. 3**A). The CT scan demonstrated the intra-articular deformity on sagittal, coronal, and axial cuts (**Fig. 3**B). Computer-generated 3D modeling of the intra-articular malunion was performed, demonstrating the correction needed to restore the anatomy (**Fig. 3**C). 3D printed custom cutting guides were prepared for the case (**Fig. 3**D). Intraoperatively, the cutting guides were used to help navigate the osteotomy precisely (**Fig. 3**E). Fluoroscopic images demonstrated restoration of the distal radius anatomy, matching the preoperative simulation (**Fig. 3**F).

The reported complication rates following 3D-assisted osteotomies of the distal radius compare favorably with those following conventional techniques.[1,9,13,18] Finally, a crucial long-term outcome parameter that is theoretically in favor of 3D technology and corresponding more accurate restoration of the anatomy is prevention in progression of post-traumatic arthritis. However, there are sparse clinical data on this. Recently, Singh and colleagues[19] reported on the intermediate-term outcome of 15

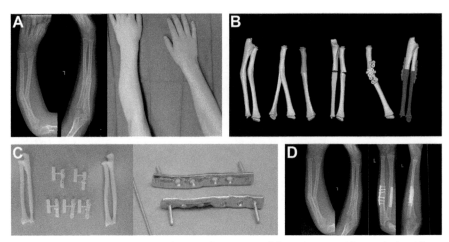

Fig. 2. Forearm malunion (*A*), 3D planning of surgical correction (*B*), patient-specific surgical guides and fixation plates (*C*), clinical outcome (*D*). (*Images copyright of* Frederik Verstreken, MD, FEBHS)

patients that underwent 3D-guided corrective osteotomies for intra-articular malunion of the distal radius with a mean follow-up of 6 years. They found excellent patient-reported outcomes measures (PROMs) and no clinically relevant progression of osteoarthritis based on the osteoarthritis grading system described by Knirk and Jupiter.

Disadvantages of 3D technology include the need for specialized computer software, radiation exposure from CT scanning of both forearms and wrists, the time and effort for preoperative planning, and, perhaps most relevant at the present time, the additional high cost of the custom-made surgical guides and implants.[9,13,20] The

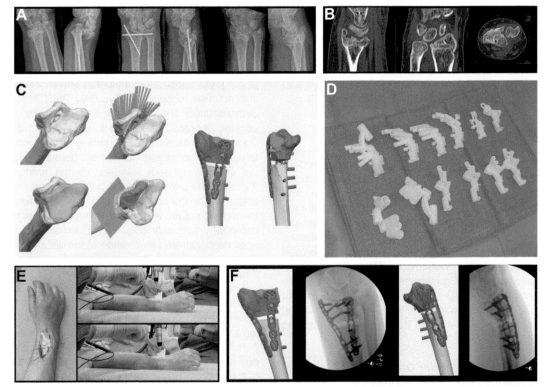

Fig. 3. Radiographs (*A*), CT scan (*B*), 3D planning of surgical correction (*C*), 3D printed patient-specific surgical guides (*D*), positioning of the drilling guide (*E*), fluoroscopic images following surgical correction (*F*). (*Images copyright of* Frederik Verstreken, MD, FEBHS)

current costs of software and engineering prevent its use in daily clinical practice. In Europe, costs for 3D planning and surgical guides generally range from $2000 for simple nonunions to $5000 for complex cases; in the United States, these costs tend to be somewhat higher. A strategy for lowering costs and improving expertise is centralizing this care in academic centers with an "in-hospital 3D laboratory." Other developments include the fact that some implant manufacturers offer 3D technology at no or very low cost to promote the use of their material in fracture fixation. Caiti and colleagues[2] have proposed a software solution to streamline the design of patient-specific instruments to make 3D technology more accessible.

FUTURE DIRECTIONS

Some of the latest developments in the field of 3D management of forearm and wrist malunions include in-hospital planning and 3D printing of guides,[21,22] navigated osteotomies,[23] and the use of printed patient-tailored plates.[24] Several investigators have reported positively on in-hospital planning and 3D printing of guides, citing the benefits of decreasing the cost of 3D technology.[21,22] To truly be cost-effective, this would, however, require centralization of these patients to tertiary referral centers to increase the volume at these sites. Recent clinical and radiographic experience on computer-navigated osteotomy for intra-articular distal radius malunion has been reported by Roner and colleagues,[23] who evaluated residual articular incongruity on CT. They reduced articular incongruity to an average step-off of 0.8 mm (range, 0.3–1.4 mm) and demonstrated overall reduction in pain and improvement of range of motion and grip strength in 36 of 37 patients. A disadvantage of navigated technology is its requirement of both specialized hardware and software, increasing setup costs. No benefit of navigated versus printed 3D technology has yet been proven. With regard to patient-specific plates, Schindele and colleagues[24] recently evaluated 15 patients with 3D planned corrective osteotomy of their distal radius, radial shaft, or ulnar shaft using a printed, anatomic, patient-tailored plate. At 1-year follow-up, they reported an improvement of the median baseline PRWE score from 47 to 7 as well as improvement in range of motion. No severe adverse advents were reported. In contrast, Dobbe and colleagues[25] published their early experience with patient-specific plating for navigation and fixation of distal radius, in a series combining a total of 10 malunion and congenital cases. They reported screws breaking in 3 of the first 4 cases. This was explained as probable fatigue because of repetitive stress, as because custom plates are more rigid than standard anatomic plates, the stress level at the plate-screw boundary is higher. They resolved the issue by changing the screw diameter from 2.4 to 3.5 mm. The other 7 cases were successful, with residual alignment error reduced by approximately 50% compared with conventional treatment and significant pain reduction.

SUMMARY

In patients with symptomatic forearm and wrist malunions, current evidence suggests the following:

- A corrective osteotomy is the treatment of choice and significantly improves functional and radiographic outcomes.
- The use of 3D technology allows better correction of radiographic parameters, including angulation, height, and rotation.
- No significant difference in functional outcome favoring 3D technology has yet been shown, but a trend toward better PROMs exists.
- Complex deformities of the forearm and wrist and those with intra-articular incongruity benefit the most from 3D planning and guidance.
- The use of 3D technology allows for a lower complication rate compared with conventional techniques.
- The use of 3D technology is expensive, and its overall cost-effectiveness has not yet been demonstrated.

CLINICS CARE POINTS

Pearls

- In patients with symptomatic complex multidirectional or intra-articular malunion of the wrist and/or forearm, the use of three-dimensional technology may be beneficial to facilitate surgical correction when indicated.

- The pros and cons of the procedure with its inherent complication rate should be discussed in detail with the patient. The additional cost needs to be taken into account.

- Virtual three-dimensional planning of corrective surgery allows the exploration of different osteotomy planes and fixation options. If needed, plates can be prebent on printed anatomic models for optimal fit on the bone. When standard plates do not allow adequate fixation, three-dimensional printed custom plates can be designed and printed in titanium.

- Clear exposure of bony landmarks is essential for a precise fit of the surgical guides, in order to obtain the planned result. The availability of three-dimensional printed anatomic models of the distal radius helps to check the correct placement of the surgical guides.

- If needed, fluoroscopy and/or intraoperative navigation can confirm the correct position of the guide. The guide itself will not show clearly, but the K-wires used to fix it will. Their position can be compared with K-wires placed in a printed anatomic model or confirmed during navigation.

Pitfalls

- The use of three-dimensional technology can facilitate complex surgical procedures but does not replace good clinical practice and standard surgical techniques.

- In the planning process, close collaboration between the engineer and treating surgeon is essential. Visualization limitations with surgical approaches and soft tissue restraints for guide placement need to be taken into account.

- Malpositioning of the patient-specific guides causes incorrect placement of drill holes and cutting planes, possibly leading to an inaccurate restoration of anatomy and a compromised clinical outcome.

- Patient-specific plating is a promising option for the most complex cases but is still an emerging field with inherent risks of failure in the development phase.

DISCLOSURE

G.A. Buijze and A. Verstreken declare no potential conflicts of interest with respect to the research, authorship, and/or publication of this article. F. Verstreken receives royalties from Materialise NV, Leuven, Belgium.

SUPPLEMENTARY DATA

Supplementary data related to this article can be found online at https://doi.org/10.1016/j.hcl.2023.09.002.

REFERENCES

1. Mulders MaM, d'Ailly PN, Cleffken BI, et al. Corrective osteotomy is an effective method of treating distal radius malunions with good long-term functional results. Injury 2017;48(3):731–7.
2. Caiti G, Dobbe JGG, Loenen ACY, et al. Implementation of a semiautomatic method to design patient-specific instruments for corrective osteotomy of the radius. Int J Comput Assist Radiol Surg 2019;14(5):829–40.
3. Cooney WP, Dobyns JH, Linscheid RL. Complications of Colles' fractures. J Bone Joint Surg Am 1980;62(4):613–9.
4. Park MJ, Cooney WP, Hahn ME, et al. The effects of dorsally angulated distal radius fractures on carpal kinematics. J Hand Surg Am 2002;27(2):223–32.
5. Bizzotto N, Tami I, Tami A, et al. 3D Printed models of distal radius fractures. Injury 2016;47(4):976–8.
6. Fernandez DL. Correction of post-traumatic wrist deformity in adults by osteotomy, bone-grafting, and internal fixation. J Bone Joint Surg Am 1982;64(8):1164–78.
7. McQueen M, Caspers J. Colles fracture: does the anatomical result affect the final function? J Bone Joint Surg Br 1988;70(4):649–51.
8. Prommersberger KJ, Van Schoonhoven J, Lanz UB. Outcome after corrective osteotomy for malunited fractures of the distal end of the radius. J Hand Surg Br 2002;27(1):55–60.
9. de Muinck Keizer RJO, Lechner KM, Mulders MaM, et al. Three-dimensional virtual planning of corrective osteotomies of distal radius malunions: a systematic review and meta-analysis. Strategies Trauma Limb Reconstr 2017;12(2):77–89.
10. von Campe A, Nagy L, Arbab D, et al. Corrective osteotomies in malunions of the distal radius: do we get what we planned? Clin Orthop Relat Res 2006;450:179–85.
11. Haghverdian JC, Hsu JWY, Harness NG. Complications of corrective osteotomies for extra-articular distal radius malunion. J Hand Surg Am 2019;44(11):987.e1.
12. Jupiter JB, Ruder J, Roth DA. Computer-generated bone models in the planning of osteotomy of multidirectional distal radius malunions. J Hand Surg Am 1992;17(3):406–15.
13. Buijze GA, Leong NL, Stockmans F, et al. Three-dimensional compared with two-dimensional preoperative planning of corrective osteotomy for extra-articular distal radial malunion: a multicenter randomized controlled trial. J Bone Joint Surg Am 2018;100(14):1191–202.
14. Michielsen M, Van Haver A, Bertrand V, et al. Corrective osteotomy of distal radius malunions using three-dimensional computer simulation and patient-specific guides to achieve anatomic reduction. Eur J Orthop Surg Traumatol 2018;28(8):1531–5.
15. Athlani L, Chenel A, Detammaecker R, et al. Computer-assisted 3D preoperative planning of corrective osteotomy for extra-articular distal radius

malunion: A 16-patient case series. Hand Surg Rehabil 2020;39(4):275–83.

16. Oka K, Shigi A, Tanaka H, et al. Intra-articular corrective osteotomy for intra-articular malunion of distal radius fracture using three-dimensional surgical computer simulation and patient-matched instrument. J Orthop Sci 2020;25(5):847–53.

17. Schweizer A, Fürnstahl P, Nagy L. Three-dimensional correction of distal radius intra-articular malunions using patient-specific drill guides. J Hand Surg Am 2013;38(12):2339–47.

18. Walenkamp MMJ, de Muinck Keizer RJO, Dobbe JGG, et al. Computer-assisted 3D planned corrective osteotomies in eight malunited radius fractures. Strategies Trauma Limb Reconstr 2015; 10(2):109–16.

19. Singh S, Jud L, Fürnstahl P, et al. Intermediate-term outcome of 3-dimensional corrective osteotomy for malunited distal radius fractures with a mean follow-up of 6 years. J Hand Surg Am 2022;47(7): 691.e1.

20. Miyake J, Murase T, Yamanaka Y, et al. Three-dimensional deformity analysis of malunited distal radius fractures and their influence on wrist and forearm motion. J Hand Surg Eur 2012;37(6):506–12.

21. Inge S, Brouwers L, van der Heijden F, et al. 3D printing for corrective osteotomy of malunited distal radius fractures: a low-cost workflow. BMJ Case Rep 2018;2018. bcr2017223996, bcr-2017-223996.

22. Temmesfeld MJ, Hauksson IT, Mørch T. Intra-articular osteotomy of the distal radius with the use of inexpensive in-house 3d printed surgical guides and arthroscopy: a case report. JBJS Case Connect 2020;10(1):e0424.

23. Roner S, Schweizer A, Da Silva Y, et al. Accuracy and early clinical outcome after 3-dimensional correction of distal radius intra-articular malunions using patient-specific instruments. J Hand Surg Am 2020;45(10):918–23.

24. Schindele S, Oyewale M, Marks M, et al. Three-dimensionally planned and printed patient-tailored plates for corrective osteotomies of the distal radius and forearm. J Hand Surg Am 2022;S0363-5023(22):00388–94.

25. Dobbe JGG, Peymani A, Roos HAL, et al. Patient-specific plate for navigation and fixation of the distal radius: a case series. Int J Comput Assist Radiol Surg 2021;16(3):515–24.

Management of Ulnar Styloid Nonunions

Maximilian A. Meyer, MD, Fraser J. Leversedge, MD*

KEYWORDS

- Ulnar styloid fracture • Distal ulna fracture • Nonunion • Triangular fibrocartilage complex
- Distal radioulnar joint • DRUJ instability

KEY POINTS

- Ulnar styloid nonunions commonly occur in the setting of distal radius fractures, but typically do not cause functional deficits or pain.
- Understanding the pertinent local and regional anatomy is critical for completing a thorough diagnostic evaluation and guiding effective treatment.
- Ulnar styloid nonunions associated with persistent ulnar-sided wrist pain despite conservative management may benefit from fragment excision; however, other potential etiologies should be evaluated.
- Ulnar styloid nonunions associated with distal radioulnar joint instability may benefit from fragment excision and triangular fibrocartilage complex repair or nonunion repair with open reduction and internal fixation, depending on the location and size of the displaced styloid fragment.

INTRODUCTION

Fractures of the ulnar styloid are common and typically do not require surgical repair as they usually do not cause long-term consequences.[1–3] Ulnar styloid fractures occur most commonly in the setting of distal radius fractures, accompanying between 50% and 60% of distal radius fractures in most series.[1,4,5] However, ulnar styloid fractures can also occur with concomitant triangular fibrocartilage complex (TFCC) injury or in isolation from direct impact.[6,7] Fracture location may influence distal radioulnar joint (DRUJ) stability; ulnar styloid fractures at the foveal base may destabilize the distal radioulnar ligament attachments and cause DRUJ instability, compared with ulnar styloid tip fractures in which DRUJ stability is maintained.[8] For nonunions causing persistent ulnar-sided wrist pain, indications for fragment excision or open reduction and internal fixation (ORIF) may be guided with a diagnostic local anesthetic injection. Management of symptomatic DRUJ instability can be more challenging, with

need for fragment ORIF versus fragment excision with concomitant TFCC repair versus DRUJ reconstruction. This article will (1) describe the pertinent anatomy of the ulnar styloid, including relevant soft tissue and osseous relationships, (2) review the clinical and radiographic evaluation of symptomatic ulnar styloid nonunions, including common ulnar styloid fracture patterns and their implications for DRUJ stability, and (3) provide an algorithm for the management of symptomatic ulnar styloid nonunions.

PERTINENT ANATOMY

The ulna is the stable fixed unit of the forearm, supporting load transfer from both the radius and the carpus and providing a base around which the radius rotates during forearm pronation and supination. The distal ulna is covered with articular cartilage on its radial, palmar, dorsal, and distal surfaces, allowing it to articulate with the sigmoid notch radially and with the articular disc of the TFCC distally.[9] The ulnar styloid projects distally

Department of Orthopedic Surgery, University of Colorado School of Medicine, 12631 E. 17th Avenue, Academic Office 1, Mail Stop B202, Aurora, CO 80045, USA
* Corresponding author.
E-mail address: fraser.leversedge@cuanschutz.edu

Hand Clin 40 (2024) 97–103
https://doi.org/10.1016/j.hcl.2023.08.003

from the ulnar aspect of the ulnar head, providing an attachment site for the extensor carpi ulnaris (ECU) tendon sheath and superficial radioulnar ligaments and supporting the origins of the ulnocarpal ligaments.[10] Together, the ulnar head and styloid assist in load transfer across the wrist. Approximately 20% of the axial load is transmitted through the ulnocarpal joint with the wrist in a neutral position, and this load is increased proportionally with progressive ulnar deviation or increased ulnar variance.[11] Incompetence of the ulnar-sided supporting structures, such as an ulnar styloid fracture, TFCC injury, or interosseous membrane injury, can alter radiocarpal joint contact pressures.[12] Just proximal and radial to the ulnar styloid, the ulnar head sits within the shallow concavity of the distal radius sigmoid notch. There is notable disparity between the radius of curvature of the sigmoid notch compared with that of the ulna and the radius of curvature of the sigmoid notch being approximately 4 to 7 mm greater than that of the ulnar head.[13] Given the discrepancies in radius of curvature and substantial variation in sigmoid notch anatomy, articular contact only accounts for approximately 20% of DRUJ stability.[14] DRUJ motion consequently involves a combination of dorsal and volar translation with rotation along a small area of articular contact.[15]

Based on the absence of substantial articular constraints, DRUJ stability depends on soft tissue attachments at the distal ulna and ulnar styloid. The volar and dorsal radioulnar ligaments, components of the TFCC, are the primary contributors to DRUJ stability.[14] The radioulnar ligaments have both superficial and deep limbs which insert at the ulnar styloid and ulnar fovea, respectively. The superficial limbs support the articular disc and its ability to sustain load via the ulnocarpal joint. Conversely, the deep fibers (also known as the ligamentum subcruentum) play a greater role in DRUJ stability for two reasons.[15] The ligamentum subcruentum has a more obtuse angle of insertion than its superficial counterpart and therefore maintains the radius seated on the ulnar head throughout the full arc of forearm rotation.[9] Second, in the extremes of pronation and supination, the radius translates along the ulna to a point beyond the confines of the superficial fibers and relies nearly exclusively on the ligamentum subcruentum to prevent dislocation.[9] Of note, in supination, the dorsal fibers of ligamentum subcruentum become taut, whereas the palmar fibers are lax. In pronation, the palmar fibers of ligamentum subcruentum become taut, whereas the dorsal fibers are lax.

Although only separated by a few millimeters, the differential attachment sites of the deep and superficial fibers of the radioulnar ligaments have significant consequences in the setting of an ulnar styloid fracture. Displaced styloid tip fractures result in discontinuity of the superficial limbs of the radioulnar ligaments, whereas displaced styloid base fractures may disrupt both the superficial and deep limbs due to proximity to the foveal attachments.[10] Secondary soft tissue contributors to DRUJ stability include the extensor carpi ulnaris (ECU) tendon and its subsheath,[15,16] the deep head of the pronator quadratus,[17] and the interosseous membrane,[18] particularly the distal oblique bundle.[19] Although isolated injury to the ligamentum subcruentum may not result in DRUJ instability, its disruption in conjunction with injury to these secondary soft tissue stabilizing structures may lead to DRUJ subluxation or dislocation.[15]

Evaluation

Evaluation of a symptomatic ulnar styloid nonunion begins with a thorough clinical history. This includes date and mechanism of injury, associated wrist injuries, presence of open fracture or substantial soft tissue injuries, and any ipsilateral elbow and/or segmental forearm injury. If the patient underwent prior treatment for the acute injury, or if the patient has a pertinent history of remote/chronic injury, then obtaining previous records (including prior operative reports and imaging studies) is important for completing a comprehensive history. Along with the trauma history, a review of the patient's medical history should include medical comorbidities and risk factors for nonunion, such as smoking status, malnutrition, and metabolic bone disease. Also, conditions affecting soft tissue stability such as collagen vascular disease may influence treatment decision-making.

Careful attention to detail regarding patient symptoms, including provocative maneuvers and activities, may assist in understanding the pathomechanics and pathoanatomy of the condition. For example, a patient describing painful clunking of the wrist, a prominent ulnar head, or deficits in forearm rotation, may be suggestive of DRUJ instability. Conversely, a patient who describes ulnar-sided wrist pain aggravated with grip and ulnar deviation may be suggestive of ulnocarpal impaction involving a displaced styloid fracture. Pain amplified by torsional activities against resistance may be suggestive of concomitant TFCC injury.

A comprehensive physical examination includes a global patient assessment including status of the soft tissue envelope and neurovascular examination of the entire extremity. Assessment of the elbow–forearm–wrist axis is essential and may be the focus of the examination; however, evaluating hand positioning and function may influence the global assessment. The key to the evaluation is localizing the anatomic site of pain through focal palpation and with provocative maneuvers. Numerous structures may contribute to ulnar wrist pain and a systematic approach to palpation may be confirmed with diagnostic injection in some instances. Specific areas of tenderness that can help the clinician elucidate the source of pain include the ulnar styloid tip or base, ulnar head, DRUJ, distal radius, lunate, dorsal triquetrum, lunotriquetral joint, TFCC, hook of hamate, pisotriquetral joint, ECU, flexor carpi ulnaris (FCU), and distal ulnar tunnel. A painful "fovea sign" involves tenderness between the ulnar styloid and flexor carpi ulnaris tendon and is suggestive of foveal disruption of the deep radioulnar ligaments as well as ulnotriquetral ligament injury.[20] Dynamic provocative testing includes attempted loading or translation of the DRUJ (ballottement), the lunotriquetral joint, and the pisotriquetral joint. An ECU synergy test may assist in evaluating contributions of the ECU to ulnar wrist pathology. Wrist motion should be assessed, including wrist flexion and extension, radioulnar deviation, and forearm rotation. Decreased motion or crepitus during forearm rotation may suggest pathology arising from the DRUJ, although the proximal radioulnar joint should be assessed.

Radiographic evaluation of an ulnar styloid nonunion begins with anteroposterior, oblique, and lateral views of the affected wrist and forearm. Fracture location and amount of displacement may be assessed. Occasionally, a fleck sign can be appreciated off the fovea, which is suggestive of an avulsion injury of the deep radioulnar ligaments.[21] Serial radiographs can be reviewed for progression of callous formation at the ulnar styloid. Contralateral films can be assessed for differences in ulnar length or rotation or presence of angular deformity. In the setting of a concomitant distal radius fracture, a critical assessment of the fracture and articular reduction, progression of fracture healing, and hardware placement is important. A computed tomography scan can improve analysis of the fracture fragments, in particular the articular surface, as well as critical assessment of hardware placement, if present. MRI arthrogram can be useful to assess for concomitant TFCC injury if clinical suspicion is high.[6]

Classification of ulnar styloid nonunion includes the Hauck classification, which separates Type 1 nonunions with a stable DRUJ from Type II nonunions with an unstable DRUJ.[22] In our experience, although radiographs and advanced imaging help to define ulnar styloid fracture pattern and displacement as well as rule out concomitant pathologies, definitive management (nonsurgical and surgical) is guided often by the clinical history and physical examination and outcomes of prior treatment.

DISCUSSION

The management of ulnar styloid nonunions is largely determined by stability of the DRUJ. Early evidence suggested that ulnar styloid fractures with greater than 2 mm of displacement in the setting of distal radius fracture may have a higher likelihood of DRUJ instability.[8] However, several clinical series have demonstrated the limited influence of ulnar styloid nonunion location or displacement on outcomes.[1,23,24] Souer and colleagues found that unrepaired ulnar styloid fractures did not influence clinical or functional outcomes in a series of distal radius fractures, even when displaced greater than 2 mm.[2] Kim and colleagues found no relationship between ulnar styloid location or displacement and subsequent DRUJ instability or patient-reported outcomes and found that subsequent nonunion did not impact functional outcomes.[1,24] In a series of 36 consecutive patients with fractures of both the distal radius and the proximal half of the ulnar styloid, Buijze and colleagues found no differences between patients with and without ulnar styloid nonunions with respect to range of motion, grip strength, pain levels, or functional outcomes.[25] Similarly, in a meta-analysis of more than 300 patients from six comparative studies, Wijffels reported no influence of ulnar styloid nonunion on grip strength, motion, DRUJ instability, pain, or functional outcomes.[3] Long-term outcomes seem similarly unaffected by ulnar styloid nonunion, as Korhonen and colleagues showed that young adults had no differences in motion nor grip strength compared with contralateral side at a mean 11 years after distal radius fracture with ulnar styloid nonunion.[26] Indeed, when the DRUJ seems clinically stable after distal radius ORIF, neither the presence nor the size of an ulnar styloid fracture seems to alter functional outcomes.[27] As such, in the setting of an acute distal radius fracture with concomitant ulnar styloid fracture, we agree with conventional treatment of addressing the distal radius fracture first, then assessing for DRUJ instability, and if unstable, treating the ulnar-sided pathology with either splinting in a position of stability or stabilizing with internal fixation for large fracture fragments.[28]

As most of the ulnar styloid nonunions do not cause functional deficits, we reserve operative

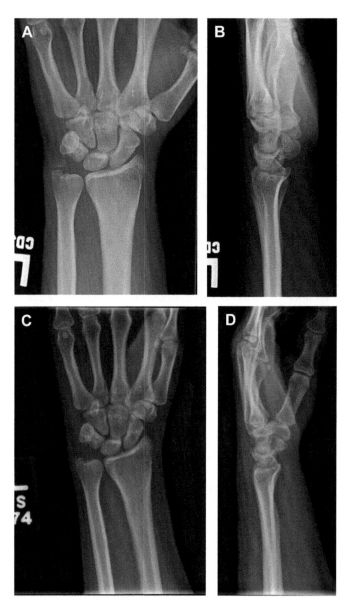

Fig. 1. Preoperative anteroposterior (AP) and lateral left wrist radiographs (*A, B*) of a 45-year-old woman who presented with longstanding ulnar-sided wrist pain and a remote history of distal radius fracture in adolescence. She had no clinical or radiographic evidence of DRUJ instability. After 6 months of conservative treatment, she underwent left wrist arthroscopy and ulnar styloid excision. Her TFCC was found to be intact. Final postoperative AP and lateral radiographs (*C, D*) demonstrate ulnar styloid excision with a stable DRUJ. Her pain resolved and she was able to return to work. (*Courtesy of* Rajshri Bolson, MD.)

intervention for symptomatic DRUJ instability or persistent ulnar wrist pain that does not resolve with conservative treatment. After fixation of a distal radius fracture and subsequent rehabilitation, persistent discomfort can be managed with splinting, hand therapy for dynamic wrist strengthening, anti-inflammatory modalities, and, occasionally, corticosteroid injection(s). If definitive treatment for the ulnar styloid nonunion is indicated, ORIF or fragment excision with or without TFCC repair is recommended based on the size of the styloid fracture and presence of DRUJ instability (**Fig. 1**).

Diagnostic wrist arthroscopy is typically performed at the time of ulnar styloid excision or fixation, as TFCC pathology is confirmed and secondary conditions such as ulnocarpal arthrosis may be evaluated. An open approach to the ulnar styloid is then performed for definitive management, using a medial mid-axial incision, immediately volar to the ECU tendon. The dorsal sensory branch of the ulnar nerve is identified and protected, including its distal branches. Alternatively, a dorsal approach to the distal ulna can be used, incorporating an existing dorsal approach from prior dorsal radius plating. However, we find that a medial mid-axial approach provides better exposure for anatomic assessment of the injury, for nonunion fracture fragment excision (if indicated) and for direct reduction and

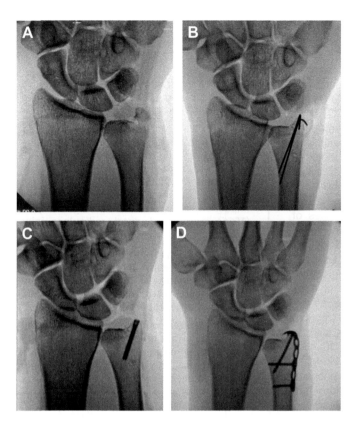

Fig. 2. Various fixation constructs exist for a patient with a symptomatic ulnar styloid nonunion amenable to open reduction and internal fixation (ORIF). (*A*) A large ulnar styloid nonunion can be repaired with a tension band construct using nonabsorbable suture tape to minimize implant prominence (*B*), a cannulated headless compression screw (*C*), or a custom pre-contoured 2.4 mm hook plate (*D*).

repair of the TFCC and/or ulnar styloid nonunion. The retinaculum and ulnocarpal joint capsule are divided, and the fracture is identified. If the styloid fragment is small, it is isolated and excised sharply. If a concomitant destabilizing TFCC injury is confirmed either on preoperative MRI or during diagnostic arthroscopy, foveal reattachment is performed using either open[29] or arthroscopic methods.[30] If the fragment is large and suitable for surgical fixation, the fracture site is debrided of fibrous tissue with care not to detach the radio-ulnar ligaments or other components of the TFCC. Fracture reduction and stabilization can be performed using Kirschner wires, tension band wiring, headless compression screws, mini-fragment plates, or suture anchors, depending on fragment size, orientation, and location of the fracture (**Fig. 2**). A bone reduction tenaculum may be used to assist the reduction. Following TFCC repair and/or ulnar styloid ORIF, DRUJ stability is evaluated in positions of forearm protonation, neutral position, and supination. Comparison to the contralateral side may be useful.

A postoperative rehabilitation protocol is individualized based on treatment provided. Patients undergoing simple fragment excision are placed into a soft dressing to facilitate early forearm and wrist motion, advancing to protected activity after the first postoperative visit. Following TFCC repair, patients are placed into a sugar-tong splint initially, transitioning to a Munster cast in a position of DRUJ stability for approximately 6 weeks before placement of a removable splint to facilitate protected forearm and wrist motion. Light-resisted activity is started at approximately 8 weeks postoperatively and graduated strengthening is introduced at 10 weeks postoperatively. Patients undergoing ORIF are typically immobilized for 4 weeks, then placed into a removable splint for an additional 4 weeks and instructed to perform gentle forearm and wrist range of motion, avoiding resisted or weight-bearing activity until fracture healing is confirmed radiographically.

Clinical Outcomes

Clinical studies after nonunion repair have demonstrated consistently good outcomes with both fragment excision and ORIF. In his initial series of ulnar styloid nonunion treatment, Hauck reported that all 11 patients with Type 1 ulnar styloid nonunions (stable DRUJ) achieved either "excellent" or "good" outcomes with fragment excision alone.[22] Of the 9 patients with Type II nonunions (unstable DRUJ), three underwent ORIF with tension band wiring or screw fixation. All three patients achieved excellent pain relief and regained full motion, but all underwent subsequent hardware removal. The remaining six patients underwent fragment excision and open TFCC repair through bone tunnels, with four "excellent," one "good," and one "fair" result. Protopsaltis and Ruch reported on arthroscopic-assisted outside-in TFCC repairs in eight patients after ulnar styloid excision and found improvements in Disabilities of the Arm, Shoulder, and Hand (DASH) and Visual Analogue Scale (VAS) scores with no cases of recurrent DRUJ instability.[6] More recent series have explored outcomes with modern locking plate technology. Nunez and colleagues reported on six patients who underwent ulnar styloid nonunion ORIF with a 2.0-mm distal ulna hook plate with or without TFCC reattachment.[7] Improvements were noted in grip strength, motion, and functional outcomes for all patients with no complications or reoperations. Similarly, Kumbuloglu and colleagues achieved bony union in 11 of 12 patients using a pin plate technique and noted improvements in forearm rotation, grip strength, QuickDASH, and VAS pain scores.[31]

SUMMARY

Ulnar styloid fractures commonly occur in conjunction with distal radius fractures but can also occur in isolation. Displaced basilar styloid fractures that involve the attachment of the ligamentum subcruentum may be associated with DRUJ instability. However, a large majority of proximal fractures involving the base of the ulnar styloid can progress to an asymptomatic nonunion. Various clinical series have reported minimal to no effect of ulnar styloid nonunion on strength, motion, or functional outcomes in the setting of a healed distal radius fracture. When an ulnar styloid nonunion remains symptomatic or causes persistent DRUJ instability, surgical intervention is warranted. Preoperative advanced imaging and/or diagnostic wrist arthroscopy can provide critical information when considering TFCC repair. Treatment options include: (1) ulnar styloid fragment excision for painful impingement; (2) ulnar styloid fragment excision and TFCC repair for DRUJ instability in the setting of a small styloid tip not amenable for repair; and (3) ulnar styloid fragment ORIF ± TFCC repair for large fragments. During ulnar styloid nonunion repair, rigid fixation can be accomplished with several implant options, selected based on fracture pattern and location.

CLINICS CARE POINTS

- Ulnar styloid fractures occur commonly in conjunction with distal radius fractures and frequently progress to asymptomatic nonunion.
- A thorough clinical history and physical examination should differentiate potential etiologies of ulnar-sided wrist pain and/or dysfunction including ECU tendonitis, hypothenar hammer syndrome, ulnocarpal impaction, triangular fibrocartilage complex (TFCC) injury, and distal radioulnar joint arthritis.
- Advanced imaging such as magnetic resonance arthrography and computed topography, and diagnostic wrist arthroscopy can be useful in assessing concomitant TFCC injury and other ulnocarpal pathology.
- Good functional outcomes can be achieved with surgical treatment with fragment excision with or without TFCC repair or open reduction and internal fixation of the ulnar styloid fragment.

DISCLOSURE

M.A. Meyer has no disclosures. F.J. Leversedge: (1) Consulting fees have been received from Axogen, Stryker, CoNextions; (2) Royalties have been received from Wolters Kluwer.

REFERENCES

1. Kim JK, Yun YH, Kim DJ, et al. Comparison of united and nonunited fractures of the ulnar styloid following volar-plate fixation of distal radius fractures. Injury 2011;42(4):371–5.
2. Souer JS, Ring D, Matschke S, et al. Effect of an unrepaired fracture of the ulnar styloid base on outcome after plate-and-screw fixation of a distal radial fracture. J Bone Joint Surg Am 2009;91(4):830–8.
3. Wijffels MM, Keizer J, Buijze GA, et al. Ulnar styloid process nonunion and outcome in patients with a distal radius fracture: a meta-analysis of comparative clinical trials. Injury 2014;45(12):1889–95.
4. Frykman G. Fracture of the distal radius including sequelae–shoulder-hand-finger syndrome, disturbance in the distal radio-ulnar joint and impairment of nerve function. A clinical and experimental study. Acta Orthop Scand 1967;Suppl 108:3+.
5. Okoli M, Silverman M, Abboudi J, et al. Radiographic Healing and Functional Outcomes of Untreated Ulnar Styloid Fractures Following Volar

Plate Fixation of Distal Radius Fractures: A Prospective Analysis. Hand (N Y) 2021;16(3):332–7.

6. Protopsaltis TS, Ruch DS. Triangular fibrocartilage complex tears associated with symptomatic ulnar styloid nonunions. J Hand Surg Am 2010;35(8):1251–5.

7. Nunez FA Jr, Luo TD, Nunez FA, et al. Treatment of symptomatic non-unions of the base of the ulnar styloid with plate osteosynthesis. J Hand Surg Eur 2017;42(4):382–8.

8. May MM, Lawton JN, Blazar PE. Ulnar styloid fractures associated with distal radius fractures: incidence and implications for distal radioulnar joint instability. J Hand Surg Am 2002;27(6):965–71.

9. af Ekenstam F, Hagert CG. Anatomical studies on the geometry and stability of the distal radio ulnar joint. Scand J Plast Reconstr Surg 1985;19(1):17–25.

10. Leversedge FJ, Adams BD. Distal Radioulnar Joint. In: Wolfe SW, Hotchkiss RN, Pederson WC, et al, editors. Green's operative hand surgery. Philadelphia, PA: Elsevier; 2017. p. 497–515.

11. af Ekenstam FW, Palmer AK, Glisson RR. The load on the radius and ulna in different positions of the wrist and forearm. A cadaver study. Acta Orthop Scand 1984;55(3):363–5.

12. Viegas SF, Pogue DJ, Patterson RM, et al. Effects of radioulnar instability on the radiocarpal joint: a biomechanical study. J Hand Surg Am 1990;15(5):728–32.

13. Tolat AR, Stanley JK, Trail IA. A cadaveric study of the anatomy and stability of the distal radioulnar joint in the coronal and transverse planes. J Hand Surg Br 1996;21(5):587–94.

14. Stuart PR, Berger RA, Linscheid RL, et al. The dorsopalmar stability of the distal radioulnar joint. J Hand Surg Am 2000;25(4):689–99.

15. Kleinman WB. Stability of the distal radioulna joint: biomechanics, pathophysiology, physical diagnosis, and restoration of function what we have learned in 25 years. J Hand Surg Am 2007;32(7):1086–106.

16. Spinner M, Kaplan EB. Extensor carpi ulnaris. Its relationship to the stability of the distal radio-ulnar joint. Clin Orthop Relat Res 1970;68:124–9.

17. Johnson R, Shrewsbury MM. The pronator quadratus in motions and in stabilization of the radius and ulna at the distal radioulnar joint. J Hand Surg Am 1976;1:205–9.

18. Hotchkiss RN, An KN, Sowa DT, et al. An anatomic and mechanical study of the interosseous membrane of the forearm: pathomechanics of proximal migration of the radius. J Hand Surg Am 1989;14(2 Pt 1):256–61.

19. Kitamura T, Moritomo H, Arimitsu S, et al. The biomechanical effect of the distal interosseous membrane on distal radioulnar joint stability: a preliminary anatomic study. J Hand Surg Am 2011;36(10):1626–30.

20. Tay SC, Tomita K, Berger RA. The "ulnar fovea sign" for defining ulnar wrist pain: an analysis of sensitivity and specificity. J Hand Surg Am 2007;32(4):438–44.

21. Szabo RM. Distal radioulnar joint instability. J Bone Joint Surg Am 2006;88(4):884–94.

22. Hauck RM, Skahen J 3rd, Palmer AK. Classification and treatment of ulnar styloid nonunion. J Hand Surg Am 1996;21(3):418–22.

23. Daneshvar P, Chan R, MacDermid J, et al. The effects of ulnar styloid fractures on patients sustaining distal radius fractures. J Hand Surg Am 2014;39(10):1915–20.

24. Kim JK, Koh YD, Do NH. Should an ulnar styloid fracture be fixed following volar plate fixation of a distal radial fracture? J Bone Joint Surg Am 2010;92(1):1–6.

25. Buijze GA, Ring D. Clinical impact of United versus nonunited fractures of the proximal half of the ulnar styloid following volar plate fixation of the distal radius. J Hand Surg Am 2010;35(2):223–7.

26. Korhonen L, Victorzon S, Serlo W, et al. Non-union of the ulnar styloid process in children is common but long-term morbidity is rare: a population-based study with mean 11 years (9-15) follow-up. Acta Orthop 2019;90(4):383–8.

27. Sammer DM, Shah HM, Shauver MJ, et al. The effect of ulnar styloid fractures on patient-rated outcomes after volar locking plating of distal radius fractures. J Hand Surg Am 2009;34(9):1595–602.

28. Wysocki RW, Ruch DS. Ulnar styloid fracture with distal radius fracture. J Hand Surg Am 2012;37(3):568–9.

29. Lee KH, Shim BJ, Gong HS. Open Foveal Repair of the Triangular Fibrocartilage Complex Tears Associated with Symptomatic Ulnar Styloid Non-union. J Hand Surg Asian Pac 2022;27(2):248–55.

30. Goorens CK, Anthonissen L, Goubau JF. Styloidectomy and reattachment of the triangular fibrocartilage complex for longstanding nonunion of the ulnar styloid. J Hand Surg Eur Vol 2020;45(7):763–5.

31. Kümbüloğlu Ö F, Cam N, Özdemir HM. Treatment with Buttress Plate Technique for Symptomatic Ulnar Styloid Base Nonunion. J Wrist Surg 2022;11(3):257–61.

Traditional Bone Grafting in Scaphoid Nonunion

Erin A. Miller, MD, MS[a],*, Jerry I. Huang, MD[b]

KEYWORDS

- Scaphoid nonunion • Delayed union • Bone grafting • Scaphoid revision
- Proximal pole avascular necrosis

KEY POINTS

- Adequate debridement of fibrous material at the nonunion site is critical for success.
- Correction of humpback deformity is critical and may be achieved with structural and nonstructural graft.
- Rigid fixation remains essential to ensure bony healing and can be obtained with various techniques

BACKGROUND

Scaphoid nonunion is a perennial problem in hand surgery. The commonly quoted nonunion rate of around 10% is cited from a 1989 study by Dias and colleagues that published a 12.3% nonunion rate for nonoperatively treated scaphoid waist fractures.[1] Multiple randomized prospective studies with relatively small patient cohorts have been published comparing union rates of nonoperative and surgically treated nondisplaced scaphoid waist fractures, and reported faster radiographic healing and return to activities with operative fixation.[1,2] However, there is a paucity of literature looking at surgical treatment of nonunions resulting from failed primary surgery. Because of the retrograde blood supply, nonunion rates are higher in proximal pole fractures. In a recent meta-analysis, Chong and colleagues reported an overall rate of nonunion in 11% of proximal pole fractures, with significantly higher nonunion rates of 18% in nonoperative fractures compared with 6% in operatively treated fractures.[3]

The definition of union in scaphoid fractures is also poorly defined. Many authors cite 50% bony bridging seen on computed tomography (CT) scan as their criterion for union.[4] Unfortunately, this criterion is not universal when reporting scaphoid outcomes, and there are no studies demonstrating that 50% bridging of the scaphoid is adequate for long-term stability. Moreover, many published studies do not cite their criteria for union, making comparison of outcomes even more difficult. Every hand surgeon has had the experience of seeing a patient in clinic presenting with a scaphoid nonunion several years out from treatment with the patient reporting they were told by their surgeon the bone was healed.

Slade and colleagues proposed a classification for scaphoid nonunions that is helpful in determining treatment. The grading focuses on time of nonunion in relation to the degree of bone resorption, which typically increases with time.[5] Grade I nonunions may be treated with fixation alone as there is minimal bone resorption present, and graft is not required. Similarly, grade II nonunions do not have significant bony resorption and often do not require grafting. Some of these nonunions can be treated with percutaneous fixation. In patients with grade III to IV nonunions and some grade V nonunions, aggressive debridement back to healthy cancellous bone followed by meticulous bone grafting and stable fixation is critical to successful repair of the nonunion.

The last point to be considered when discussing scaphoid nonunion is the argument over avascular

[a] Department of Surgery, Division of Plastic Surgery, University of Washington Medical Center, 325 9th Avenue, Seattle, WA 98013, USA; [b] Department of Orthopaedics and Sports Medicine, University of Washington Medical Center, 4245 Roosevelt Way Northeast, Seattle, WA 98105, USA
* Corresponding author.
E-mail address: erinmill@uw.edu

Hand Clin 40 (2024) 105–116
https://doi.org/10.1016/j.hcl.2023.08.001

necrosis (AVN). Although many leaders in the hand surgery world cite AVN as an indication for vascularized bone grafting, there is no standard for assessing AVN. Studies have shown that imaging, including MRI, and intraoperative findings of punctate bleeding do not correlate with histologic findings of trabecular bone necrosis.[6,7] Despite the retrograde vascular supply of the scaphoid playing a critical role in healing, it has been demonstrated repeatedly that proximal pole fractures can heal with traditional bone grafting. Although rigid fixation remains a key principle of nonunion surgery, equivalence has been shown between both k-wires and compression screws.[8] The authors believe that additional factors, such as aggressive debridement, rigid fixation, and meticulous surgical technique, are critical in achieving fracture union. Thus, when considering repair in scaphoid nonunions, the authors do not use AVN as a criterion for their treatment algorithm.

FRACTURE ANATOMY

The role of the scaphoid in kinematics of the wrist plays a role in its propensity to go on to nonunion. As the link between the proximal and distal rows, the scaphoid is subjected to shearing, bending, and pronating forces. In cadaveric studies of scaphoid fractures, during wrist motion, there is significantly increased motion of the distal fragment relative to the proximal fragment, leading to interfragmentary motion and shear across the fracture. These increased forces predispose the scaphoid to development of nonunion and subsequent collapse across the bone, which in turn further alters carpal kinematics and exacerbates the fracture instability.[9]

In discussion of scaphoid nonunion, it is important to review the bony anatomy. Scaphoid fractures are typically classified as distal pole, waist, or proximal pole (**Fig. 1**). Tubercle fractures are not uncommon. However, as this portion of the bone does not participate in load bearing, these fractures are often considered inconsequential and treated conservatively. In addition, because of the robust blood supply of the distal pole and the wide surface area, nonunion at the distal pole is an uncommon entity.

The waist of the scaphoid is generally accepted to be the central third of the bone; however, there is no widely accepted break point between the waist and proximal pole. This thirds division is additionally muddied as the location of the fracture appears differently in the various radiographic projections.[10] In a recent meta-analysis performed to define nonunion rate of proximal pole fractures, the authors found there to be 12 different definitions of proximal pole fractures, leading to a heterogenous group, which precluded robust aggregate data.[3] To circumvent this, a proposed definition of scaphoid fracture site based on the ratio of the proximal pole fragment to the overall length of the scaphoid has been studied. This is measured on plain radiographs on either the ulnarly deviated posterior anterior (often termed scaphoid view) view or the semi-pronated oblique. Smaller proximal pole fragment size was directly correlated to increased risk of nonunion on multivariate analysis. Distal fractures – ratio greater than 0.75 – had a 100% union rate compared with a 27% union rate in the 0.15 to 0.3 group. This classification provides significantly more granularity than the simple thirds classification (see **Fig. 1**).[10] Unfortunately, despite the ease of calculation, use of the ratio to describe fracture location has yet to be widely adopted into the literature of clinical practice since initial publication over 15 years ago.

The lateral intrascaphoid angle is a key factor in any scaphoid fracture or nonunion. It is measured by selecting the most complete lateral view of the bone on tomography and marking lines parallel to the proximal and distal articular surfaces. A perpendicular line is then drawn from each articular surface, and the angle between these 2 lines is the intrascaphoid angle (**Fig. 2**A). The normal range for lateral intrascaphoid angle is 15° to 34°; angulation greater than 34° is considered a malunion with a humpback deformity, as coined by Amadio and colleagues in their landmark study from 1989 (**Fig. 2**B).[11,12] Additional radiographic parameters such as dorsal intercalated segmental instability (DISI) deformity with increased scapholunate and radiolunate angles and decreased carpal height ratio are important to consider and correlate with the bony reduction and correction of the internal anatomy of the collapsed scaphoid. Simply achieving union of the scaphoid can lead to disappointing functional results if normal anatomy is not restored. Scaphoid malunion with residual humpback deformity has been correlated with worse clinical outcomes. In Amadio's study of 46 scaphoid fractures with long term follow-up and adequate data, the clinical results in range of motion, grip strength, and wrist pain were most closely predicted by the lateral intrascaphoid angle.[11] In over 60% of fractures with a humpback deformity, defined as intrascaphoid angle greater than 45°, patients had either a fair or poor outcome on the Cooney scale. Three of their malunions were treated with corrective osteotomy and subsequent improvement to a good clinical outcome.[11] Lynch and Linscheid published a case series of 5 patients with corrective osteotomy of a scaphoid malunion with improvement in grip

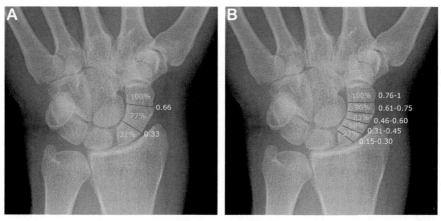

Fig. 1. Representation of union rate of scaphoid fractures based on data by Ramamurthy and colleagues.[10] (*A*) Union rates based on traditional 1/3 classification – proximal pole, waist, and distal pole - of scaphoid regions. (*B*) Union rates based on ratio classification – the distance of the fracture from the proximal extent divided by the overall length of the scaphoid – gives a more granular risk of nonunion for discussion with patients.

strength and range of motion, as well as wrist score in all patients (J Hand Surg 1997).

The degree of arthritis present should be evaluated during the preoperative planning phase. Although an increased scapholunate angle and resultant dorsal intercalated segment instability (DISI) deformity can often be corrected with proper reduction of the scaphoid, loss of carpal height or other evidence of significant radioscaphoid or scaphocapitate arthritis should be seen as a relative contraindication to nonunion repair.

SCAPHOID PREPARATION

In established nonunions in the scaphoid waist, the standard volar approach allows ideal visualization

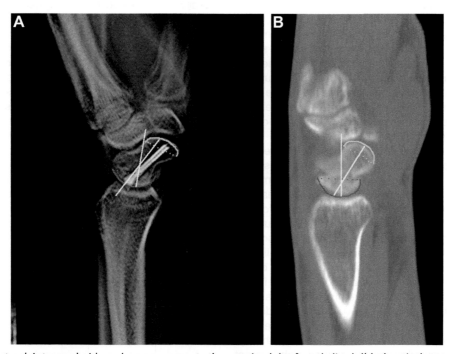

Fig. 2. Lateral intrascaphoid angle measurement; the proximal (*red*) and distal (*blue*) articular surfaces are marked and a perpendicular line drawn from each of them (*yellow*); the angle of intersection of these lines is the lateral intrascaphoid angle. (*A*) Normal lateral intrascaphoid angle. (*B*) Increased lateral intrascaphoid angle representing humpback deformity.

of the fracture nonunion to ensure appropriate debridement and bone grafting can be accomplished This is critical in cases of severe humpback deformity in which the distal pole of the scaphoid needs to be extended to restore the height, followed by aggressive decortication of the sclerotic surfaces. Aguilella and colleagues describe a volar approach radial to the flexor carpi radialis tendon, between the tendon and the radial artery to decrease scarring in the tendon.[12] In proximal pole fracture nonunions, a dorsal approach should be used to allow better visualization and reduction.

Some fractures are easily visible upon approach, while others have a fibrous union that initially precludes direct visualization. Use of fluoroscopy and a blunt instrument, such as a Freer elevator, is essential to correctly identify the fracture location so as not to create a secondary fracture plane. Luchetti and colleagues recommended using radio-opaque dye on an angiocatheter to inject into the nonunion site, for identification and to guide the extent of debridement that is needed.[13]

Aggressive debridement is the most critical step in nonunion repair. Without adequate debridement, no rigid fixation or amount of bone grafting will coax osteocytes to grow across a fibrous union or through a sclerotic margin. The senior surgeon should be the one performing the debridement. K-wires may be inserted into the proximal and distal poles to use as joysticks to assist in opening the fracture site. Using a curette or ronguer, cysts and fibrous tissue are removed from the nonunion site. The curette should sound harsh as it scrapes again the sclerotic bone. The change in pitch and sound quality is an auditory cue that the debridement is adequate. The bone should then be visually inspected to ensure there is no sclerosis remaining that would block osteocyte migration. If healthy cancellous bone is not visualized, further debridement with a curette or a high-speed burr under copious irrigation should be used. The authors do not drop the tourniquet to evaluate for punctate bleeding, as this has not been shown to be a reliable marker for proximal pole vascularity. The authors find other auditory and visual cues to be more helpful and adequate.

There has been a recent trend toward limited debridement of the dorsal distal margin of the scaphoid, leaving the volar radial margin intact. The authors feel it is important to clarify this technique refers the total area of bone debrided as opposed to the aggression used in debridement. In a retrospective review of 12 patients with nonunions repaired using this limited debridement technique, where only the dorsal distal 50% of the bone was debrided, there was a 100% union rate confirmed by CT.[14] The authors' definition of

union was 50% bone bridging or fully healing of one cortex. They noted that the portion of the bone that was not debrided remained a nonunion even at final follow-up. It is important to note that this technique is not appropriate for scaphoids with a humpback deformity that need restoration of length and extension of the distal scaphoid.

After debridement, the fracture fragments should be adequately mobile to accomplish appropriate reduction. The authors recommend use of 0.045 K-wires as joysticks in the proximal and distal fragments. The distal fragment is extended, while the proximal fragment is flexed, to correct the humpback deformity (**Fig. 3**). In addition, it is important to supinate the distal fragment to correct the rotational deformity. Alternatively, humpback deformity may be corrected by the Linscheid maneuver. First, the wrist is flexed until the lunate is aligned on the radius and a radiolunate K-wire is passed percutaneously through the dorsal radius to hold the lunate in neutral position. The wrist is then extended until the capitate is in anatomic alignment over the lunate; this extension brings the scaphoid back into alignment and opens the fracture gap to allows accurate measurement of the defect.[15] Following reduction with correction of the shortening and humpback and protonation deformities, a provisional K-wire is placed across the scaphoid nonunion to hold the bone in appropriate reduction. These maneuvers all allow the full extent of the bony defect to be visualized and measured to ensure an appropriate sized graft is placed to fully correct the deformity.

Arthroscopy has also been described for scaphoid nonunions. Although technically more challenging, for the experienced arthroscopist, it may allow improved visualization of the debridement and better preservation of the scaphoid's tenuous vascularity. Visualization of the nonunion site is accomplished via a radial midcarpal portal. Percutaneous K-wires are inserted into the proximal and distal fragments as joysticks to aid in reduction of the fracture. An arthroscopic burr is introduced to complete debridement with arthroscopic visualization of the debrided bone surfaces. With dry arthroscopy, bone graft is then inserted through a cannula at a portal adjacent to the nonunion site and firmly impacted; it is then sealed in placed with fibrin glue. Fixation is obtained percutaneously with either K-wires or a compression screw. Wong and colleagues reported a series of 125 scaphoid nonunions treated with arthroscopic debridement and grafting and reported a 90% union rate.[16]

BONE GRAFT SELECTION

The traditional doctrine of using corticocancellous bone in scaphoid nonunions stems from the

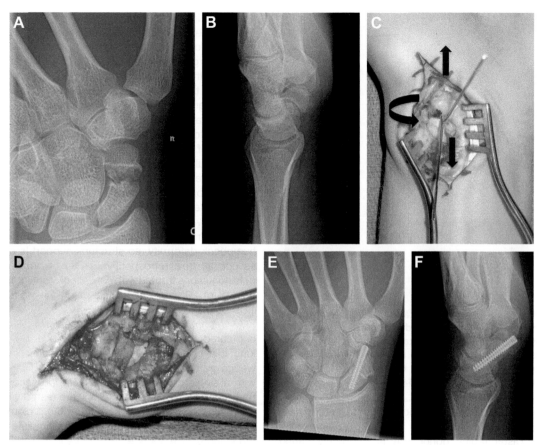

Fig. 3. Humpback deformity and correction with ICBG (*A*) Preoperative radiographs of a scaphoid nonunion with humpback deformity, AP image. (*B*) Lateral image demonstrating increased intrascaphoid angle and moderate DISI pattern. (*C*) K-wire placement into proximal and distal poles of the scaphoid. The distal fragment is extended while the proximal pole is flexed (*arrows*) with additional supination force across the distal pole to correct the humpback deformity and open the defect for bone grafting. (*D*) Iliac crest bone graft inset into scaphoid defect. (*E*) Postoperative radiographs at 3 months demonstrating union, AP image. (*F*) Lateral image, note correction of humpback and improvement of DISI deformity.

Russe modification of the Matti procedure, which used a wedge-shaped bone graft from the iliac crest placed as an inlay graft from the volar approach.[17] Dozens of modifications have been described, including the Fisk-Fernandez modification that included use of internal fixation in addition to the iliac crest inlay graft.[18] Essentially, these modifications all rely on a strut or match-stick of cortical bone for structural support surrounded by cancellous bone for its osteogenic factors. More recently, Lee and colleagues described the "modified hybrid Russe procedure" using a cortical strut internally in the scaphoid to restore scaphoid length with the addition of compression screw fixation, followed by cancellous bone grafting in the nonunion site. A series of 17 patients had a 100% union rate at 3.6 months with correction of the preoperative humpback and DISI deformities.[19]

Iliac crest provides a large amount of available harvestable bone, cortical and cancellous, significantly more than even the largest scaphoid defects can hold (**Fig. 4**). Although a reliable donor, it hampers recovery by increasing postoperative pain and necessitates the need for a general anesthetic. It was once thought to contain high-quality bone that would speed union; however, this has been disproven. In a retrospective cohort of 68 cases using iliac crest graft and 24 cases with distal radius graft, the overall union rate was 66% and not statistically significant between groups.[20] Additionally, there were no differences in SL angle or carpal height index in the fractures that went on to union. Jarrett and colleagues published a biomechanical study comparing bone wedges from the distal radius with iliac crest followed by headless compression screw fixation in an osteotomy model.[21] There was a trend toward greater strength in the iliac crest

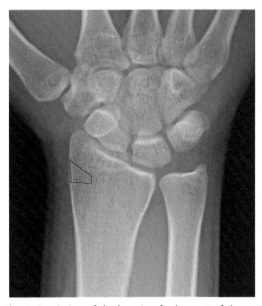

Fig. 4. Depiction of the location for harvest of the anterolateral corner of radius graft; a trapezoidal shaped graft can be obtained of the appropriate size. The curvature of the radial cortex at this point closely matches the radial curvature of the scaphoid as seen in cadaver sections.

group, but the difference was not statistically significant.

Distal radius donor site is frequently varied based on surgeon preference. Many use volar graft from underneath the pronator quadratus; however, harvest of a wedge shape graft to correct the humpback deformity can be difficult, as the cancellous bone is relatively thin at the volar wall. Aguilella and Garcia-Elias described a corticocancellous graft from the anterolateral corner of the distal radius for ease of harvest, dense subchondral bone, and similar size and shape to the scaphoid waist that requires next to no contouring when harvested appropriately (see **Fig. 4**).

The size limit of the anterolateral corner is typically 15 mm wide by 10 mm long and deep; if a larger graft is needed, iliac crest is recommended.[12]

Cortical bone takes significantly longer to heal, as more remodeling must occur to incorporate the structural bone graft. The dogma that cortical bone is needed to restore scaphoid anatomy has been challenged in recent years, in part because of the advent of compression screws that provide rigid structural support and may assist in maintaining length to the scaphoid. Cohen and colleagues retrospectively reviewed 12 patients with nonunions and average lateral intrascaphoid angle of 49° treated with distal radius cancellous graft and intramedullary screw for fixation with a minimum of 2-year follow-up. All nonunions healed, with an average intrascaphoid angle of 32°.[4] A prospective study of 17 nonunions treated with corticocancellous iliac crest and 18 treated with cancellous grafting was published in 2018. One patient from the corticocancellous group went on to nonunion; the remainder of the patients healed without significant differences in radiographic or clinical parameters. Additionally, the authors found the cancellous group to have faster healing by an average of 4 weeks.[22] A meta-analysis found similar results with no statistically significant difference between union rate or humpback deformity between cortical and cancellous grafts, with significantly faster healing in the cancellous bone graft group, 11 weeks compared with 16 weeks.[23] Proximal pole fractures less frequently present with a humpback deformity, so structural support is not as critical. In a retrospective series of proximal pole nonunions treated with cancellous bone grafting, 18 of 20 went on to heal at an average of 11.5 weeks.[13]

A recent cadaveric biomechanical study compared the modified Russe technique with a long thin cortical strut with a corticocancellous wedge graft on rotational stability.[24] All were fixated with a single compression screw. In the second part of the study, the specimens were tested with removal of all cancellous bone from the proximal and distal poles of the scaphoid to simulate a more aggressive debridement. In the initial model, there was no significant difference in the 2 constructs with respect to load to failure or maximal torque. However, in the second model, the strut graft provided improved rotational stability. The authors postulated that the additional graft may be able to compensate for decreased screw purchase from poor bone quality.[24]

Additional technical tips for cancellous graft alone have been described including packing the graft into a syringe to create more compact, moldable filler.[4,13] Careful patient selection is also required when using nonstructural graft. If only cancellous bone graft is used, it is important to ensure the screw will have appropriate bites proximally and distally in the scaphoid, as it is serving as the sole structural support for the bone.

FIXATION

Creating bony stability at the grafted site is key to achieving successful union. Stable bony contact prevents shearing of new vessels that are essential vascular ingrowths to facilitate healing.[5] The surgeon's graft choice also alters healing biology and should be considered. Cancellous bone grafts heal through resorption and substitution as opposed to cortical bone healing, which uses cutting cones that require absolute stability. Therefore, with cancellous bone grafting, less rigid fixation with K-wires can be successful in achieving union.[16]

Compression screw fixation is the most common modality used in the literature. Placing the screw along the central axis of the bone leads to the greatest stability given the ability to place the longest length screw. In proximal pole fractures and vertical oblique fractures, frequently, compression is of greater importance than stability. Placement of the screw perpendicular to the fracture plane best achieves this.[25,26] Although several studies suggest lower union rates with K-wires compared with compression screws, a meta-analysis from 2015 did not find a statistically significant difference in union rate between the two.[27] When using K-wires alone, a minimum of 2 K-wires should be placed in a divergent fashion to prevent rotation; maximal separation of K-wires at the fracture plane provides the highest degree of stability[28] (**Fig. 5**).

Rotational instability is the most common mode of failure in scaphoid waist nonunions. Multiple methods have been trialed to increase the rotational stability of scaphoid fixation. Placement of a derotational K-wire placement with a single compression screw can provide additional stability.[29] Ruch and colleagues described the safe use of 2 screws in the scaphoid with superior stability compared to a single screw.[30] However, there is yet to be any data-based literature detailing the optimal placement of the 2 screws. In addition, there are concerns with the small cross-sectional area of the scaphoid and increased diameter of 2 screws and risk of iatrogenic fragmentation. In a cadaveric biomechanical study of fixation comparing single screw fixation, double screw fixation, and plate fixation, both the double screw and plate constructs had statistically significantly increased loads to failure than the single screw group, with the most common mode of failure in rotation.

Although biomechanically stronger, the surgeon must take into account the balance between increased stability and potentially increased hardware-related complications related to 2 screws or plate screw constructs. The challenge with using a plate stems from the large area of articular cartilage of the scaphoid leaving limited area for plate placement to avoid hardware contact with the cartilage of the scaphoid facet during motion. However, in cases of revision surgery with significant bone loss where there are concerns of inadequate purchase of the compression screw or extrusion of the bone graft, plating from a volar approach should be considered (**Fig. 6**). Overall union rates are similar to those of compression screws.[31]

Compression staples have also been described with 5 reports in the literature; a meta-analysis

found similar union rates to compression screws, and the subgroup analysis of nonunions treated with staples found a 92% union rate.[32]

OUTCOMES

Despite the copious literature on scaphoid nonunion, evidence supporting superiority of 1 technique over another is lacking. Most reports on scaphoid nonunion are retrospective in nature and relatively small case series. The best data come from meta-analyses, which still lack definitive data because of the heterogeneity of procedures and lack of consistent definition of outcomes or characterization of the nonunion. Many studies do not report CT evidence of bony healing, use criteria other than 50% bridging to declare union, inconsistently designate proximal pole versus waist fractures, and fail to provide long term follow-up. A retrospective review of 462 scaphoid nonunion cases treated with bone grafting from 19 centers highlighted the difficulty in evaluating union status; 9% of their cases had uncertain union status. The overall union rate of 69%, significantly lower than other published series, was partially attributed to the categorization of all patients with uncertain union status as failures. On subgroup analysis, smoking status significantly decreased union rate, with a 2 times increased risk of nonunion, similar to previous reports.[33]

There are good data showing that time from injury significantly affects the success of nonunion repair. Patients who had surgery completed within 12 months of injury had a 90% union rate as opposed to 80% in those patients whose surgery was performed more than a year after injury.[8] Further evaluation of time to surgery found a 40% increased chance of persistent nonunion for fractures treated between 1 and 2 years after injury and a 140% increased risk in those repaired more than 2 years from injury.[33]

The evidence remains inconclusive on fixation method. When examining individual studies, there are several series that report superiority of either K-wire or screw fixation. However, pooled data from a 2015 meta-analysis found no statistically significant difference in union rate; 91% union was found in the K-wire group, and 88% union was found in the screw group. Additionally, the K-wire group was composed of fractures with factors indicating poorer prognosis.[27] Given the differences in fracture characteristic, bone quality, prior surgery, and surgeon experience, the decision to fixate with either K-wires or compression screws should be made on an individual basis, often intraoperatively. Despite the trend toward use of screws in recent years, if wires allow more

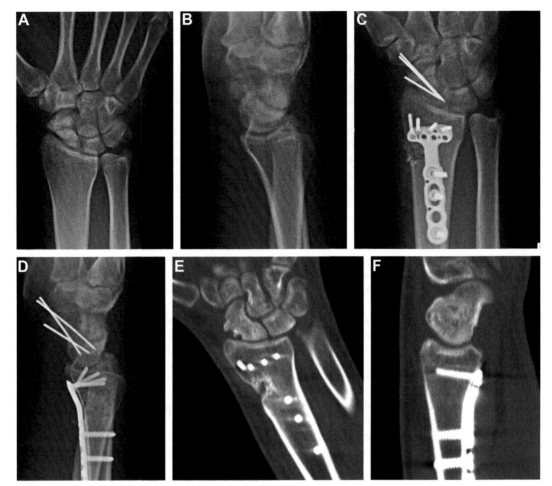

Fig. 5. Correction of humpback deformity using distal radius corticocancellous bone graft and K-wire fixation. (*A*) Scaphoid waist nonunion with sclerosis and resorption at the fracture line, AP radiographs. (*B*) Lateral radiograph with notable humpback deformity and significant DISI. (*C*) 2-week postoperative images demonstrating K-wire position and prophylactic plating of the distal radius after harvest of a large-sized graft. (*D*) Lateral image with notable correction of DISI and humpback. (*E*) 3-month postoperative CT scan notable for complete union of the scaphoid. (*F*) Sagittal view of the healed scaphoid demonstrating improvement of the lateral intrascaphoid angle and resolution of humpback.

purchase on a small corticocancellous graft or if prior screw tracks leave concern that a compression screw may not provide adequate fixation, there should be no hesitation on the surgeon's part to leave wires as the definitive fixation or for supplemental fixation.

Bone graft choice – iliac crest or distal radius – did not significantly affect union rates in any study. Similarly, graft choice of corticocancellous or cancellous bone had no effect on union rate.[12,20,22,23] In Sayegh's 2014 review, union rates were equivalent between graft choice. However, there were improved Mayo wrist scores in patients with corticocancellous grafts[23]; In reviewing the information available, it is likely that these outcomes depend on surgical technique. It is known that

failure to restore scaphoid length and correct the intrascaphoid angle leads to worse wrist function, and in cases with cancellous bone grafts, surgeons either may not recognize the scaphoid collapse or may not work as aggressively to re-establish normal anatomy. Cohen and colleagues have reliably demonstrated that cancellous graft alone can correct the intrascaphoid angle and lead to excellent functional outcomes.[4]

WHAT IS THE ROLE OF VASCULARIZED GRAFTS?

When comparing traditional bone grafting to vascularized bone, outcomes are similar. Rancy and colleagues reviewed the literature to compare

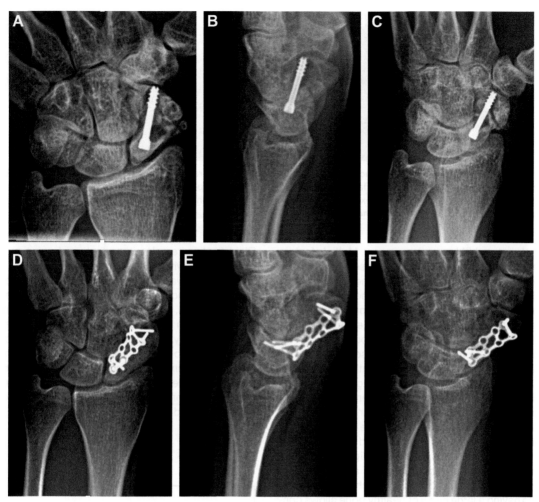

Fig. 6. Plate fixation for revision of scaphoid nonunion with significant cystic changes using cancellous bone graft. (*A*) Preoperative AP view. (*B*) Preoperative lateral view. (*C*) Preoperative oblique view. (*D*) 3-month postoperative AP view. (*E*) 3-month postoperative lateral view. (*F*) 3-month postoperative oblique view.

outcomes between type of bone graft. The non-vascularized grafts had a union rate of 87%. Further subgroup analysis of patients with compression screw fixation and union confirmed on CT showed a 96% union rate. The vascularized bone graft group had an 86% union rate, with the aforementioned subgroup analysis yielding a 93% union rate.[7] A recent database review from 2020 evaluated 4177 patients with nonunion treated with traditional bone graft and vascularized bone graft (both pedicled and free). Persistent nonunion was present in 6% of traditional bone graft patients and 5% of vascularized grafts, which was not statistically significant.[34]

Given that the studies reported have similar union rates for vascularized and nonvascularized graft, many surgeons have recently asked if vascularized bone grafting is ever needed. Traditional

teaching is that scaphoids with avascular necrosis should be treated with vascularized grafts; however, AVN is difficult to identify clinically. A prospective study performed by Rancy and colleagues demonstrated that even in cases of AVN, traditional bone grafting is adequate to achieve union. In 35 nonunions treated with nonvascularized bone graft (both corticocancellous and cancellous), histology was sent at the time of operation to evaluate for AVN; 14 had trabecular loss, and 3 had frank tissue necrosis confirming AVN in more than half the patients. In 32 of the 35 patients, 91%, had healing demonstrated on CT scan at 12 weeks, showing that healing may be achieved in patients with AVN even without vascularized bone grafting.[35]

These results, however, do not necessarily mean that vascularized bone grafting does not have any

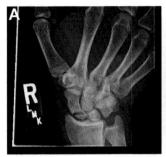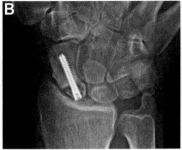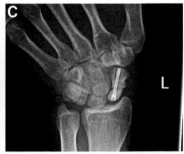

Fig. 7. Demonstration of proximal pole characteristics that have a low rate of union and authors prefer to replace with free osteocartilagenous bone flaps. (*A*) Extremely small proximal pole where a headless compression screw is unlikely to have a solid bite. (*B*) Proximal pole with significant cystic changes, again expecting inadequate screw purchase. (*C*) Significant sclerosis and shrinkage of the proximal pole.

role in scaphoid nonunion surgery. Multiple factors play into the surgeon's choice to use a vascularized graft. It is readily apparent in the literature that increasingly small proximal pole fragments, increased time from injury, and previous surgery decrease the union rate. Consideration of these factors and the increased risk of poor healing may often lead to the choice for a vascularized graft.[6] In scaphoids that have fragmentation of the proximal pole, a small proximal pole fragment that is unlikely to have adequate purchase on a compression screw, extreme cystic changes, or sclerosis of the bone on radiography, complete osteochondral reconstruction with a vascularized medial femoral trochlea flap may be necessary (**Fig. 7**). By replacing the entire proximal pole, the achievement of robust rigid fixation becomes technically simpler, as having a large piece of healthy bone allows confidence in screw placement. Replacement of the unhealthy bone additionally forces the surgeon to aggressively debride the native scaphoid to make room for the flap, bypassing the natural instinct to be cautious and conservative when debriding the proximal pole.

SUMMARY

Scaphoid nonunion remains a difficult problem for the hand surgeon. Attention to technical details is likely of greater importance than bone graft choice in achieving union and in overall functional outcome of the patient. Aggressive debridement before grafting is often glossed over, as this is a difficult factor to evaluate, but the authors believe it to be the most critical step in the operation. Correction of scaphoid collapse, although not necessary to achieve union, improves postoperative wrist function and may be achieved with either corticocancellous or cancellous grafting. When cancellous grafting is used, pairing with a compression screw may help hold the reduction.

Rigid fixation remains important, and union may be achieved with either K-wires or compression screws. As always with surgery, patient selection is crucial; in those with diminutive or fragmented proximal poles, or other risk factors for recurrent nonunion such as smoking status or increased time from injury, replacement with a vascularized bone flap should be considered. Studies on scaphoid nonunions will remain limited until there are standardized criteria for describing fracture location, outcomes in wrist motion, definition of union, and modality to assessing union.

CLINICS CARE POINTS

- Most scaphoid nonunions can be treated successfully with nonvascularized bone grafts.
- Preoperative prediction of vascularity with advanced imaging is unreliable. Aggressive debridement to healthy cancellous bone is critical to achieving union of the nonunion.
- Evaluation of the defect and correction of the humpback deformity are critical to a good clinical outcome with satisfactory pain relief and range motion.
- Outcomes do not differ in the literature when comparing screw and K-wire fixation, but stable osteosynthesis is critical to bone healing given the forces around the scaphoid.
- Destroyed proximal poles that cannot be rigidly fixated warrant reconstruction with free osteochondral bone grafts.

FUNDING

None.

DISCLOSURE

The authors have no relevant disclosures to report.

REFERENCES

1. Dias J, Brenkel I, Finlay D. Patterns of union in fractures of the waist of the scaphoid. J BONE Jt Surg 1989;71B(2):307–10.
2. Bond CD, Shin AY, Mcbride MT, et al. Percutaneous screw fixation or cast immobilization for nondisplaced scaphoid fractures. J Bone Joint Surg Am 2001. https://doi.org/10.2106/00004623-200104000-00001.
3. Chong HH, Kulkarni K, Shah R, et al. A meta-analysis of union rate after proximal scaphoid fractures: terminology matters. J Plast Surg Hand Surg 2022;56(5):298–309.
4. Cohen MS, Jupiter JB, Fallahi K, et al. Scaphoid waist nonunion with humpback deformity treated without structural bone graft. J Hand Surg 2013;38(4):701–5.
5. Slade JF, Dodds SD. Minimally invasive management of scaphoid nonunions. Clin Orthop 2006;445:108–19.
6. Higgins JP, Giladi AM. Scaphoid nonunion vascularized bone grafting in 2021: is avascular necrosis the sole determinant? J Hand Surg 2021;46(9):801–6.e2.
7. Rancy SK, Schmidle G, Wolfe SW. Does anyone need a vascularized graft? Hand Clin 2019;35(3):323–44.
8. Merrell GA, Wolfe SW, Slade JF. Treatment of scaphoid nonunions: quantitative meta-analysis of the literature. J Hand Surg 2002;27(4):685–91.
9. Smith DK, Cooney WP, An KN, et al. The effects of simulated unstable scaphoid fractures on carpal motion. J Hand Surg 1989;14(2):283–91.
10. Ramamurthy C, Cutler L, Nuttall D, et al. The factors affecting outcome after non- vascular bone grafting and internal fixation for nonunion of the scaphoid. J BONE Jt Surg 2007;89(5).
11. Amadio P, Berquist T, Smith D, et al. Scaphoid malunion. J Hand Surg 1989;14A(4):679–87.
12. Aguilella L, Garcia-Elias M. The anterolateral corner of the radial metaphysis as a source of bone graft for the treatment of scaphoid nonunion. J Hand Surg 2012;37(6):1258–62.
13. Luchetti TJ, Rao AJ, Fernandez JJ, et al. Fixation of proximal pole scaphoid nonunion with non-vascularized cancellous autograft. J Hand Surg Eur 2018;43(1):66–72.
14. McInnes CW, Giuffre JL. Fixation and grafting after limited debridement of scaphoid nonunions. J Hand Surg 2015;40(9):1791–6.
15. Lynch NM, Linscheid RL. Corrective osteotomy for scaphoid malunion: technique and long-term follow-up evaluation. J Hand Surg 1997;22(1):35–43.
16. Wong WYC, Ho PC. Arthroscopic management of scaphoid nonunion. Hand Clin 2019;35(3):295–313.
17. Russe O. Therapeutic results with cancellous bone filling in pseudoarthrosis of the navicular bone. Z Orthop Ihre Grenzgeb 1951;81(3):466–73.
18. Fernandez DL. A technique for anterior wedge-shaped grafts for scaphoid nonunions with carpal instability. J Hand Surg 1984;9(5):733–7.
19. Lee SK, Byun DJ, Roman-Deynes JL, et al. Hybrid Russe procedure for scaphoid waist fracture nonunion with deformity. J Hand Surg 2015;40(11):2198–205.
20. Tambe AD, Cutler L, Murali SR, et al. In scaphoid non-union, does the source of graft affect outcome? Iliac crest versus distal end of radius bone graft. J Hand Surg 2006;31(1):47–51.
21. Jarrett P, Kinzel V, Stoffel K. A biomechanical comparison of scaphoid fixation with bone grafting using iliac bone or distal radius bone. J Hand Surg Am 2007. https://doi.org/10.1016/j.jhsa.2007.06.009.
22. Kim JK, Yoon JO, Baek H. Corticocancellous bone graft vs cancellous bone graft for the management of unstable scaphoid nonunion. Orthop Traumatol Surg Res 2018;104(1):115–20.
23. Sayegh ET, Strauch RJ. Graft choice in the management of unstable scaphoid nonunion: a systematic review. J Hand Surg 2014;39(8):1500–6.e7.
24. Gire JD, Thio T, Behn AW, et al. Rotational stability of scaphoid waist nonunion bone graft and fixation techniques. J Hand Surg 2020;45(9):841–9.e1.
25. Faucher GK, Golden ML, Sweeney KR, et al. Comparison of screw trajectory on stability of oblique scaphoid fractures: a mechanical study. J Hand Surg 2014;39(3):430–5.
26. Luria S, Hoch S, Liebergall M, et al. Optimal fixation of acute scaphoid fractures: finite element analysis. J Hand Surg 2010;35(8):1246–50.
27. Pinder RM, Brkljac M, Rix L, et al. Treatment of scaphoid nonunion: a systematic review of the existing evidence. J Hand Surg 2015;40(9):1797–805.e3.
28. Ezquerro F, Jiménez S, Pérez A, et al. The influence of wire positioning upon the initial stability of scaphoid fractures fixed using Kirschner wires. Med Eng Phys 2007;29(6):652–60.
29. Adams BD, Blair WF, Reagan DS, et al. Technical factors related to Herbert screw fixation. J Hand Surg 1988;13(6):893–9.
30. Garcia RM, Leversedge FJ, Aldridge JM, et al. Scaphoid nonunions treated with 2 headless compression screws and bone grafting. J Hand Surg 2014;39(7):1301–7.

31. Wu F, Ng CY, Hayton M. The authors' technique for volar plating of scaphoid nonunion. Hand Clin 2019;35(3):281–6.

32. Dunn J, Kusnezov N, Fares A, et al. The scaphoid staple: a systematic review. Hand 2017;12(3):236–41.

33. Ammori MB, Elvey M, Mahmoud SS, et al. The outcome of bone graft surgery for nonunion of fractures of the scaphoid. J Hand Surg Eur 2019;44(7):676–84.

34. Ross PR, Lan WC, Chen JS, et al. Revision surgery after vascularized or non-vascularized scaphoid nonunion repair: a national population study. Injury 2020;51(3):656–62.

35. Rancy SK, Swanstrom MM, DiCarlo EF, et al. Success of scaphoid nonunion surgery is independent of proximal pole vascularity. J Hand Surg Eur 2018;43(1):32–40.

Scaphoid Nonunions
Local Vascularized Bone Flaps

Justin C. McCarty, DO, MPH, Ryoko Hamaguchi, MD, Kyle R. Eberlin, MD*

KEYWORDS

- Scaphoid nonunion • Vascularized bone graft/Flap • Local vascularized bone flaps

KEY POINTS

- Local vascularized bone flaps (VBFs) are options to treat scaphoid nonunions and do not require microsurgical techniques. They may have higher union rates than nonvascularized grafts, especially in the setting of proximal pole avascular necrosis (AVN).
- The choice of local vascularized bone flap is based on the location of the nonunion with distinction made between proximal pole nonunion (with or without AVN) and waist nonunion with or without humpback deformity or carpal instability.
- Dorsal-based flaps are commonly used for proximal pole scaphoid nonunion, whereas volar-based VBFs are more commonly used to address nonunions with humpback deformity or carpal instability.

BACKGROUND

Scaphoid fractures are the most common carpal bone fracture, and the second most common fracture of the wrist following distal radius fractures. Among carpal fractures, scaphoid fractures account for 66% of fractures and have a pooled incidence of 23.0 per 100,000 person-years.[1] The incidence varies according to the population observed with the highest incidence seen in men aged 20 to 29 years.[2,3] The importance of the scaphoid stems from its role as a mechanical linkage between the proximal and distal carpal rows, a "tie rod," which enable normal carpal mechanics.

The anatomy of the scaphoid, which is composed of 80% articular cartilage on its surface, complicates fracture management because it is at high risk for nonunion and is second only to the femoral head for risk of posttraumatic avascular necrosis (AVN).[4] Gelberman's research describing the vascularity of the scaphoid demonstrated the external vascular supply is via the radial artery perfusing branches on the volar and dorsal sides that enter on the limited nonarticular surfaces. The volar scaphoid artery branches off the

radial or superficial palmar arch and account for 20% to 30% of internal vascularity in the region of the distal pole. The dorsal scaphoid arteries branch off the radial artery and enter the dorsal oblique ridge on the distal aspect of the scaphoid, accounting for the remaining 70% of blood supply to the scaphoid. The internal vascularity of the proximal 70% to 80% of the scaphoid is based almost exclusively on branches that enter on the dorsal oblique ridge. The vascular supply partly accounts for the nonunion rate differences observed based on fracture location.

The rate of nonunion for nondisplaced proximal pole fractures managed nonoperatively is 34%, which is 7.5 times that of waist and tubercle fractures.[5] Initial operative management, however, may substantially decrease proximal pole nonunion rates to as low as 1%.[6] The rate of nonunion for scaphoid fractures displaced greater than 1 mm is significantly higher, up to 55%.[7] Once nonunion occurs, commonly defined as lack of bony healing persisting for 6 months or longer, there may be a predictable cascade of changes including the following:

Division of Plastic Surgery, Massachusetts General Hospital, Harvard Medical School, Boston, MA, USA
* Corresponding author. Division of Plastic Surgery, Massachusetts General Hospital, Harvard Medical School, 55 Fruit Street, Boston, MA 02135.
E-mail address: keberlin@mgh.harvard.edu

Hand Clin 40 (2024) 117–127
https://doi.org/10.1016/j.hcl.2023.08.004

- Carpal instability
- AVN
- Humpback deformity (intrascaphoid angle >35°)
- Scaphoid collapse
- Scaphoid nonunion advanced collapse (SNAC)

SNAC wrist may occur in 80% to 90% of cases within 10 years[8] and the subsequent resulting pain, decreased strength, and diminished function that would otherwise require salvage procedures such as partial carpal fusion or proximal row carpectomy. Once nonunion is identified, the goal of surgery is to restore both the bony structure and alignment to avoid these aforementioned consequences.

Management for scaphoid nonunions is determined by the anatomic location as well as patient factors. Nonvascularized bone grafts and internal fixation can be used effectively when there is no evidence of AVN with union rates of 80% to 100%.[9–11] The method of healing for nonvascularized grafts is via creeping substitution and resorption.[12,13] This is in contrast to vascularized bone grafts, technically considered flaps (vascularized bone flap [VBF]), which heal via primary bone healing which decreases time to healing and bony union.[14,15] Free VBFs are able to transfer a larger amount of bone than local flaps but are more technically demanding. Local, pedicled VBFs should be within the armamentarium of most hand surgeons because they do not require formal microsurgical techniques. The aim of scaphoid nonunion operations is to restore carpal alignment and avoid the progressive arthritic changes of SNAC wrist. This article will describe indications and technical aspects of various local vascularized bone flap options for scaphoid nonunion.

PRESENTATION AND EVALUATION

Patients with scaphoid fractures often present with wrist pain, tenderness at the distal pole of the scaphoid or anatomic snuffbox, and pain with axial compression of the thumb. Some patients with nonunions present with a distant history of wrist trauma, although several patients with nonunion may not recall a history of wrist trauma. Some patients with incidentally discovered nonunions on imaging may not have symptoms. The physical examination should also take note of any earlier incisions or lacerations because many patients have undergone earlier operations that could compromise potential vascular pedicles for local or regional osseous flaps.

The initial evaluation should include the standard 3-view x-ray of the wrist and a scaphoid view. Unlike the presentation of acute scaphoid

fractures, which may not be apparent on early x-ray, a scaphoid nonunion will be readily visible radiographically with signs, including cystic changes, bone resorption at the fracture site, sclerosis, and if previously fixated hardware loosening or failure (**Fig. 1**A). Once identified, a CT scan may be helpful to more accurately delineate the presence of humpback deformity, structure and exact measurements of the scaphoid fragments, and joint congruity (**Fig. 2**). A CT should be oriented in the plane of the scaphoid with 1 mm cuts. The lateral intrascaphoid angle should be assessed to look for collapse and any associated humpback deformity. The progressive arthritis that develops in SNAC should be noted as patients who have progressed onto SNAC stages 2, 3, or 4 are generally no longer a candidate for VBF. MRI has moderate sensitivity and specificity for identifying AVN—71% and 82%, respectively—but no gold standard exists for diagnosing AVN.[16] Contrast-enhanced MRI may be beneficial but evidence is variable.

PRINCIPLES OF SURGICAL INTERVENTION

The most reliable method to identify the presence and extent of AVN is at the time of operation. The approach to the scaphoid may be either volar or dorsal depending on the anatomic location of the nonunion and presumed risk of AVN. A dorsal approach may be more advantageous for proximal nonunions, whereas the volar approach may be more ideal for distal pole or waist nonunions with significant humpback deformities. Exposure of the scaphoid is followed by comprehensive debridement of any sclerotic bone and fibrous tissue until punctate bleeding is seen from both the proximal and distal poles; debridement is a critical aspect of the procedure. The size of the defect to be reconstructed can then be measured to assess its 3-dimensional size for length, width, and depth. Each bone flap should be templated to fill the defect.

As with any bone graft/flap reconstruction, the VBF should ideally be secured with rigid fixation and maintenance of bony contact while healing. The choice of fixation depends on the size of the fragments present.[10] Most often, fixation is achieved with K-wires or headless compression screws. Scaphoid-specific locked volar buttress plating represents an additional option although with less evidence specifically for when used in conjunction with VBF.[17] The union rates are not significantly different between K-wires and screws (88%–91%, respectively) although this is based on retrospective, nonrandomized control data.[10] Cannulated headless compression screws may

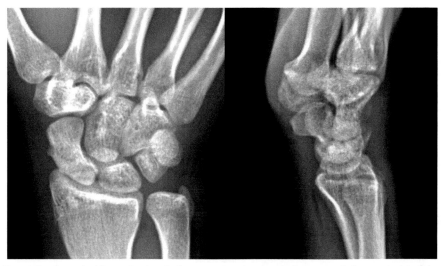

Fig. 1. Radiograph of scaphoid proximal pole fracture. Proximal pole fracture of the scaphoid without notable sclerotic changes and no evidence of humpback deformity.

be preferred for their more rigid fixation combined with the compression they provide to maintain bony contact but are not always feasible given anatomic constraints and the geometry of the intercalated graft. Volar plates can be used in multifragmentary or recalcitrant scaphoid nonunions and have similar union rates to other fixation methods (90%) but require removal in up to 20% of patients at 1 year.[18] Additionally, plate fixation may be associated with longer time to union and lower modified Mayo wrist scores when compared with screw fixation.[19] Thus, the choice of fixation is left to the surgeon and individualized based on surgeon experience, planned approach, and anatomy of the nonunion for each patient.

LOCAL VASCULARIZED BONE FLAPS

Local bone flaps are pedicled and, given this vascularity, are more appropriately called "flaps" as opposed to the traditional nomenclature "grafts." Multiple local VBF options exist from both the volar and dorsal side of the wrist. Sheetz and colleagues in their detailed anatomic study in 1995 showed the available pedicled flaps from the distal radius and ulna based on the extraosseous and intraosseous blood supply.[20] They found relatively consistent anatomy across 41 cadaveric specimens with consistent spatial relationships to anatomic landmarks. The dorsal blood supply of the radius is described in relation to the extensor

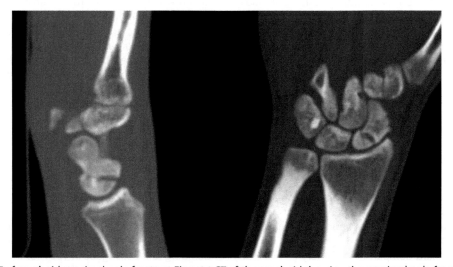

Fig. 2. CT of scaphoid proximal pole fracture. Fine cut CT of the scaphoid showing the proximal pole fracture with greater than 2 mm displacement but no evidence of humpback deformity.

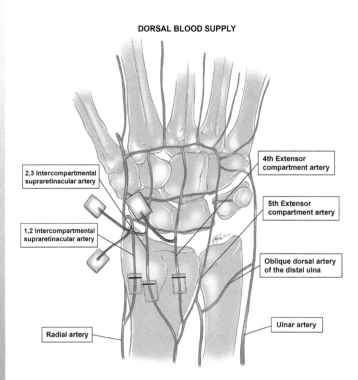

DORSAL BLOOD SUPPLY

2,3 Intercompartmental supraretinacular artery

1,2 Intercompartmental supraretinacular artery

Radial artery

4th Extensor compartment artery

5th Extensor compartment artery

Oblique dorsal artery of the distal ulna

Ulnar artery

Fig. 3. Vascular pedicles for the dorsal VBFs. Demonstration of the relative anatomic locations, arc of rotation, and location of several common dorsal VBFs for scaphoid nonunion. (Image courtesy of Ryoko Hamaguchi, MD)

compartments and extensor retinaculum; flaps are considered compartmental when lying within an extensor compartment and intercompartmental when located between compartments.

The anatomic location of each pedicle and accompanying description of the surgical technique is described below. Additional local flaps are possible based on an understanding of the vascular anatomy. Flap choice should take note of any and all earlier procedures that could disrupt the normal anatomy and potentially compromise the pedicle. Each VBF is typically harvested with the tourniquet insufflated with or without Esmarch exsanguination to help with visualization of the vasculature.

Dorsal Vascularized Bone Flaps

Dorsal VBFs are the most commonly used flaps for scaphoid nonunions because of their proximity to proximal third fractures where AVN is most common. Flaps with appropriate pedicle reach to the scaphoid are as follows:

1. 1,2 intercompartmental supraretinacular artery (1,2 ICSRA)
2. 2,3 intercompartmental supraretinacular artery (2,3 ICSRA)
3. 4 + 5 extra compartmental artery (4 + 5 ECA) **(Fig. 3)**
4. Dorsal capsular flap

It is difficult to correct humpback deformity from a dorsal approach and is generally a contraindication. Multiple authors have, however, described their successful use of the 1,2 ICSRA VBF for both humpback deformities and dorsal intercalated segmental instability (DISI) deformities by volarly inserting the flap a wedge-shaped 1,2 ICSRA flap and supporting it with a headless compression screw with union rates of 93% to 100% in their small series.[21–23] The approach described requires a radial styloidectomy of 5 mm to enable pedicle reach.[23] The utility of the dorsal flaps to address humpback deformities and cases of carpal instability outside of experienced hands may be better approached with a volar pedicled bone flap, medial femoral condyle, or medial femoral trochlea flap as the literature supporting these approaches is stronger.[24,25]

Dorsal VBFs are most useful for the following:

1. Nonunion without humpback deformity
2. AVN of the proximal scaphoid pole
3. Persistent nonunion after an earlier nonvascularized bone flap procedure

1,2 intercompartmental supraretinacular artery

The 1,2 ICSRA VBF was first described by Zaidemberg and colleagues in 1991 for the treatment of scaphoid nonunion.[26] The 1,2 ICSRA VBF is among the most commonly used local pedicled

VBF for scaphoid nonunion. Contraindications include damage to the pedicle from any prior operations or trauma based on its anatomic location as described below. The rate of damage to the pedicle from prior operations is not described in the literature. Humpback and DISI deformity is a relative contraindication and requires adjustment to the technique.[23]

The 1,2 ICSRA branches originate from the radial artery approximately 5 cm proximal to the radiocarpal joint or 1.9 mm proximal to the tip of the radial styloid.[27] The pedicle courses deep to the brachioradialis muscle before becoming more superficial at the extensor retinaculum where it runs in the septum between the first and second dorsal compartments.[20] Distal to the retinaculum, the 1,2 ICSRA has an anastomosis with either radial artery in the snuffbox (52%), the radiocarpal arch (52%), and/or the intercarpal arch (19%). This distal connection may be used as the pedicle if the proximal vessel is ligated to allow the VBF to rotate into the scaphoid defect. The length of the pedicle is on average 22.5 mm. It is described as having a separate, combined, or shared origin with the dorsal scaphoid branch in anatomic latex studies by Waitayawinyu and colleagues.[27] Taking a flap 8 to 18 mm proximal to the articular surface of the distal radius incorporates the most bony perforators with the largest branch at 10 mm proximal to the radial styloid.[27] The superficial position in the retinaculum and directly on the bony tubercle facilitates dissection.

A curvilinear, zig-zag, or linear incision over the dorsoradial wrist is made after tourniquet inflation with arm elevation (**Fig. 4**A and B). This incision will allow access to the dorsum of the scaphoid and the VBF. The vascular pedicle of the 1,2 ICSRA should be visible over the extensor retinaculum between the first and second compartments (**Fig. 5**A). Parallel incisions at least 5 mm apart are made adjacent to the pedicle to allow for mobilization and rotation of the VBF (**Fig. 5**B). The associated bone flap is harvested from the radial metaphysis approximately 8 to 18 mm proximal to the radial styloid using osteotomes (**Fig. 5**C).[27] It is best to slightly oversize the flap and it is taken with its periosteum to preserve the vascular supply of the bone. The VBF can then be rotated 180° and tunneled under the extensor tendons to press fit into the prepared nonunion site (**Fig. 5**D). Allograft cancellous bone chips may be used to fill the defect from the VBF harvest (**Fig. 5**E). Finally, the flap is fixated in place with K wires or screws.

The 2 to 3 intercompartmental supraretinacular artery vascularized bone flap

The 2,3 ICSRA is less commonly used compared with the 1,2 ICSRA but carries similar indications.[28] It has a wider arc of rotation based on the location of its pedicle compared with the 1,2 ICSRA, which enables it to reach the more volar carpus. There is less literature regarding its efficacy likely because the 1,2 ICSRA carries similar indications with more familiar anatomy.

The technique is similar to the 1,2 ICSRA for all aspects except for the expected anatomic location of the pedicle (**Fig. 6**A–D): the 2,3 ICSRA originates proximally from the anterior interosseous artery or its divisions after they pierce the interosseous membrane just proximal the pronator quadratus (PQ) before coursing superficial to the extensor retinaculum directly on Lister tubercle.[20] It runs in the septum between the second and third compartments then anastomoses distally to the dorsal intercarpal arch in 94% of cases, the dorsal radiocarpal arch (52%), and/or the fourth extensor compartment artery. The 2,3 ICSRA flap is anatomically reliable because it has a nutrient artery in the septum, which penetrates the bone in 92% of specimens.

The 4 + 5 extra compartmental vascularized bone flap

The 4 + 5 ECA VBF is harvested using a dorsal approach to the fourth extensor compartment.[29]

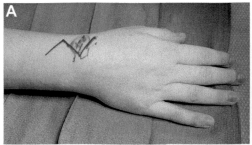
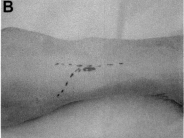

Fig. 4. Depiction of dorsal incisions for scaphoid nonunion. These are made ulnar to Lister tubercle to center them over the planned flap. (*A*) Incision for a 1,2 ICSRA flap. (*B*) Incision for a 2,3 ICSRA flap.

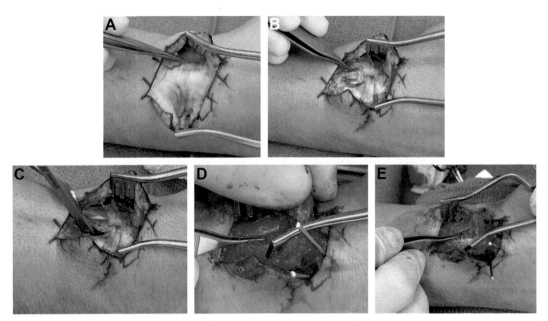

Fig. 5. ICSRA flap for scaphoid nonunion. (*A*) The 1,2 ICSRA pedicle can be seen coursing over the extensor retinaculum between the first and second compartments. (*B*) Precise incisions through the periosteum are made 5 mm apart adjacent to the vascular pedicle. (*C*) The VBF is lifted carefully after all osteotomies have been made. (*D*) The donor defect from the VBF is filled with cancellous bone allograft. (*E*) The VBF is rotated and inset into the prepared scaphoid nonunion site.

The arterial pedicle is 0.4 mm in diameter.[20] The vascularity of this pedicle may not be reliable in patients who have had prior dorsal approach operations or those with an earlier significant trauma to the area. This VBF is more often used for treating Kienbock disease but is able to reach the proximal pole of the scaphoid if needed.

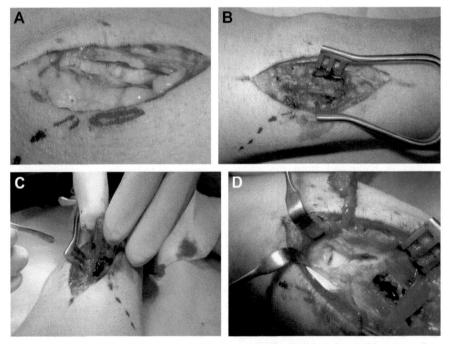

Fig. 6. The 2,3 ICSRA flap for scaphoid nonunion. (*A*) The 2,3 ICSRA pedicle is located between the second and third compartment and courses directly over Lister tubercle. (*B*) The osteotomies parallel the pedicle. (*C*) The VBF fully mobilized on its vascular supply. (*D*) Rotation of the pedicle into the scaphoid nonunion site.

Capsular-based/fourth extensor compartment flap

The capsular-based bone flap is based on the fourth extensor compartment artery, which runs under the dorsal retinaculum extending between the anterior or posterior interosseous arteries and the radiocarpal arch.[30] The advantage of this flap is it avoids the need for a microvascular pedicle dissection because the vascular pedicle is included with the capsule attached to the bone graft. It is approached via a 4-cm dorsal incision just ulnar to Lister tubercle. At the base of the fourth compartment, a 1 × 1 cm bone harvest is performed from the distal aspect of the dorsal radius just ulnar and distal to Lister tubercle leaving 2 to 3 mm of distal radius cortex to avoid propagation into the radiocarpal joint cartilage. The flap is harvested with its capsule attached with a base of the capsule measuring 1.5 cm where it rotates 10° to 30° to insert into the nonunion site.

Volar Vascularized Bone Flaps

The Volar VBFs are useful for cases of scaphoid nonunion with humpback deformity or dorsal intercalated segment instability because they allow for a more direct approach compared with the dorsal VBFs. Additionally, by approaching the scaphoid volarly, they protect the dorsal side of scaphoid where the dominant native blood supply is located. There are 4 primary options on the volar aspect of the wrist (**Fig. 7**).

1. Volar carpal artery or palmar radiocarpal (PRCA) VBF
2. PQ VBF
3. Pisiform VBF

Volar carpal artery/palmar radiocarpal vascularized bone flap

The volar carpal artery or PRCA VBF, first described in 1987 by Kuhlmann and colleagues for use in scaphoid nonunions, and later refined by Mathoulin in 1998, is a local VBF option for those cases with unstable humpback deformity.[31]

The PRCA VBF harvest technique, as described by Sommerkamp, uses a modified extensile Russe approach measuring approximately 8 cm in length centered over the ulnar aspect of the radius.[32] The PRCA runs along the volar aspect of the carpus along the distal border of the PQ. It courses from the radial to the ulnar artery and in 98% of patients is radial artery dominant. The dissection is kept radial to the flexor carpi radialis (FCR) tendon and distal to the volar rim of the radius to expose the scaphoid nonunion as the pedicle of the

PRCA originates off the radial artery on the radius just proximal. Because the indication for this flap is for the correction of humpback deformity, time must be spent to distract and place the scaphoid into anatomic position. Once this is done, the size of the defect is measured so the appropriate size flap may be harvested.

To harvest the PRCA VBF, the dissection begins ulnar to the FCR tendon, which is retracted radially to expose the volar aspect of the distal radius and the PQ. The PRCA pedicle originates just distal to the PQ edge. The flap is centered based on the pedicle encompassing an area just proximal to the lunate fossa and radial to the sigmoid notch. The ulnar extension of the PRCA pedicle is ligated where it crosses the distal radial ulnar joint (DRUJ). A trapezoidal-shaped flap is harvested in a similar manner to other VBFs using a saw and osteotomes. To avoid entry into the lunate fossa or sigmoid notch, they can be marked with a 25-gauge needle or K-wires along the angle of their articular inclination. The PRCA VBF is rotated 30° to 40° on its pedicle into the defect. Typically, additional dissection toward the pedicle's origin off the radial artery is necessary to allow the VBF to reach the waist of scaphoid. The VBF and the pedicle are tunneled underneath the FCR and inset into the scaphoid. The flap is then fixated as a structural interposition flap with a headless compression screw or K wires.

Pronator quadratus vascularized bone flap

The PQ VBF was first described for use in scaphoid nonunion by Kawai and Yamato in 1988.[33] It is based on maintaining the PQ muscle with limited manipulation because it has rich vascular anastomoses between the anterior interosseous, radial, and ulnar artery branches and perfuses the bone it is adherent to. It has similar indications as the PRCA VBF, and the exposure is similar. Notably, it has a shorter arc that can be rotated compared with the PRCA VBF. It has a relatively straightforward harvest because it does not require dissecting out a vascular pedicle.

A volar incision is made similar to the PRCA. After exposing and reducing the scaphoid nonunion, the flap is harvested by first identifying the leading edge of the PQ. A block measuring approximately 15 to 20 mm is outlined at the distal radial insertion of the PQ near the abductor pollicis tendon. An L-shaped incision is made in the PQ and the bone flap is taken from the radial styloid while ensuring that the muscle remains attached to the VBF. It can then be rotated on the muscle pedicle into the volar scaphoid.

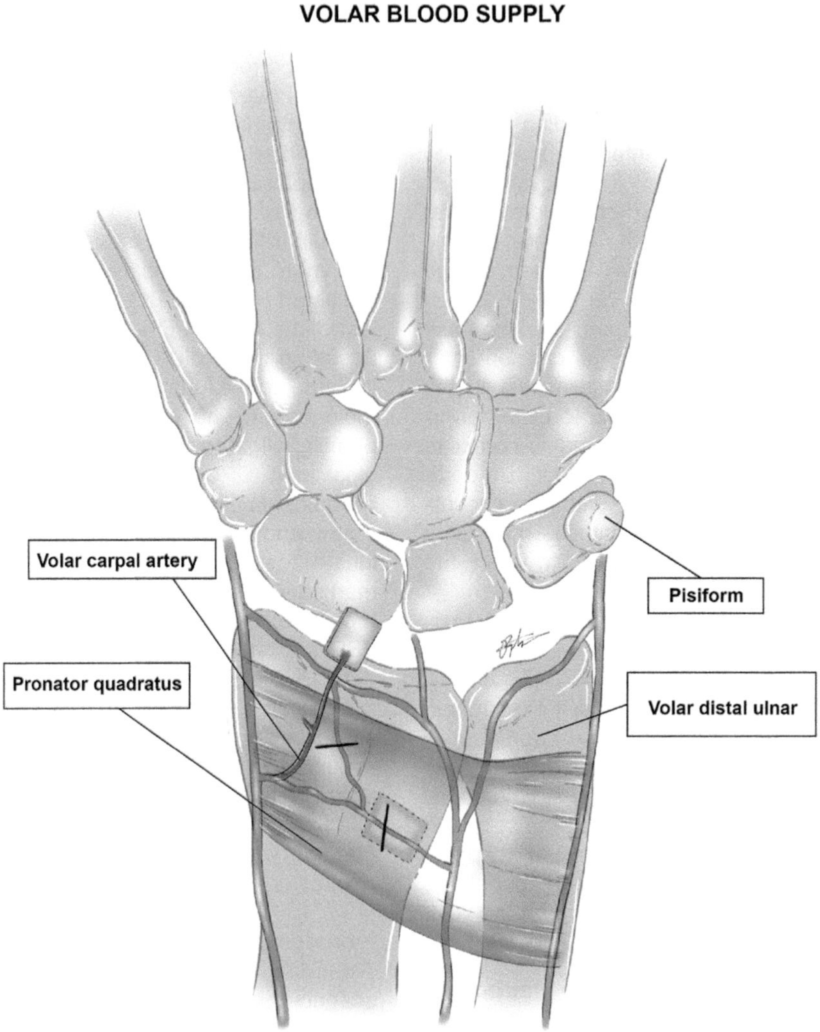

VOLAR BLOOD SUPPLY

Fig. 7. Vascular pedicles for volar VBFs. Demonstration of the relative anatomic locations, arc of rotation, and location of the bone flap for the common volar VBFs for scaphoid nonunion. (Image courtesy of Ryoko Hamaguchi, MD)

Pisiform vascularized vascularized bone flap

The pisiform VBF can be used to reconstruct the proximal pole of the scaphoid with AVN.[34] Its arterial pedicle is off the dorsal branch of the ulnar artery with a 4-cm pedicle length.[20,35] One of its key advantages is that it is covered by articular cartilage on its surface. This is counterbalanced by its relatively small size, which results in some loss of height of the scaphoid.

The approach as described by Kuhlmann is via a longitudinal zig-zag incision over the volar wrist radial to the flexor carpi ulnaris (FCU) tendon directed toward the ring finger to avoid the palmar cutaneous nerves.[34] The pisiform is freed from the FCU and pisohamate ligament. The only soft tissue attachments left in place are on the ulnar border where the dorsal branch of the ulnar artery enters.

The VBF is then passed underneath the FCU tendon to reach the proximal pole of the scaphoid, inset and fixated per surgeon preference.

OUTCOMES

A large comparative meta-analysis of 54 studies of both dorsal and volar VBFs for treating scaphoid nonunions found union rates between 83.3% and 94.9% for all the various flaps.[36] Within this meta-analysis, the 1,2 ICSRA flap was the most commonly assessed flap, and out of 463 patients with 1,2 ICSRA flaps, 83.3% healed their nonunion compared to other dorsal flaps which healed in 85.3% of cases. The scaphoid union rate following repair with following 1,2 ICSRA is variable in the literature based on the treated population with union rates of 27% to 100% with much of the variability stemming from its use as salvage after an earlier failed operation or use in patients with a humpback deformity.[25,37,38] Among the volar radius VBFs, 87.7% went on to heal the nonunion. The functional outcome scores were within a similar range of 79 for the 1,2-ICSRA, 83 for other dorsal radius, and 89 for volar radius VBFs. Generally, there was not a notable clinically significant difference even the few instances when statistical significance was achieved.

Sommerkamp and colleagues using the PRCA VBF successfully treated a series of 15 consecutive patients with AVN of the proximal pole and concomitant instability and achieved 100% union rate and correction of the humpback deformity during a 22-month follow-up.[32] There are no comparative studies between the PQ VBF and other volar VBFs, whereas several cases series demonstrate between 85% and 100% union rates for patients with scaphoid nonunion and humpback deformity.[36] For the pisiform VBF, Kuhlmann presented a 14 patient series with 7 patients having AVN of the proximal scaphoid and the other 7 patients with Kienbock disease. Six of 7 cases were effective in treating scaphoid AVN with improved pain, with the one failure being presumed secondary to a technical error with poor placement of the VBF necessitating wrist fusion for resolution of pain.[34]

SUMMARY

Multiple different local VBF are available to the hand surgeon treating scaphoid nonunions. The choice of which flap to use is individualized based on the anatomy of the patient's fracture coupled with the surgeon's familiarity with the anatomy. There is considerable overlap in the indications for vascularized and traditional bone grafting, and the hand surgeon should carefully consider all options when deciding on technique.

CLINICS CARE POINTS

- Local VBFs achieve union rates of 83% to 100% for scaphoid nonunion with AVN in appropriately selected patients while avoiding microsurgical techniques. Union rates for VBFs are higher and achieved faster than non-VBFs by allowing primary bone healing.
- The choice of which local vascularized bone flap is based on the location of the nonunion with distinction made between proximal pole nonunion with or without AVN and waist

nonunion with or without humpback deformity or carpal instability.

- Dorsal-based flaps, with the 1,2 ICSRA being the most common, are advantageous for proximal pole scaphoid nonunion because they easily reach the proximal pole. Volar-based VBFs are more commonly used to address nonunions with humpback deformity or carpal instability because the volar approach simplifies the anatomic reduction of nonunion and allows the VBF pedicle to easily reach the defect after nonunion debridement.

ACKNOWLEDGMENTS

The authors would like to acknowledge and thank Sang Gil Lee, MD, who provided the clinical photos of the 1,2 ICSRA scaphoid nonunion repair and Chaitanya Mudgal, MD, who provided the clinical photos of the 2,3 ICSRA scaphoid nonunion repair.

DISCLOSURES

K.R. Eberlin-consultant for AxoGen, Integra, Checkpoint.

REFERENCES

1. Ponkilainen V, Kuitunen I, Liukkonen R, et al. The incidence of musculoskeletal injuries: a systematic review and meta-analysis. Bone Joint Res 2022; 11(11):814–25.
2. Wolf JM, Dawson L, Mountcastle SB, et al. The incidence of scaphoid fracture in a military population. Injury 2009;40(12):1316–9.
3. Van Tassel DC, Owens BD, Wolf JM. Incidence estimates and demographics of scaphoid fracture in the U.S. population. J Hand Surg Am 2010;35(8): 1242–5.
4. Berger RA. The anatomy of the scaphoid. Hand Clin 2001;17(4):525–32.
5. Eastley N, Singh H, Dias JJ, et al. Union rates after proximal scaphoid fractures; meta-analyses and review of available evidence. J Hand Surg Eur Vol 2013;38(8):888–97.
6. Slade JF 3rd, Gillon T. Retrospective review of 234 scaphoid fractures and nonunions treated with arthroscopy for union and complications. Scand J Surg 2008;97(4):280–9.
7. Szabo RM, Manske D. Displaced fractures of the scaphoid. Clin Orthop Relat Res 1988;230:30–8.
8. Duppe H, Johnell O, Lundborg G, et al. Long-term results of fracture of the scaphoid. A follow-up study of more than thirty years. J Bone Joint Surg Am 1994;76(2):249–52.

9. Sayegh ET, Strauch RJ. Graft choice in the management of unstable scaphoid nonunion: a systematic review. J Hand Surg Am 2014;39(8):1500–1506 e7.

10. Pinder RM, Brkljac M, Rix L, et al. Treatment of Scaphoid Nonunion: A Systematic Review of the Existing Evidence. J Hand Surg Am 2015;40(9):1797–1805 e3.

11. Yasuda M, Ando Y, Masada K. Treatment of scaphoid nonunion using volar biconcave cancellous bone grafting. Hand Surg 2007;12(2):135–40.

12. Sgromolo NM, Rhee PC. The Role of Vascularized Bone Grafting in Scaphoid Nonunion. Hand Clin 2019;35(3):315–22.

13. Sunagawa T, Bishop AT, Muramatsu K. Role of conventional and vascularized bone grafts in scaphoid nonunion with avascular necrosis: A canine experimental study. J Hand Surg Am 2000;25(5):849–59.

14. Arata MA, Wood MB, Cooney WP 3rd. Revascularized segmental diaphyseal bone transfers in the canine. An analysis of viability. J Reconstr Microsurg 1984;1(1):11–9.

15. Berggren A, Weiland AJ, Dorfman H. Free vascularized bone grafts: factors affecting their survival and ability to heal to recipient bone defects. Plastic and Reconstructive Surgery 1982;69(1):19–29.

16. Fox MG, Wang DT, Chhabra AB. Accuracy of enhanced and unenhanced MRI in diagnosing scaphoid proximal pole avascular necrosis and predicting surgical outcome. Skeletal Radiol 2015;44(11):1671–8.

17. Dodds SD, Halim A. Scaphoid Plate Fixation and Volar Carpal Artery Vascularized Bone Graft for Recalcitrant Scaphoid Nonunions. J Hand Surg Am 2016;41(7):e191–8.

18. Dodds SD, Williams JB, Seiter M, et al. Lessons learned from volar plate fixation of scaphoid fracture nonunions. J Hand Surg Eur Vol 2018;43(1):57–65.

19. Van Nest DS, Reynolds M, Warnick E, et al. Volar Plating versus Headless Compression Screw Fixation of Scaphoid Nonunions: A Meta-analysis of Outcomes. J Wrist Surg 2021;10(3):255–61.

20. Sheetz KK, Bishop AT, Berger RA. The arterial blood supply of the distal radius and ulna and its potential use in vascularized pedicled bone grafts. J Hand Surg Am 1995;20(6):902–14.

21. Henry M. Collapsed scaphoid non-union with dorsal intercalated segment instability and avascular necrosis treated by vascularised wedge-shaped bone graft and fixation. J Hand Surg Eur 2007;32(2):148–54.

22. Waitayawinyu T, McCallister WV, Katolik LI, et al. Outcome after vascularized bone grafting of scaphoid nonunions with avascular necrosis. J Hand Surg Am 2009;34(3):387–94.

23. Tsumura T, Matsumoto T, Matsushita M, et al. Correction of Humpback Deformities in Patients With Scaphoid Nonunion Using 1,2-Intercompartmental Supraretinacular Artery Pedicled Vascularized Bone Grafting With a Dorsoradial Approach. J Hand Surg Am 2020;45(2):160 e1–e160 e8.

24. Chang MA, Bishop AT, Moran SL, et al. The outcomes and complications of 1,2-intercompartmental supraretinacular artery pedicled vascularized bone grafting of scaphoid nonunions. J Hand Surg Am 2006;31(3):387–96.

25. Hirche C, Heffinger C, Xiong L, et al. The 1,2-intercompartmental supraretinacular artery vascularized bone graft for scaphoid nonunion: management and clinical outcome. J Hand Surg Am 2014;39(3):423–9.

26. Zaidemberg C, Siebert JW, Angrigiani C. A new vascularized bone graft for scaphoid nonunion. J Hand Surg Am 1991;16(3):474–8.

27. Waitayawinyu T, Robertson C, Chin SH, et al. The detailed anatomy of the 1,2 intercompartmental supraretinacular artery for vascularized bone grafting of scaphoid nonunions. J Hand Surg Am 2008;33(2):168–74.

28. Woon Tan JS, Tu YK. 2,3 intercompartmental supraretinacular artery pedicled vascularized bone graft for scaphoid nonunions. Tech Hand Up Extrem Surg 2013;17(2):62–7.

29. Karaismailoglu B, Fatih Guven M, Erenler M, et al. The use of pedicled vascularized bone grafts in the treatment of scaphoid nonunion: clinical results, graft options and indications. EFORT Open Rev 2020;5(1):1–8.

30. Sotereanos DG, Darlis NA, Dailiana ZH, et al. A capsular-based vascularized distal radius graft for proximal pole scaphoid pseudarthrosis. J Hand Surg Am 2006;31(4):580–7.

31. Kuhlmann JN, Mimoun M, Boabighi A, et al. Vascularized bone graft pedicled on the volar carpal artery for non-union of the scaphoid. J Hand Surg Br 1987;12(2):203–10.

32. Sommerkamp TG, Hastings H 2nd, Greenberg JA. Palmar Radiocarpal Artery Vascularized Bone Graft for the Unstable Humpbacked Scaphoid Nonunion With an Avascular Proximal Pole. J Hand Surg Am 2020;45(4):298–309.

33. Kawai H, Yamamoto K. Pronator quadratus pedicled bone graft for old scaphoid fractures. J Bone Joint Surg Br 1988;70(5):829–31.

34. Kuhlmann JN, Kron C, Boabighi A, et al. Vascularised pisiform bone graft. Indications, technique and long-term results. Acta Orthop Belg 2003;69(4):311–6.

35. Elzinga K, Chung KC. Volar Radius Vascularized Bone Flaps for the Treatment of Scaphoid Nonunion. Hand Clin 2019;35(3):353–63.

36. Ditsios K, Konstantinidis I, Agas K, et al. Comparative meta-analysis on the various vascularized bone flaps used for the treatment of scaphoid nonunion. J Orthop Res 2017;35(5):1076–85.

37. Lim TK, Kim HK, Koh KH, et al. Treatment of avascular proximal pole scaphoid nonunions with vascularized distal radius bone grafting. J Hand Surg Am 2013;38(10):1906–19012 e1.

38. Malizos KN, Dailiana Z, Varitimidis S, et al. Management of scaphoid nonunions with vascularized bone grafts from the distal radius: mid- to long-term follow-up. Eur J Orthop Surg Traumatol 2017;27(1):33–9.

Metacarpal and Phalangeal Nonunions

Stefan Czerniecki, MD, MSc, Mark Mishu, MD, Ryan Schmucker, MD*

KEYWORDS

• Nonunion • Phalangeal • Metacarpal

KEY POINTS

• Phalangeal and metacarpal fractures comprise 18% and 23% of all hand and forearm fractures, respectively.
• Mostly, fractures can be treated with great success with closed reduction and immobilization or minimally invasive percutaneous fixation procedures and techniques. Due to the well-vascularized nature of metacarpals and phalanges, nonunion is very rare.
• Rates of metacarpal nonunion are between 0.5% and 1.5%, and phalangeal nonunion rates are similarly low. Despite the low rates of nonunion, given the high incidence of these fractures, it is important to understand the causes, risk factors, and management strategies for this complication.

INTRODUCTION

Phalangeal and metacarpal fractures comprise 18% and 23% of all hand and forearm fractures, respectively.[1] The majority of fractures can be treated successfully with closed reduction and immobilization or minimally invasive percutaneous fixation techniques. Due to the well-vascularized nature of metacarpals and phalanges, nonunion is rare. Metacarpal nonunion rates are between 0.5% and 1.5%, and phalangeal nonunion rates are similarly low. Despite the low rates of nonunion, given the high incidence of these fractures, it is important to understand the causes, risk factors, and management strategies for this complication.

BASIC SCIENCE OF FRACTURE HEALING

Fractures heal either through direct or indirect means. Direct healing requires cortical apposition, compression, and absolute stability of fracture fragments. When this occurs, cutting cones of osteoclasts form at the osteons bordering the fracture and tunnel across the fracture to create new Haversian canals. These cavities are subsequently filled by osteoblasts. Indirect healing will occur with approximation and relative stability of fracture fragments.[2] This process can be subdivided into 4 stages: hematoma formation/inflammation, soft callus formation, hard callus formation, and bone remodeling.[3] In contrast to direct fracture healing, micromotion and loading will promote rather than impede indirect fracture healing.

VASCULAR ANATOMY OF THE METACARPALS AND PHALANGES

For bone healing to occur after a fracture, there must be both stability of fracture fragments and adequate blood supply. Adequate blood supply delivers the osteogenic precursors, oxygen, and growth factors that are necessary for fracture healing. Both the initial trauma itself and surgical intervention can disrupt the blood supply to the fractured bone fragments, leading to delay or failure of fracture healing. Open injuries with soft tissue trauma and periosteal stripping are at high risk of nonunion. The blood supply to metacarpals and phalanges originates from the superficial and deep palmar arches and the dorsal carpal arch. Blood supply to the phalanges and metacarpals comes from 3 systems: the periosteal system, the metaphyseal/epiphyseal system, and the nutrient artery system. While there has not been

Department of Plastic and Reconstructive Surgery, The Ohio State University Columbus, OH, USA
* Corresponding author. 915 Olentangy River Road, Suite 2100, Columbus, OH 43212.
E-mail address: Ryan.Schmucker@osumc.edu

Hand Clin 40 (2024) 129–139
https://doi.org/10.1016/j.hcl.2023.09.003
0749-0712/24/© 2023 Elsevier Inc. All rights reserved.

a named nutrient artery consistently identified in cadaver studies, the metaphyseal/epiphyseal and periosteal blood supply of the metacarpals has been well described (**Fig. 1**). The dorsal metacarpal arteries give off segmental branches to the interosseous muscle and periosteal branches to the ulnar border of the bone as they course from the dorsal carpal arch to form the dorsal digital branches. Palmarly, 3 metacarpal arteries arise from the deep palmar arch and course distally, providing blood supply to the volar aspect of the metacarpals before contributing to the common digital arteries.[4] Blood supply of the phalanges via the proper digital arteries has a regular branching pattern along each phalanx from proximal to distal: condylar vessels, metaphyseal vessels, dorsal skin vessels, and distal transverse palmar arch (**Fig. 2**).[5]

TYPES OF NONUNION

Nonunion can occur if there is failure to maintain fracture stability, failure to maintain adequate blood supply, or infection. Nonunion is the cessation of fracture healing with a persistent bone gap and can be subdivided into hypertrophic and atrophic nonunions (**Table 1**).[6] Hypertrophic nonunion is thought to occur secondarily to inadequate fracture stabilization, while atrophic nonunion is thought to be more related to poor vascularity or impaired biologic healing. On imaging, hypertrophic nonunion can be distinguished by an overgrowth of callus without bridging bone between fracture fragments. In contrast, atrophic nonunion demonstrates absent callus on radiographs. Hypertrophic nonunions typically heal with improved fracture stability. Atrophic nonunions proceed to union if the underlying biologic cause is addressed, or a local biologic stimulus is provided.[7] Some references also describe a third type, oligotrophic nonunion, which has an incomplete callus, and is often due to inadequate reduction combined with unstable fixation. Finally, septic nonunion is a subtype of atrophic nonunion caused by persistent infection of the bone, which impedes fracture healing. Surgical debridement is required before fracture healing can occur.

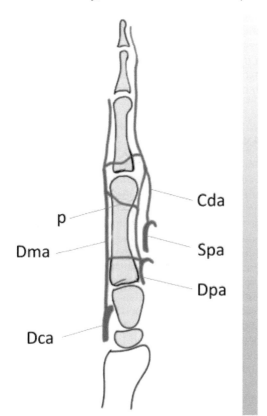

Fig. 1. Metacarpal blood supply. Cda, common digital artery; Dca, dorsal carpal arch; Dma, dorsal metacarpal artery; Dpa, deep palmar arch; p, perforator from deep palmar circulation; Spa, superficial palmar arch. (*From* Tan RES, Lahiri A. Vascular Anatomy of the Hand in Relation to Flaps. Hand Clin. 2020;36(1):1 to 8.

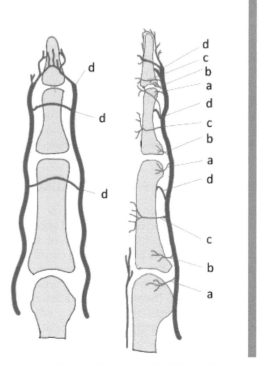

Fig. 2. Phalangeal blood supply. (*A*) condylar vessel; (*B*) metaphyseal vessel; (*C*) dorsal skin vessel; (*D*) transverse palmar arch. (*From* Tan RES, Lahiri A. Vascular Anatomy of the Hand in Relation to Flaps. Hand Clin. 2020;36(1):1 to 8.

Table 1 Descriptions of types of nonunion and pseudoarthrosis	
Atrophic Nonunion	• Caused by inadequate blood supply to the fractured bone • Seen radiographically as absent callus formation
Hypertrophic Nonunion	• Caused by inadequate mechanical stability • Seen radiographically as abundant callus formation but without bridging bone
Oligotrophic Nonunion	• Caused by incomplete reduction of fracture fragments and inadequate fixation with or without compromised blood supply • Seen radiographically with characteristics of both atrophic and hypertrophic nonunion
Septic/Infectious Nonunion	• Infection precludes bone healing • Clinical signs of infection • Seen radiographically as absent callus formation with possible signs of osteomyelitis
Pseudoarthrosis	• Caused by excessive and persistent motion at the fracture site • A false joint subsequently forms, lined with synovium that allows for unstable axial and rotational deformities.

DIAGNOSIS OF AND EVALUATION OF NONUNION

Diagnosis of a nonunion is made clinically (pain, instability, or deformity on examination) and radiographically (evidence of a persistent fracture gap). Delayed union implies that bone healing is occurring, albeit at a slower than normal pace for a given fracture and patient age. There is no consensus on criteria with respect to timing for delayed union and nonunion for metacarpal and phalangeal fractures. Delayed union of a metacarpal or phalanx has been defined as 2 months without bony consolidation.[8,9] Other studies have used 3 and 6 months without bony consolidation on radiographs to define delayed union and nonunion, respectively.[10] Historically, some argued that nonunion should not

be diagnosed until at least 1 year has elapsed from the time of the fracture.[11] Our preference is to use 3 months as a marker for delayed union and 6 months to diagnose nonunion as proven by a lack of bridging bone on computed tomography (CT) scan.

When evaluating a patient with a nonunion, it is important to first determine the underlying cause, beginning with a detailed history and physical examination. Special attention should be paid to the surrounding soft tissue and vascularity of the entire extremity. Radiography with multiple views including anteroposterior, lateral, and oblique is standard, although determination of radiographic nonunion has high inter-rater variability.[12] Multiple radiographic scoring systems have been developed to assess union more objectively in the upper extremity fractures, including distal radius[13] and humeral shaft;[14] however, none have yet been validated for the assessment of union in metacarpal or phalangeal fractures. There is limited data regarding the use of CT for evaluation of nonunions in the hand, and data are mixed for other fractures. Some studies suggested improvement in diagnostic accuracy with the use of CT scans, and others suggested no change.[15,16] CT certainly has a role in the assessment of complex fracture patterns and preoperative planning. It is our preference to obtain CT scans preoperatively for all nonunions in preparation for surgical intervention. If there is concern for infection as the cause of nonunion, MRI is the most sensitive tool; however it can be limited by artifact from existing hardware.[17] Laboratory testing including complete blood count, erythrocyte sedimentation rate, and C-reactive protein are useful in the assessment of possible infected nonunion, and calcium, vitamin D, and thyroid hormone levels may be helpful if there is concern for nutritional deficiency.[18]

NONUNIONS OF THE METACARPALS AND PHALANGES
Incidence of Nonunion

Nonunion of the metacarpals and phalanges occur very infrequently due to the ample vascular supply to the hand. Reported rates of metacarpal nonunion across all methods of treatment are between 0.45% and 1.5% in 2 large population-level studies.[19,20] Rates of phalangeal fracture nonunion are similarly low at approximately 0.7% across 148 fractures treated with a variety of methods including splinting, pinning, and internal fixation.[21] When nonunions do occur, they are most commonly a sequela of open fractures with a crush/avulsion mechanism but can also occur iatrogenically as a complication of operative treatment from vascular injury or inappropriate reduction and/or fixation. Injury and treatment factors that increase rates of nonunion include open injuries, multiple fractures, infection, soft tissue trauma with periosteal stripping, and vascular injury.[10,22,23] Patient systemic factors that increase rates of nonunion include diabetes, smoking or nicotine use, noncompliance with weight-bearing restrictions, neuropathy, and nutrition/metabolic factors.[20,24,25]

Incidence by Fixation Method

No large-scale studies comparing rates of nonunion with different fixation have been performed; thus, no technique has conclusively been demonstrated to have lower rates of nonunion. Kirschner wire (K-wire), intramedullary (IM) pins, and external fixators allow fracture opposition with minimal disruption of the soft tissue envelope and fracture vascularity. However, this fixation has less mechanical stability than other methods and does not allow for compression at the fracture site. Jupiter and colleagues reviewed 25 consecutive phalangeal and metacarpal delayed unions and found that the initial form of stabilization was K-wire fixation in 17 patients and closed reduction with plaster immobilization in 8.[26] In 6 of the 17 patients with K-wires, radiographs demonstrated distraction at the fracture site. Grundberg examined 27 metacarpal and phalangeal fractures treated with IM Steinmann pins, and found only 1 nonunion in a proximal phalanx which resolved with placement of a large diameter pin and bone graft.[27] External fixation has been hypothesized to carry a slightly higher risk of nonunion from inadvertent over-distraction of the bone fragments.[28] A retrospective cohort study by Ashmead and colleagues found a 90% union rate with external fixation of acute hand fractures.[29]

Plate and screw constructs allow compression and rigid fixation to promote direct bone healing. However, open reduction and internal fixation require some amount of periosteal stripping which compromises the vascularity, theoretically increasing the risk of atrophic nonunion. This theoretic risk is not borne out in several small case series or in our experience if judicious dissection and careful exposure techniques are used. O'Sullivan and colleagues found no nonunions with miniplate fixation of 36 metacarpals and 8 phalanges.[30] Similarly, Ouellette and Freeland treated 41 metacarpal and 27 phalangeal fractures with condylar plates and had no nonunions.[31] Similarly, Page and Stern analyzed 66 metacarpal and 39 phalangeal fractures treated with low-profile titanium Association of Osteosynthesis (AO) mini-fragment plates, with only 2 cases of nonunion (1 metacarpal, 1 phalangeal).[32] Finally, Fusetti and colleagues reported on 129 consecutive patients with 157 metacarpal fractures with open reduction and internal fixation with miniplates and found 12 cases with impaired fracture healing, with 6 delayed unions and 6 nonunions.[10] IM headless compression screw fixation of metacarpal and phalangeal fractures also provides compression across the fracture site and requires less disruption of the external vascularity of the fractured bone. Evidence for use of IM screws in nonunion is limited; however, 1 small case series by del Pinal and colleagues found 100% union of 21 phalangeal fractures managed by headless compression screw fixation.[33] When osteotomies were performed in the setting of malunion, a near 100% union rate was achieved when utilizing plate and screw fixation, or IM screws.[34–36] No cases series have described union rates with lag screw or IM nail fixation techniques.

It should be noted, that in the case of a distal phalanx tuft fracture where soft tissue approximation alone is usually sufficient to reduce bony fragments, fibrous union will result. Despite the persistent radiographic nonunion of the bony fragments, most patients have good to excellent clinical outcomes.[37–39]

TREATMENT OF NONUNION
Timing and Overall Strategy

If a nonunion is left untreated, patients will continue to have fracture site pain and impaired function of not only the involved digit but likely the entire hand. Moreover, prolonged immobilization will lead to stiffness that can be difficult to correct. Therefore, although there is variability in the timing criteria of delayed union and nonunion, some argue that operative intervention for delayed union or nonunion should happen no later than 4 months from injury.[26] The authors' preference is to allow mobilization at 3 to 4 months even in delayed unions to avoid stiffness in the fingers. If the patient does go on to a nonunion, surgical treatment is initiated no later than 6 months. When treating a nonunion, 4 key questions must be considered to help guide operative planning:

1. What was the initial fixation technique, and did this provide adequate stabilization?
2. Is infection present?
3. Is a bone gap present and if so, how large is the gap?
4. Is there a healthy, vascularized soft tissue envelope present?

Fracture Stabilization

If an infection or a bone gap is not present and there is a hypertrophic callus on the radiograph, then the most likely culprit for nonunion is a lack of stability at the fracture site. In these situations, a more stable fixation method is required. Those fractures initially treated with a splinting or other nonrigid interventions such as K-wires may benefit from a technique that utilizes a more stable construct and provides compression at the fracture site such as compression plating or, IM screws. It should be noted that IM screws differ from IM K-wires in their ability to provide more rigid fixation as well as potential compression across the fracture site.

Biomechanical studies in cadaver metacarpals have shown that techniques that provide compression (eg, plates, interfragmentary screws, and IM screws) to be superior to K-wires and IM nails in both bending and torsional strength.[40,41] Comparisons of plates and IM screws have conflicting evidence. One biomechanical study found that plate fixation, regardless of locking or compression capabilities, exhibited more stiffness and a higher load to failure rate than IM screws.[42] A separate study reported that IM screws provide equivalent stability compared to plate and screws when used for short oblique proximal phalanx fractures.[43] A third study compared IM screws, titanium plates, and K-wires for distal epiphyseal fractures of proximal phalanges and found that IM screws had significantly less displacement at the fracture site in torsional testing and were significantly more stable in bending testing. K-wires were significantly less stable than either plating or screw fixation.[44] Although the relative instability of K-wire fixation is not ideal in the setting of nonunion, there have been several cases of distal phalanx shaft nonunion treated successfully with crossed K-wires.[45,46] Interfragmentary and IM screws have also been used to successfully treat nonunions of the distal phalanx.[47,48] In the senior author's practice, plate fixation is the most commonly utilized technique when treating established nonunions in the metacarpals and phalanges, given the inherent rigidity and higher load to failure of other available options (**Figs. 3A–C–5A and B**).

Management of Infected Nonunion

Infection present at a fracture site will preclude callus formation or ossification regardless of the fixation stability. Infection must be surgically treated with thorough debridement and appropriate culture-directed antibiotics. Local delivery of antibiotics can be achieved with absorbable calcium sulfate beads and is commonly used in our practice with infected nonunions. Any involved hardware is likely colonized and will typically require explantation. External fixation can be used to stabilize septic nonunions when it is necessary to remove infected bone and colonized hardware.[29] Following aggressive debridement of infected soft tissue and bone, there is often a significant bone gap surrounded by fibrotic and poorly vascularized tissue bed. For these situations, the Masquelet technique can be successfully utilized to achieve union in phalanges and metacarpals.[49] This is a 2-step procedure involving initial debridement and placement of an antibiotic spacer, followed by a second stage in which the vascularized membrane is peeled back, and the cement spacer is replaced with cancellous bone graft (**Fig. 6A–C**). The second stage is optimally performed at 4 to 8 weeks after the initial surgery for the most optimal concentration of growth factors. Moris and colleagues retrospectively evaluated 18 patients using the Masquelet technique in fractures of the metacarpals (8 cases) and phalanges (10 cases) and demonstrated union by 4 months in 16 of 18 patients with a mean 145° of total active digital motion.[50] The Masquelet technique has been described to achieve union in bone gaps up to 24 cm in various long bones throughout the body.[51]

Management of Bone Gaps

Aseptic nonunions will also require debridement of devascularized or poor-quality bone and decortication of any pseudoarthrosis back to healthy bleeding bone. Compression of the freshly debrided bone edges without grafting is a theoretic treatment option; however, the shortening will lead to a weakness of grip due to the resulting decreased length of the musculotendinous unit, as well as extensor lag. There is an estimated 7° of extensor lag for every 2 mm of metacarpal shortening.[52] Excessive shortening of the metacarpals is limited by the relatively immobile carpometacarpal joints and transverse intermetacarpal ligaments. Proximal phalangeal shortening produces anywhere from 2.5° to 12° of extension lag for every millimeter of shortening.[53,54]

Given these drawbacks, the recommended treatment of small to moderate-sized bone gaps consists of corticocancellous or cancellous bone grafting with stable fixation.[55–57] Corticocancellous grafting can be helpful in treating large intercalary defects due to its ability to provide better structural support than cancellous bone grafts. Corticocancellous grafts also allow the use of compressive fixation techniques that further increase stability and bony apposition and possibly allow earlier initiation of rehabilitation.[58] Common donor sites for bone graft

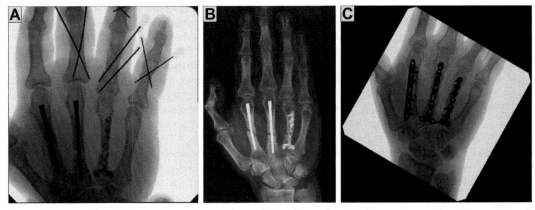

Fig. 3. Treatment of multiple metacarpal nonunions with revision plate fixation and cancellous bone autograft. This patient initially presented with multiple open fractures of the metacarpals and phalanges. (*A*) Intraoperative radiograph after K-wire fixation of the phalangeal fractures, retrograde intramedullary screw placement for second and third metacarpal shaft fractures, and plate fixation for a fourth metacarpal shaft fracture. (*B*) The patient unfortunately discontinued splinting against medical advice and was in an altercation soon after fixation. He ultimately went on to nonunion of all metacarpal fractures, with 1 bent screw and a fractured plate. (*C*) Intraoperative radiograph after intramedullary screw and plate removal, cancellous bone autograft, and subsequent fixation with larger 2.4-mm plates. Union was ultimately achieved in all 3 metacarpals.

include the distal radius, olecranon, iliac crest, and proximal tibia.

Moderate-sized bone gaps (<2–3 cm) can be treated successfully with nonvascularized bone grafting. However, for defects larger than 3 cm, nonvascularized bone grafting may result in incomplete healing.[59,60] Vascularized bone grafts should be considered in these scenarios. The most common vascularized bone grafts include the fibula based on branches of the peroneal artery, the medial femoral condyle based on the descending genicular artery, and iliac crest based on deep circumflex iliac artery. The fibula is rarely utilized except in cases of very large bone gaps in the metacarpals (**Fig. 7**), whereas the medial femoral condyle is more versatile for use in the hand and carpus, given the ability to tailor this into a wider array of bone graft sizes while maintaining excellent vascularity.

Restoration of Vascularity and Soft Tissue

The presence of a well-vascularized soft tissue envelope is critical to bony healing in patients with open fractures and high-energy trauma. There are many flap options (local, regional, and free) that can provide coverage for metacarpal and phalangeal soft tissue defects. Osteocutaneous radial forearm and medial femoral condyle flaps can provide both soft tissue coverage and vascularized bone grafts for large soft tissue and bone defects.[61,62] Periosteal flaps have been shown to

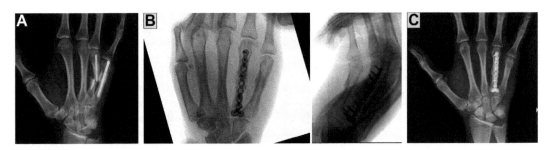

Fig. 4. Treatment of metacarpal nonunion with revision plate fixation and cancellous bone autograft. This patient initially presented with fourth and fifth metacarpal shaft fractures which were treated with retrograde IM screws at an outside facility. (*A*) At time of initial evaluation in our clinic he had sustained hardware failure and nonunion of the fourth metacarpal after a physical altercation. (*B*) Intraoperative radiograph after removal of the intramedullary screw from the healed fifth metacarpal and fractured hardware from the fourth metacarpal. The fourth metacarpal was then treated with plate fixation and distal radius cancellous autograft. (*C*) Postoperative radiographs at 12 weeks that showing union of the fourth metacarpal.

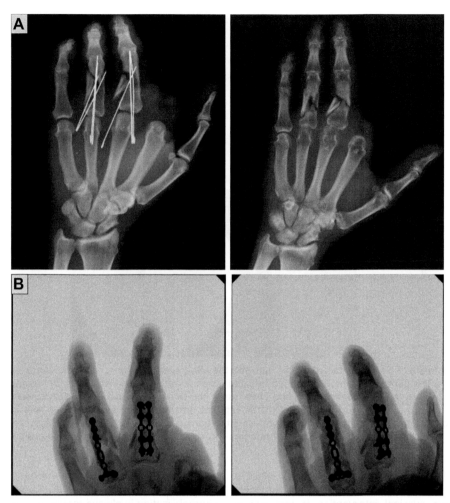

Fig. 5. Treatment of phalangeal nonunion with revision plate fixation and cancellous bone autograft. This patient presented with nonunion of his long and ring finger proximal phalanges secondary to a significant crush injury. (*A*) He initially underwent revision amputation of his index finger, as well as fixation and revascularization of his middle and ring fingers. Pins were maintained for 6 weeks before removal, unfortunately the patient went on to nonunion of both proximal phalanges. (*B*) The patient underwent debridement of his fractures with cancellous autografting and plate fixation and ultimately achieved union of his fractures.

promote bone healing in other parts of the upper extremity.[63] These can be harvested locally or distantly from the medial femoral condyle.

Adjunct Treatments

Electromagnetic field stimulation is used as an adjunct method to promote bone healing in both acute fractures and delayed unions or nonunions. High-quality evidence focusing on nonunion is limited; however, several small randomized, sham-controlled trials demonstrate increased union rates with active treatment.[64–67] These studies were performed in tibial or other long-bone nonunion. There are no randomized trials that target metacarpal or phalangeal fractures.

One nonrandomized, retrospective cohort study evaluating delayed union of phalangeal fractures found increased radiographic density of healing fractures with bone stimulation, but did not discuss overall union rates.[68] It is the senior author's preference to use bone stimulation as an adjunct on all nonunions after surgical intervention.

Postoperative Care

Postoperative care after nonunion repair must be tailored to the individual patient, type of bone graft, and rigidity of the chosen fixation. Significant tendon adhesions and adjacent joint stiffness are common in patients with metacarpal and phalangeal nonunions due to prolonged immobilization

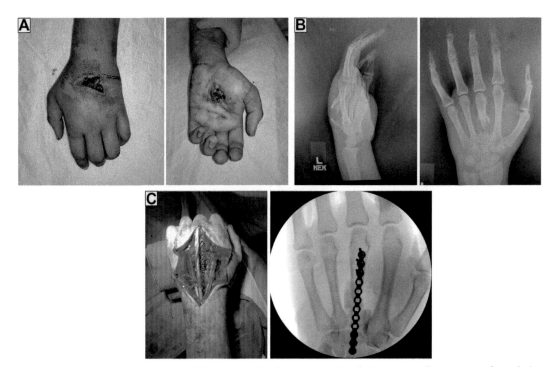

Fig. 6. Treatment of a large metacarpal bone gap with the Masquelet technique, cancellous autograft, and plate fixation. (*A*) This patient presented with a self-inflicted gunshot wound to the left hand. (*B*) Preoperative radiographs showing significant comminution and bone loss of the third metacarpal shaft. (*C*) A dorsal bridge plate was used from the distal third metacarpal to the capitate proximally, and the bone gap was initially filled with antibiotic impregnated bone cement. In this case the bone gap was treated using the Masquelet technique with distal radius cancellous bone grafting, although a corticocancellous block is also a good option in this case.

to allow for bone healing. Optimizing the passive range of motion of the surrounding joints with therapy before surgical intervention is ideal when possible. Flexor or extensor tenolysis, as well as joint capsulotomy can be performed at the time of nonunion repair. However, some period of immobilization is always required postoperatively, and thus tendon adhesions and joint stiffness may

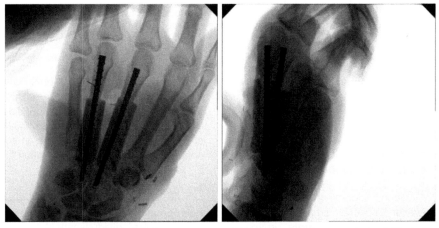

Fig. 7. Treatment of a combined multiple large metacarpal bone gaps with a vascularized fibula flap. Another option for treating significant bone gaps in the metacarpals is free vascularized bone grafts. Although this is not a case of nonunion, it illustrates a double-barrel vascularized fibula with a skin paddle used to reconstruct a third and fourth metacarpal combined bone and soft tissue defect (in this case following osteosarcoma resection). Intramedullary compression screws were utilized for fixation.

recur. It is the authors' preference to advise all patients that they may need another secondary surgery after bony union has been achieved to mobilize the surrounding tendons and joints to achieve their desired function. Our preference is to obtain CT scans routinely at 3 months after surgery to evaluate bony healing and trabecular bridging.

SUMMARY

Nonunion of the metacarpals and phalanges are uncommon but can have a devastating effect on hand function when not appropriately treated. Nonunions typically occur due to inadequate reduction and stabilization of the fracture fragments, inadequate blood supply, or infection. Successful treatment of nonunion requires that all these factors are addressed. Fractures that were initially treated with less stable constructs (splinting, K-wires, IM nails) will benefit from more stable fixation (plates, interfragmentary screws, and IM compression screws). Well-vascularized soft tissue may be brought in through local flaps or free tissue transfer. Infection should be thoroughly debrided and treated with culture-directed antibiotics. Bone gaps can be addressed with cancellous autograft, corticocancellous autograft, or vascularized bone grafts. When larger bone gaps are present, the Masquelet technique and vascularized bone grafting should be utilized.

CLINICS CARE POINTS

- Hypertrophic nonunions are best treated with more stable fixation methods (plates, interfragmentary screws, and IM compression screws).
- Restoration of healthy well-vascularized soft tissue through local or free flaps can be imperative for bone healing in the setting of significant soft tissue injury with compromised blood supply to the bone.
- Infection must be eradicated through aggressive debridement followed by local and systemic antibiotics prior to definitive fixation.
- Bone gaps less than 3 cm can be addressed effectively with cancellous and corticocancellous bone graft in conjunction with fixation.
- Bone gaps greater than 3 cm should be addressed with either the Masquelet technique or vascularized bone grafts.
- Bone stimulation is a useful adjunct following surgical treatment of nonunions.

DISCLOSURE

Commercial and financial: Trimed Ortho Inc, Speaker's Bureau.

REFERENCES

1. Chung KC, Spilson SV. The frequency and epidemiology of hand and forearm fractures in the United States. J Hand Surg 2001;26(5):908–15.
2. Marsell R, Einhorn TA. The biology of fracture healing. Injury 2011;42(6):551–5.
3. Bahney CS, Zondervan RL, Allison P, et al. Cellular biology of fracture healing. J Orthop Res 2019; 37(1):35–50.
4. Uysal AC, Alagoz MS, TÜCcar E, SensÖZ Ö. Vascular Anatomy of the Metacarpal Bones and the Interosseous Muscles. Lippincott Williams & Wilkins; 63-68.
5. Strauch B, de Moura W. Arterial system of the fingers. J Hand Surg 1990;15(1):148–54.
6. Nicholson JA, Makaram N, Simpson A, et al. Fracture nonunion in long bones: A literature review of risk factors and surgical management. Injury 2021; 52(Suppl 2). https://doi.org/10.1016/j.injury.2020. 11.029. S3-S11.
7. Simpson AHRW, Robiati L, Jalal MMK, et al. Nonunion: Indications for external fixation. Injury 2019; 50(Suppl 1):S73–8.
8. Chen S, Wei F-c, Chen H-c, et al. Miniature plates and screws in acute complex hand injury. J Trauma 1994; 37(2):237–42.
9. Beris A, Soucacos P. Delayed union and nonunion: treatment modalities. In: Bruser P, Gilbert A, editors. Finger bone and joint injuries. Martin Dunitz; 1999. p. 113–9.
10. Fusetti C, Meyer H, Borisch N, et al. Complications of Plate Fixation in Metacarpal Fractures. J Trauma Inj Infect Crit Care 2002;52(3):535–9.
11. Smith FL, Rider DL. A study of the healing of one hundred consecutive phalangeal fractures. J Bone Jt Surg Am Vol 1935;17:91–109.
12. Corrales L, Morshed S, Bhandari M, et al. Variability in the assessment of fracture-healing in orthopaedic trauma studies. J Bone Jt Surg Am Vol 2008;90(9): 1862–8.
13. Patel SPMD, Anthony S, Zurakowski DP, et al. Radiographic scoring system to evaluate union of distal radius fractures. J Hand Surg 2014;39(8):1471–9.
14. Oliver WM, Smith TJ, Nicholson JA, et al. The Radiographic Union Score for HUmeral fractures (RUSHU) predicts humeral shaft nonunion. Journal of Bone and Joint Surgery British 2019;101-B(10):1300–6.
15. Bhattacharyya T, Bouchard K, Phadke A, et al. The accuracy of computed tomography for the diagnosis of tibial nonunion. J Bone Jt Surg Am Vol 2006;88(4):692–7.

16. Kleinlugtenbelt YV, Scholtes VAB, Toor J, et al. Does computed tomography change our observation and management of fracture non-unions? Archives of Bone And Joint Surgery 2016;4(4):337–42.

17. Nicholson JA, Yapp LZ, Keating JF, et al. Monitoring of fracture healing. Update on current and future imaging modalities to predict union. Injury 2021;52:S29–34.

18. Stucken C, Olszewski D, Creevy W, et al. Preoperative diagnosis of infection in patients with nonunions. J Bone Jt Surg Am Vol 2013;95(15):1409–12.

19. Hayes DS, Cush C, El Koussaify J, et al. Defining nonunion for metacarpal fractures: a systematic review. Journal of Hand Surgery Global Online 2023. https://doi.org/10.1016/j.jhsg.2023.04.014.

20. Zura R, Xiong Z, Einhorn T, et al. Epidemiology of fracture nonunion in 18 human bones. JAMA Surgery 2016;151(11):e162775.

21. Barton NJ. Fractures of the shafts of the phalanges of the hand. Hand 1979;11(2):119–33.

22. Stern PJ, Wieser MJ, Reilly DG. Complications of plate fixation in the hand skeleton. Clin Orthop Relat Res 1987;214(214):59–65.

23. Van Oosterom FJT, Brete GJV, Ozdemir C, et al. Treatment of phalangeal fractures in severely injured hands. Journal of Hand Surgery, British volume 2001;26(2):108–11.

24. Gaston MS, Simpson AHRW. Inhibition of fracture healing. Journal of Bone and Joint Surgery British 2007;89(12):1553–60.

25. Zura R, Mehta S, Della Rocca GJ, et al. Biological Risk Factors for Nonunion of Bone Fracture. JBJS Rev. Jan 05 2016;4(1). https://doi.org/10.2106/JBJS.RVW.O.00008.

26. Jupiter JB, Koniuch MP, Smith RJ. The management of delayed union and nonunion of the metacarpals and phalanges. J Hand Surg 1985;10(4):457–66.

27. Grundberg AB. Intramedullary fixation for fractures of the hand. Journal of Hand Surgery (American ed) 1981;6(6):568–73.

28. Hastings H. Open fractures and those with soft tissue damage: treatment by external fixation. In: Barton N, editor. Fractures of the hand and wrist. Churchill Livingstone; 1988. p. 145–72.

29. Ashmead D, Rothkopf DM, Walton RL, et al. Treatment of hand injuries by external fixation. J Hand Surg 1992;17(5):956–64.

30. O'Sullivan ST, Limantzakis G, Kay SPJ. The role of low-profile titanium miniplates in emergency and elective hand surgery. Journal of Hand Surgery, British volume 1999;24(3):347–9.

31. Ouellette EA, Freeland AE. Use of the minicondylar plate in metacarpal and phalangeal fractures. Clin Orthop Relat Res 1996;327(327):38–46.

32. Page SM, Stern PJ. Complications and range of motion following plate fixation of metacarpal and phalangeal fractures. Journal of Hand Surgery (American ed) 1998;23(5):827–32.

33. del Piñal FMDP, Moraleda EMD, Rúas JSMD, et al. Minimally invasive fixation of fractures of the phalanges and metacarpals with intramedullary cannulated headless compression screws. J Hand Surg 2015;40(4):692–700.

34. Thurston AJ. Pivot osteotomy for the correction of malunion of metacarpal neck fractures. Journal of Hand Surgery, British volume 1992;17(5):580–2.

35. Gollamudi S, Jones WA. Corrective osteotomy of malunited fractures of phalanges and metacarpals. Journal of Hand Surgery, British volume 2000;25(5):439–41.

36. Lucas GL, Pfeiffer CM. Osteotomy of the metacarpals and phalanges stabilized by AO plates and screws. Ann Hand Surg 1989;8(1):30–8.

37. Schneider LH. Fractures of the Distal Phalanx. Hand Clin 2023;4(3):537–47.

38. Weeks PM. Acute bone and joint injuries of the Hand and wrist: a clinical guide to management. Mosby; 1981.

39. Lucas G, Pfeiffer C. Osteotomy of the metacarpals and phalanges. In: Weeks P, editor. Acute Bone and joint Injuries of the Hand and wrist. CV Mosby; 1981. p. 547.

40. Curtis BD, Fajolu O, Ruff ME, et al. Fixation of metacarpal shaft fractures: biomechanical comparison of intramedullary nail crossed k-wires and plate-screw constructs. Orthop Surg 2015;7(3):256–60.

41. Oh JR, Kim DS, Yeom JS, et al. A comparative study of tensile strength of three operative fixation techniques for metacarpal shaft fractures in adults: a cadaver study. Clin Orthop Surg 2019;11(1):120–5.

42. Melamed E, Hinds RM, Gottschalk MB, et al. Comparison of dorsal plate fixation versus intramedullary headless screw fixation of unstable metacarpal shaft fractures. Hand (New York, NY) 2016;11(4):421–6.

43. Miles MR, Krul KP, Abbasi P, et al. Minimally invasive intramedullary screw versus plate fixation for proximal phalanx fractures: a biomechanical study. Journal of Hand Surgery (American ed) 2021;46(6):518.e1.

44. Rausch V, Harbrecht A, Kahmann SL, et al. Osteosynthesis of phalangeal fractures: biomechanical comparison of kirschner wires, plates, and compression screws. Journal of Hand Surgery (American ed) 2020;45(10):987.e1–8.

45. Read L. Non-union in a fracture of the shaft of the distal phalanx. Hand 1982;14(1):85–8.

46. Wray RC, Glunk R. Treatment of Delayed Union, Nonunion, and Malunion of the Phalanges of the Hand. Ann Plast Surg 1988;21(5):498.

47. Chim H, Teoh LC, Yong FC. Open reduction and interfragmentary screw fixation for symptomatic nonunion of distal phalangeal fractures. Journal of Hand Surgery, European Volume 2008;33(1):71–6.

48. Meijs CMEM, Verhofstad MHJ. Symptomatic nonunion of a distal phalanx fracture: treatment with a percutaneous compression screw. J Hand Surg 2009;34(6):1127–9.

49. Pruzansky M, Lee Y, Pruzansky J. Masquelet technique for phalangeal reconstruction and osteomyelitis. Tech Hand Up Extrem Surg 2020;25(1):52–5.

50. Moris V, Loisel F, Cheval D, et al. Functional and radiographic evaluation of the treatment of traumatic bone loss of the hand using the Masquelet technique. Hand Surgery and Rehabilitation 2016; 35(2):114–21.

51. Masquelet ACMD, Begue TMD. The Concept of Induced Membrane for Reconstruction of Long Bone Defects. Orthop Clin N Am 2010;41(1):27–37.

52. Strauch RJ, Rosenwasser MP, Lunt JG. Metacarpal shaft fractures: The effect of shortening on the extensor tendon mechanism. Journal of Hand Surgery (American ed) 1998;23(3):519–23.

53. Vahey JW, Vegas L, Wegner DA, et al. Effect of proximal phalangeal fracture deformity on extensor tendon function. Journal of Hand Surgery (American ed) 1998;23(4):673–81.

54. Beekman RA, Abbot AE, Taylor NL, et al. Extensor mechanism slide for the treatment of proximal interphalangeal joint extension lag: An anatomic study. J Hand Surg 2004;29(6):1063–8.

55. Itoh Y, Uchinishi K, Oka Y. Treatment of pseudoarthrosis of the distal phalanx with the palmar midline approach. J Hand Surg 1983;8(1):80–4.

56. Freeland AE, Jabaley ME, Hughes JL. Stable Fixation of the Hand and Wrist. Springer; 1986.

57. Heim U. The treatment of nonunion in bones of the hand. In: Chapchal G, editor. Pseudarthroses and their treatment. Georg Thieme; 1979. p. 168–9.

58. Babushkina A, Edwards S. Corticocancellous Olecranon Autograft for Metacarpal Defect Reconstruction: A Case Report. Hand (New York, NY) 2012; 7(4):457–60.

59. Hertel R, Gerber A, Schlegel U, et al. Cancellous bone graft for skeletal reconstruction. Muscular versus periosteal bed–preliminary report. Injury 1994;25(Suppl 1):A59–70.

60. Weiland AJ, Phillips TW, Randolph MA. Bone grafts: a radiologic, histologic, and biomechanical model comparing autografts, allografts, and free vascularized bone grafts. Plast Reconstr Surg (1963) 1984; 74(3):368–79.

61. Yajima H, Tamai S, Yamauchi T, et al. Osteocutaneous radial forearm flap for hand reconstruction. J Hand Surg Am 1999;24(3):594–603.

62. Rodriguez JR, Chan JKK, Huang R-W, et al. Free Medial Femoral Condyle Flap for Phalangeal and Metacarpal Bone Reconstruction. J Plast Reconstr Aesthetic Surg 2022;75(12):4379–92.

63. Barrera-Ochoa S, Sapage R, Alabau-Rodriguez S, et al. Vascularized Ulnar Periosteal Pedicled Flap for Upper Extremity Reconstruction in Adults: A Prospective Case Series of 11 Patients. The Journal of hand surgery (American ed) 2022;47(1):86.e11. https://doi.org/10.1016/j.jhsa.2021.02.027.

64. Sharrard WJ. A double-blind trial of pulsed electromagnetic fields for delayed union of tibial fractures. J Bone Joint Surg Br 1990;72(3):347–55.

65. Scott G, King JB. A prospective, double-blind trial of electrical capacitive coupling in the treatment of non-union of long bones. J Bone Joint Surg Am 1994;76(6):820–6.

66. Simonis RB, Parnell EJ, Ray PS, et al. Electrical treatment of tibial non-union: a prospective, randomised, double-blind trial. Injury 2003;34(5):357–62.

67. Shi HF, Xiong J, Chen YX, et al. Early application of pulsed electromagnetic field in the treatment of postoperative delayed union of long-bone fractures: a prospective randomized controlled study. BMC Musculoskelet Disord 2013;14:35.

68. De Francesco F, Gravina P, Varagona S, et al. Biophysical Stimulation in Delayed Fracture Healing of Hand Phalanx: A Radiographic Evaluation. Biomedicines 2022;10(10). https://doi.org/10.3390/biomedicines 10102519.

Metacarpal and Phalangeal Malunions-Is It all About the Rotation?

Jeremy E. Raducha, MD, Warren C. Hammert, MD*

KEYWORDS

• Metacarpal • Phalanx • Malunion • Deformity • Osteotomy

KEY POINTS

- Metacarpal and phalangeal malunions are best prevented, but when they occur, early intervention allows easier correction.
- Malunion corrections should be considered with severe angulation or malrotation resulting in finger overlap or impingement, intra-articular deformities, and patient functional deficits.
- There are many surgical options available for finger osteotomies with similar outcomes, so the treatment course can be dictated by injury pattern, concurrent injuries, and surgeon preference.
- Malunion can occur as deformities in single plane or multiplanes and the treatment involves correction of deformities in all planes.
- Outcomes of surgical correction are good, but patients should be counseled that their finger will likely not regain pre-injury function or cosmesis.

INTRODUCTION

Phalanx and metacarpal fractures are common, accounting for approximately 10% of all fractures, more than 50% of hand fractures, and 1% of emergency department visits in the United States.[1–5] They occur most commonly in younger patients, males, and are often related to athletic events.[1,6,7] Given the hand's excellent vascularity and the common demographics, these fractures tend to heal well with callus usually visible in 4 to 6 weeks and low rates of non-union.[1] The most common bony complication of phalanx and metacarpal fractures is malunion.[5,8] Phalanx and metacarpal malunions can essentially be broken down into 4 categories of deformity: angular, rotational, intra-articular, and multiplanar. The functional impact of the malunion varies by location, type, severity, chronicity, and patient functional demand.[9] Significant extra-articular malunions can cause crossing over of the digits, pain due to joint distortion, decreased grip strength, or tendon and muscle imbalance. Intra-articular malunions can lead to synovitis and post-traumatic arthritis.[9] Concomitant soft tissue injuries can further complicate function, particularly flexor and extensor tendon adhesions and joint stiffness. Throughout this manuscript, we will discuss the anatomic and biomechanical reasoning behind the different types of malunions, the functional impact of each deformity, and the treatment options available.

Relevant Anatomy/Biomechanics

It is important to understand ligamentous and tendonous attachments on the metacarpals and phalanges as they contribute to fracture deformities. The 4 non-thumb metacarpals are connected via the strong deep transverse intermetacarpal ligament.[1] This helps maintain length in isolated metacarpal fractures and prevents >3 to 4 mm of shortening in central digits.[4] The border metacarpals, however, are more susceptible to shortening as they only have the intermetacarpal ligament on

Department of Orthopaedic Surgery, Hand, Upper Extremity and Microsurgery, Duke University Medical Center, Durham, NC 27710, USA
* Corresponding author.
E-mail address: warren.hammert@duke.edu

Hand Clin 40 (2024) 141–149
https://doi.org/10.1016/j.hcl.2023.08.005

one side. It is important to recognize that intermeta-carpal ligaments can limit the amount of distal correction of rotational deformities, particularly if trying to correct a phalangeal malunion in the metacarpal. The carpometacarpal joints of the index and middle finger are more rigid due to their bony and ligamentous anatomy.[1] As such, patients are less able to compensate for malunion in these metacarpals than they are in the thumb, ring, and small fingers, with more mobile carpometacarpal joints.

Metacarpal fracture deformity is affected by the natural apex dorsal curve of the metacarpal shaft as well as the tendinous attachments. When the metacarpal shaft is fractured, the interosseous muscles' contracture applies a volar force in the distal fragment, which leads to apex dorsal fracture deformities.[4,6,8] This deformity also causes an effective shortening of the metacarpal and digit overall.

Each phalanx is subject to different fracture deforming forces due to its tendinous insertions. The interosseous and lumbrical tendon complex have insertions onto the proximal phalanx base and are the primary metacarpophalangeal (MP) joint flexors. The central slip inserts on the dorsal base of the middle phalanx exerting an extension force, in conjunction with the remaining extensor complex, at the proximal interphalangeal (PIP) joint and distal. Due to these forces, proximal phalanx fractures commonly result in apex volar deformity due to flexion of the proximal fragment and extension of the distal fragment.[1] (**Fig. 1**) In the middle phalanx, the flexor digitorum superficialis (FDS) insertion exerts a powerful flexion force and is balanced by the extensor complex. These fractures have a less predictable deformity, as it depends on the fracture location relative to the broad FDS insertion on the volar middle phalanx diaphysis. Extra-articular fractures proximal to the FDS insertion result in apex dorsal angulation as the distal fragment is pulled into flexion by the FDS while the proximal fragment is extended by the central slip. In fractures distal to the FDS insertion, apex volar angulation is more common as the FDS now becomes a flexor of the proximal fragment, while the distal fragment extends with the lateral bands/terminal tendon.[4]

Clinical Effect of Malunion

Strauch and colleagues have shown in a cadaver model that 2 mm of metacarpal shortening results in a 7° extensor lag at the MP joint and an 8% loss of grip strength.[10] Also, the shortening of the intrinsic muscles with >30° of apex dorsal angulation affects the force tension relationship and contributes to the loss of grip strength.[4] Metacarpal

angulation >30° can also result in loss of prominence of the metacarpal head, compensatory hyperextension at the metacarpophalangeal joint, and a palpable bony deformity.[4,6] However, the MP joints typically hyperextend approximately 10° and the slight loss of intrinsic muscle force usually compensates with time, so 3 to 5 mm of metacarpal shortening is usually well tolerated.[5,6,8] Coronal plane angulation in the metacarpals is not as common due to the previously described soft tissue attachments but it is usually well tolerated as long as it does not cause impingement.[1,4] This is especially true in border digits and the thumb metacarpal due to their greater range of motion. This is supported by a retrospective cohort study comparing outcomes in non-operative versus operative management of small finger metacarpal shaft and neck fractures. There were no differences in metacarpal neck fracture outcomes with or without surgery, even with >40° of angulation, and Disabilities of the Arm, Shoulder, and Hand (DASH) and aesthetic outcome scores were better in the non-operative metacarpal shaft fracture group at any level of residual angulation.[11]

While angulation and shortening are well tolerated in metacarpal shaft malunions, rotation is not. Each degree of metacarpal rotation can result in 5° of rotation at the fingertip. Therefore, 10° of rotation can result in 2 cm of finger overlap.[4,6,12] This overlap can inhibit range of motion of the effected digit as well as the adjacent digit, and interfere with activities. For this reason, it is important to pay close attention to finger rotation when deciding on the course of treatment.

Phalanx fracture malunion can result in both angular and rotational deformity. Proximal phalanx apex volar angulation >15° to 25° shortens the extensor mechanism, resulting in decreased motion.[4,13,14] Shortening up to 6 mm may be well tolerated due to the natural viscoelastic properties of the extensor mechanism before the sagittal bands tighten. However, for anything greater than this, every 1 mm of shortening results in an average of 12° of extensor lag at the PIP joint. The PIP joint is less able to compensate for this lag than the MP joint.[14] In addition, this can result in compensatory hyperextension at the distal interphalangeal (DIP) joint with decreased DIP range of motion. Chronic PIP extensor lag can also result in dorsal capsule and central slip attenuation, leading to a boutonniere deformity.[15] This recurvatum deformity can also angulate the floor of the flexor tendon sheath, leading to irritation with tendon gliding or potentially cause a pseudoclaw deformity.[4,13] Coronal angulation and rotation at proximal or middle phalanx fractures can also cause

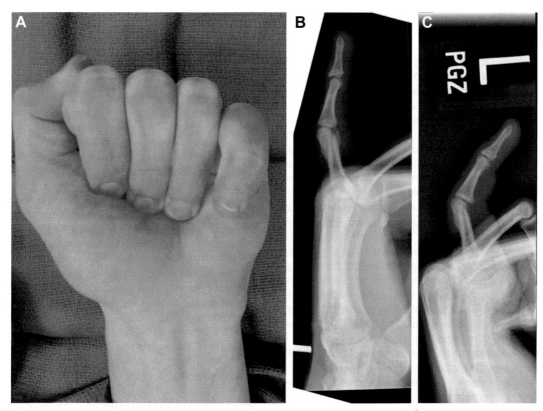

Fig. 1. Proximal phalanx apex volar malunion of the small finger. This resulted in flexion block but may be well tolerated. (A) Clinical photo, (B, C) oblique and lateral radiographs.

scissoring with overlap of the fingers, which can again affect function. Extra-articular fractures of the distal phalanx typically do not result in problematic malunion, and although fibrous non-union is relatively common, it is typically stable and asymptomatic.[1]

PRE-OPERATIVE EVALUATION AND PLANNING

When assessing phalanx and metacarpal fracture malunions for potential corrective surgery, it is important to remember that not all radiographic malunions have clinical deformities or functional deficits. A detailed history should be obtained to determine the timing of the initial injury, the patient's functional limitations with their deformity, and their goals for recovery. In addition to clinical deformity, the surgeon needs to assess for function of the flexor and extensor tendons, presence or absence of infection, nerve function, finger perfusion, digit range of motion, bony healing, quality of the soft tissues for another operation, and if any additional surgical interventions are indicated.[4,9] When assessing clinical deformity, careful assessment of digit rotation is paramount. The

fingernails should be aligned in both full flexion and full extension. With full composite flexion, all fingers should point toward the scaphoid tubercle. There should also not be any cross over or convergence.[7] Many patients can adjust to small deformities, and surgical correction is imperfect. Although function is generally improved with surgical correction, patients rarely return to pre-injury function, and we should be cautious when considering surgical intervention purely for cosmetic reasons.

For phalanx fractures, finger-specific radiographs with posterior to anterior (PA), oblique, and lateral views of the digit can help to fully assess the fracture deformity and articular alignment.[4,6] Metacarpal fractures are best assessed with 3-view radiographs (PA, oblique, and lateral) of the hand, with the oblique view obtained dictated by which metacarpal is involved. A 10° to 15° pronated view can demonstrate the second and third metacarpals while a 10° to 15° supinated view can better show the fourth and fifth metacarpals.[6] If the thumb is involved, a Robert's view should also be obtained in addition to a true lateral of the thumb.[16] Computed tomography (CT) scans can sometimes be helpful to rule out non-union, assess intra-articular deformity, and assist for preparation for a 3-dimensional (3D)-printed osteotomy guide, but it is not necessary in all cases.

There are numerous definitions of what is considered "acceptable" fracture alignment,[4–6,9] with some general consensus found in **Table 1**. Overall, the authors feel this decision should be based on the clinical deformity and the patient's functional deficits in a shared decision-making manner. Once the decision is made to proceed with operative intervention, range of motion as well as intrinsic and extrinsic strength should be maximized preoperatively.

The timing of surgical intervention is dictated by the time since injury, type of malunion, and the soft tissue considerations. If the soft tissues are amenable, extra-articular malunions are ideally operated on early (within 6–10 weeks post-injury) to allow osteoclasis through the soft callus at the original fracture site. If this early intervention is not feasible or the patient presents late, it is preferable to wait until > 3 months from injury, to allow the patient to maximize motion and determine if the malunion truly causes a functional deficit, as the fracture callus has already matured and a new osteotomy cut will be required.[4,9] Intra-articular osteotomies should be corrected as soon as possible to allow osteoclasis through the prior fracture site. However, if the patient presents greater than 10 weeks after injury, it may be better to consider an alternative treatment such as arthrodesis or arthroplasty as correcting late intra-articular malunions can be very difficult and fraught with complications.[9]

SURGICAL OPTIONS

In general, prevention of malunion is the best option, but if you cannot avoid them, various surgical methods have been described based on the deformity present. They can be broken down into categories based on the deformity correction.

Rotational Deformities

Correction of rotational deformity is a common reason for operative intervention, as scissoring and finger overlap can be quite disabling. When the malunion is in the metacarpal bone, the osteotomy is performed at the site of the original metacarpal fracture.[4,8] However, there is more controversy for phalanx malunions. There are proponents of performing the osteotomy though the metacarpal[17–23] and others promoting correction through the phalanx itself.[4,9,24,25] Osteotomies performed through the metacarpal for phalanx malunions allow for correction outside of the zone of injury, allowing for an easier dissection, as well as a lower risk of tendon adhesions compared to operations involving the phalanx.[4,8] However, while these osteotomies correct the overall finger rotation, they do not truly correct the malunion and can create a more clinically complex deformity. The correction obtained through the metacarpal is also limited by the deep transverse intermetacarpal ligaments. A cadaver study demonstrated the maximal rotation to be 19° in the index, middle, and ring fingers and 30° in the small finger when transverse osteotomies were performed through the metacarpal bases.[26] Osteotomies within the phalanx have the benefit of being at the site of malunion and can allow for multiplanar corrections. They also allow for concomitant tenolysis and capsulotomy procedures through the same incision if needed. However, there is a higher risk of post-operative tendon adhesions and subsequent stiffness.[4,9]

The step-cut osteotomy has been described in the literature for correction of rotational deformities.[17,18,23] It is most commonly performed in the metacarpal but can also be performed in the proximal phalanx (**Fig. 2**) to correct more distal rotational malunions. Two hemi-transverse cuts are made in the bone, approximately 2 to 3 cm apart. The 2 cuts are then connected with a longitudinal dorsal wedge cut, sized depending on the

Deformity	Fingers		Thumb	Metacarpal
	Proximal Phalanx	Middle Phalanx	Proximal phalanx	
Coronal	>10°	>15°	>15°	
Sagittal	>20°		>20°	>30°
Rotation	>15°	>20°		>10°
Pronation			>40°	
Supination			>15°	
Intra-articular	>2 mm	>2 mm	>2 mm	>2 mm
Shortening	>6 mm	>6 mm	>6 mm	>6 mm

Table 1
Suggested surgical cut-offs for malunion correction

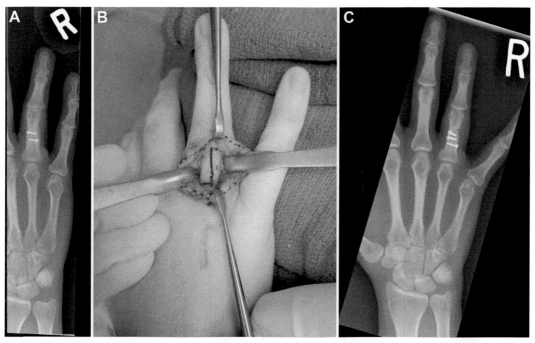

Fig. 2. Example of step-cut rotational osteotomy on a proximal phalanx. (*A*) Pre-operative radiograph following original open reduction and internal fixation (ORIF) with rotational deformity. (*B*) Planned osteotomy cuts. (*C*) Post-operative radiograph with mini lag screw fixation.

amount of rotation correction needed, to complete the step cut design (**Fig. 3**). Every 1° of metacarpal correction provides 0.7° of phalangeal rotation correction, for example, 2 mm of resection achieves a 20° or 2 cm correction at the fingertip. The third longitudinal cut is only performed through the dorsal cortex to allow the volar cortex to be broken when the 2 dorsal bone ends are reduced with a pointed reduction clamp. This maneuver cracks the volar cortex, instead of losing bone with a saw cut, and maintains the volar periosteum to improve stability. The step cut is then fixed with two or three 1.5 mm or 2.0 mm screws (**Fig. 4**). Patients are typically allowed to start early active range of motion.[17] This technique has the benefit of affording precise intra-operative control at the osteotomy site, a large surface area for bony healing and rigid fixation for early digital motion, as well as avoiding prominent hardware by using lag screws only and no plating. This technique is limited to correction of rotational deformities only.

Transverse osteotomies can be performed directly at the malunion site or through the proximal metaphysis. The digit is then rotated at the

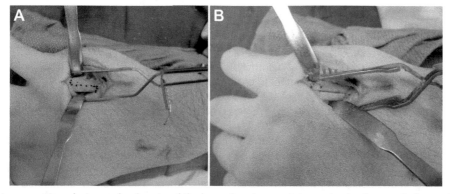

Fig. 3. Intra-operative photographs showing (*A*) planned metacarpal step cut osteotomy cut sites and (*B*) after cuts have been made and dorsal bone wedge resected.

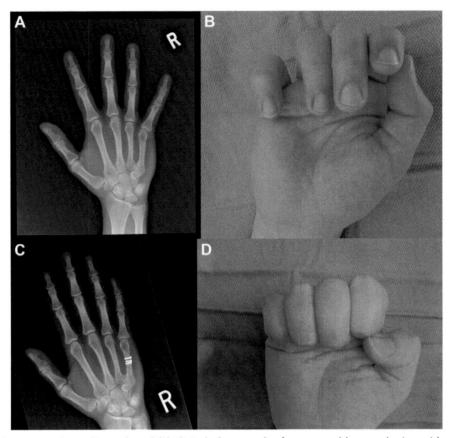

Fig. 4. (*A*) Pre-operative radiograph and (*B*) clinical photograph of metacarpal base malunion with rotational deformity. (*C*) Post-operative radiograph and (*D*) clinical photo following step cut rotational osteotomy of the small finger metacarpal.

osteotomy site and can be fixed with plates or K-wires. Plate fixation is more stable and allows for early motion at the cost of a higher tendon adhesion risk. In contrast, K-wire fixation allows for simpler insertion and hardware removal, but has the disadvantages of risk of pin site infections and delayed mobilization.[4,8,19,25]

Angular Deformities

The 2 workhorses of angular deformity correction are the opening and closing wedge osteotomies. The closing wedge osteotomy entails excision of a wedge of bone at the apex of the bony deformity. The far cortex and periosteum are left intact to preserve stability and improve healing potential.[4,8] The closing wedge benefits from only having 1 bone junction to heal, does not require graft, and can allow simultaneous correction of rotational deformity. However, it does shorten the bone and can cause extensor lag if there was already prior shortening.[4,8]

The opening wedge osteotomy is performed on the concave side of the malunion deformity. It involves a transverse cut followed by reduction of

the angular deformity followed by the insertion of structural distal radius or iliac crest bone autograft in the defect. The osteotomy can be stabilized with a plate or K-wires. As with other treatment options, correction through the malunion site is easier if performed early. In chronic deformities, a metaphyseal osteotomy provides better healing potential than diaphyseal bone.[4] When performing an opening wedge, it is important not to over lengthen the digit, as this can tighten tendons and cause stiffness.

Intra-articular Deformities

Intra-articular malunions can cause angular deformity of the finger and post-traumatic arthritis. As with all malunions, the best course of treatment is prevention, but this is particularly true in this case as intra-articular malunion corrections are very difficult and some authors suggest avoiding them altogether.[8] If correction is going to be attempted, it is strongly suggested that this be done <10 weeks after the initial injury, when the original fracture fragments can be delineated and more easily mobilized.[4,9] Once bony fragments have consolidated, options become more limited. An extra-articular opening or closing wedge osteotomy can be used to improve finger angulation and joint alignment. Harness and colleagues described a technique to treat unicondylar malunions with an extra-articular osteotomy. In these malunions, there is angulation toward the malunion (collapsed side). Their technique involves a closing wedge osteotomy to shorten the phalanx and level the joint by aligning the noninjured with the injured side, providing fixation with a K-wire and tension band.[27] (**Fig. 5**) They reported on 5 patients with correction of angular deformity and improvement in PIP and total digital motion. Arthrodesis or arthroplasty are salvage options in the setting of debilitating pain and dysfunction, but arthrodesis will limit digit total arc of motion and arthroplasty may require eventual revision in younger patients.[4,9] In the event the surgeon wishes to proceed with an intra-articular osteotomy in a consolidated fracture, the intercondylar wedge resection technique combined with a sliding osteotomy will provide a larger bony fragment for fixation.[28] In this technique, the condyle is cut in the intercondylar plane and then a second perpendicular cut is made proximal to the depressed condyle. The whole condyle and proximal bone is advanced to correct the alignment of the articular surface. The long cut allows fixation of

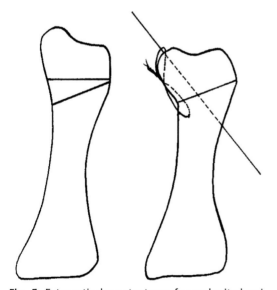

Fig. 5. Extra-articular osteotomy for malunited unicondylar fractures of proximal phalanx. Diagram depicting the extra-articular osteotomy technique for treatment of unicondylar malunions. The fixation is completed with a K-wire and tension band. (Harness et al. Extra-Articular Osteotomy for Malunited Unicondylar Fractures of the Proximal Phalanx. The Journal of Hand Surgery, 2005 30(3): 566-72.)

the bone with transverse screws and avoidance of a plate, which minimizes the chance of tendon adhesions. The gap will generally heal without the need for bone graft (**Fig. 6**).

Multiplanar Deformities

Malunions are not always simple, uni-planar deformities. They sometimes occur as a combination of angular and rotational deformities, requiring a more complicated correction. These deformities are typically corrected using a variation of the opening or closing wedge osteotomy, where if planned correctly, you can adjust angulation in multiple planes as well as the rotational alignment. This is a challenging process for more complicated deformities and requires extensive planning. One newer advancement that can be beneficial in those scenarios are 3D-printed osteotomy guides. They require pre-operative CT scans of both the affected and contra-lateral hand, for planning. Those CT scans can then be used to computer model the deformity and plan osteotomy location and resection needed to correct the deformity to match the contra-lateral side. Once the planning is completed, an osteotomy guide can be 3D printed to allow for precision cuts, and some systems will also include wedges and/or a plate to aid the correction and fixation. This can reduce the required intra-operative decision-making and make these cases more straightforward and more precise. However, it does require extensive pre-operative planning that is time consuming depending on the case complexity. In addition to a learning curve for using these systems, some of the negatives of the procedure include the increased radiation exposure from the extra CT scan as well as the increased costs from planning by the engineers and manufacturing of the custom cutting guides.[29] The main advantages are the potential decreased operative times and more precise corrections.

OUTCOMES

Overall, osteotomy outcomes are favorable, with high rates of union and satisfactory correction.[4,9] The results differ slightly based on the type of malunion and subsequent surgical correction. Buchler, and colleagues, investigated 57 patients who underwent proximal phalanx opening or closing wedge osteotomies through the malunion site. They found an average correction of 22°, all fractures healed, and they reported 76% satisfaction rate. When stratified, 96% of the patients with single malunions without concurrent complications (eg, adhesions) had excellent or good results while only 65% of the complex malunions with tenolysis had excellent or good results. With concomitant

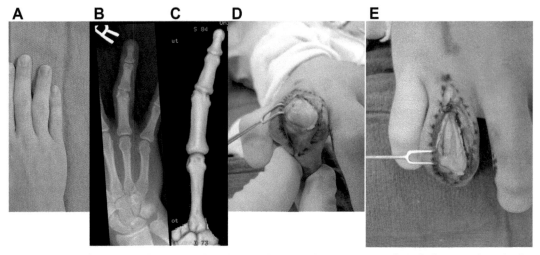

Fig. 6. Example of intra-articular proximal phalanx malunion. (*A*) Pre-operative clinical photograph with ulnar angulation at the proximal interphalangeal (PIP) joint. (*B*) Radiograph and (*C*) 3-dimensional computed tomography (CT) scan reconstruction showing the bony deformity. (*D, E*) Intra-operative photograph demonstrating the articular step off.

tenolysis, 89% gained active range of motion.[9] Other studies looking at the results of phalangeal osteotomies to correct angulation or multiplanar deformities have shown similar results, with satisfaction rates ranging from 86% to 89% and high rates of osseous union.[24,30–33] Potenza and colleagues reported mean DASH scores of 5 following proximal phalanx osteotomies performed at the site of malunion, reinforcing the high patient satisfaction and acceptable functional results.[24]

Isolated rotation deformities corrected through the metacarpal or phalanx have similar results as well. Jawa, and colleagues, performed step-cut osteotomies in 12 patients for rotational deficits in 7 metacarpals and 5 phalanges. All of these osteotomies resulted in bony union, correction of the original deformity, and maintained or improved motion without complications.[17]

Intra-articular osteotomy results are more guarded but can still have good outcomes. Light performed intra-articular osteotomies of the proximal phalanx head and showed good results in 9/10 patients, with 1 requiring conversion to arthrodesis because of fixation failure.[34] Other authors have shown similar results and despite theoretic concerns for avascular necrosis of the osteotomized articular fragment, this has not been reported frequently.[4,28,34,35] Despite this, the extra-articular osteotomy to correct intra-articular deformity was developed to decrease the risk of avascular necrosis and make the procedure less complicated. Harness performed 5 subcondylar closing wedge osteotomies which were stabilized with tension band constructs. All healed within 12 weeks and had an average angulation deformity correction from 25°

to 1°. The average range of motion at the PIP joint and total arc of motion both improved.[27]

COMPLICATIONS

Complications are reportedly low within the published studies on phalanx and metacarpal malunions, but suboptimal results may still occur. These include persistent deformity, delayed bone healing, non-union, implant failure, infection, persistent or increased stiffness, dystrophy, and chronic pain.[4] Modern mini locking plates for osteotomy fixation seem to be associated with earlier mobilization with less tendon adhesions and stiffness compared to other constructs.[4]

SUMMARY

Metacarpal and phalanx fracture are common injuries and have the risk of developing into malunions if not properly managed. Finger rotation, angulation, and intra-articular deformities are all important and can cause functional deficits which benefit from operative intervention in the circumstances described above. There are numerous surgical options to correct these deformities and the best treatment varies based on the injury pattern, concurrent injuries/complications, and surgeon's preference. While these surgeries can be technically demanding, most options report good results with satisfactory deformity correction and patient function.

DISCLOSURES

The authors have nothing to disclose.

REFERENCES

1. Cotterell IH, Richard MJ. Metacarpal and phalangeal fractures in athletes. Clin Sports Med 2015; 34(1):69–98.
2. Chung KC, Spilson SV. The frequency and epidemiology of hand and forearm fractures in the United States. J Hand Surg Am 2001;26(5):908–15.
3. Merkel D. Youth sport: positive and negative impact on young athletes. Open access J Sport Med 2013;4:151.
4. Freeland AE, Lindley SG. Malunions of the finger metacarpals and phalanges. Hand Clin 2006;22(3): 341–55.
5. Balaram AK, Bednar MS. Complications after the fractures of metacarpal and phalanges. Hand Clin 2010;26(2):169–77.
6. Lee SG, Jupiter JB. Phalangeal and metacarpal fractures of the hand. Hand Clin 2000;16(3):323–32.
7. Gaston RG, Chadderdon C. Phalangeal Fractures. Displaced/Nondisplaced. Hand Clin 2012;28(3): 395–401.
8. Ring D. Malunion and nonunion of the metacarpals and phalanges. Instr Course Lect 2006;55:121–8.
9. Buchler U, Gupta A, Ruf S. Corrective osteotomy for post-traumatic malunion of the phalanges in the hand. J Hand Surg Br 1996;21(1):33–42.
10. Strauch RJ, Rosenwasser MP, Lunt JG. Metacarpal shaft fractures: the effect of shortening on the extensor tendon mechanism. J Hand Surg Am 1998;23(3):519–23.
11. Westbrook AP, Davis TRC, Armstrong D, et al. The clinical significance of malunion of fractures of the neck and shaft of the little finger metacarpal. J Hand Surg Eur 2008;33(6):732–9.
12. ROYLE SG. Rotational deformity following metacarpal fracture. J Hand Surg Br 1990;15(1):124–5.
13. Coonrad RW, Pohlman MH. Impacted fractures in the proximal portion of the proximal phalanx of the finger. J Bone Joint Surg Am 1969;51(7):1291–6.
14. Vahey JW, Wegner DA, Hastings H. Effect of proximal phalangeal fracture deformity on extensor tendon function. J Hand Surg Am 1998;23(4):673–81.
15. Hardy MA. Principles of metacarpal and phalangeal fracture management: a review of rehabilitation concepts. J Orthop Sports Phys Ther 2004;34(12):781–99.
16. Robert M. The classic: Radiography of the trapeziometacarpal joint. Degenerative changes of this joint. 1936. Clin Orthop Relat Res 2014;472(4):1095–6.
17. Jawa A, Zucchini M, Lauri G, et al. Modified step-cut osteotomy for metacarpal and phalangeal rotational deformity. J Hand Surg Am 2009;34(2):335–40.
18. Manktelow RTMJ, Mahoney JL. Step osteotomy: a precise rotation osteotomy to correct scissoring deformities of the fingers. Plast Reconstr Surg 1981;68(4):571–6.
19. WECKESSER EC. Rotational osteotomy of the metacarpal for overlapping fingers. J Bone Jt Surg Am 1965;47:751–6.
20. Botelheiro JC. Overlapping of fingers due to malunion of a phalanx corrected by a metacarpal rotational osteotomy-Report of two cases. J Hand Surg Am 1985;10(3):389–90.
21. Menon J. Correction of rotary malunion of the fingers by metacarpal rotational osteotomy. Orthopedics 1990;13(2):197–200.
22. Pieron AP. Correction of rotational malunion of a phalanx by metacarpal osteotomy. J Bone Joint Surg Br 1972;54(3):516–9.
23. Pichora DR, Meyer R, Masear VR. Rotational step-cut osteotomy for treatment of metacarpal and phalangeal malunion. J Hand Surg Am 1991;16(3):551–5.
24. Potenza V, Luna V De, Maglione P, et al. Post-Traumatic Malunion of the Proximal Phalanx of the Finger. Medium-Term Results in 24 Cases Treated by "In Situ" Osteotomy. Open Orthop J 2012;6(1):468.
25. Jenkins CW, Smith AJ, Giddins GEB. Percutaneous corrective osteotomy for rotational malunion of metacarpal and phalangeal fractures. J Hand Surg Eur 2021;46(4):420–2.
26. Gross MS, Gelberman RH. Metacarpal rotational osteotomy. J Hand Surg Am 1985;10(1):105–8.
27. Harness NG, Chen A, Jupiter JB. Extra-articular osteotomy for malunited unicondylar fractures of the proximal phalanx. J Hand Surg Am 2005;30(3): 566–72.
28. Teoh LC, Yong FC, Chong KC. Condylar advancement osteotomy for correcting condylar malunion of the finger. J Hand Surg Am 2002;27 B(1):31–5.
29. Hirsiger S, Schweizer A, Miyake J, et al. Corrective Osteotomies of Phalangeal and Metacarpal Malunions Using Patient-Specific Guides: CT-Based Evaluation of the Reduction Accuracy. Hand 2018; 13(6):627–36.
30. Lucas GL, Pfeiffer CM. Osteotomy of the metacarpals and phalanges stabilized by AO plates and screws. Ann Chir Main 1989;8(1):30–8.
31. Sanders RAFH, Frederick HA. Metacarpal and phalangeal osteotomy with miniplate fixation. Orthop Rev 1991;20(5):449–56.
32. Van Der Lei B, Jonge J De, Robinson PH, et al. Correction osteotomies of phalanges and metacarpals for rotational and angular malunion: a long-term follow-up and a review of the literature. J Trauma 1993;35(6):902–8.
33. Trumble T, Gilbert M. In situ osteotomy for extra-articular malunion of the proximal phalanx. J Hand Surg Am 1998;23(5):821–6.
34. LIGHT T. Salvage of Intraarticular Malunions of the Hand and Wrist The Role of Realignment Osteotomy. Clin Orthop Relat Res 1987;214(January):130–5.
35. Duncan KH, Jupiter JB. Intraarticular osteotomy for malunion of metacarpal head fractures. J Hand Surg Am 1989;14(5):888–93.

Vascularized Medial Femoral Condyle Flap Reconstruction for Osseous Defects of the Hand and Wrist

James P. Higgins, MD

KEYWORDS

- Medial femoral condyle flap • Metacarpal nonunion • Phalanx nonunion • Scaphoid nonunion
- Vascularized bone

KEY POINTS

- The medial femoral condyle flap (MFC) has become a very valuable tool in the treatment of upper extremity nonunions.
- The MFC has applications is treating nonunions of tubular bones of the hand, carpal bones, long bones of the upper limb, and challenging arthrodesis.
- The upper extremity reconstructive surgeon should be familiar with the diverse sites where the MFC may be utilized and the surgical considerations for each.

INTRODUCTION

Free vascularized flaps utilizing the descending genicular artery system have become increasingly utilized over the past few decades.[1–13] Prior to the popularity of the medial femoral condyle flap (MFC), the most widely used source of vascularized bone was the vascularized fibula flap. Surgeons around the globe have become facile with applications of the MFC flap for many locations about the human skeleton. It is recognized to possess numerous beneficial characteristics:

- Ease of harvest: the flap is harvested in the supine position. This permits the use of a two-team surgical approach for efficiency and speed of the procedure.
- Lack of sacrifice of major peripheral artery: unlike the requirement of harvesting the peroneal artery for the fibula flap, the medial femoral condyle flap spares all of the major vessels providing perfusion to the distal extremity.
- Versatility: while the fibular flap provides a cylindrical long bone and is advantageous in lengthy osseous reconstructive cases, the MFC can provide corticocancellous segments of different widths, lengths, and shapes making useful for long bone, tubular bone, and joint reconstruction.
- Pliability: unlike the fibular flap, the MFC can be harvested as a thin corticoperiosteal flap with a pliable cortical surface. This enables the surgeon to fashion contoured onlay flap around atrophic nonunions without bone loss. Alternatively, the flap may be harvested as a corticocancellous flap for intercalary osseous defects.
- Length of pedicle: the descending genicular artery provides generous pedicle length enabling ease of anastomosis remote from the site of bony reconstruction.
- Chimeric tissue harvest: the descending genicular artery pedicle enables the harvest of corticocancellous bone, osteochondral bone, a reliable skin segment, and vascularized tendon as dictated by the reconstructive needs of the surgical defect.

Curtis National Hand Center, MedStar Union Memorial Hospital, 3333 North Calvert Street, Johnston Professional Building, Mezzanine Level, Baltimore, MD 21218, USA
E-mail address: higgins@curtishand.com

Hand Clin 40 (2024) 151–159
https://doi.org/10.1016/j.hcl.2023.06.003

- Ease of postoperative care: unlike the fibular flap, the osteocutaneous MFC does not typically require a skin graft applied to the donor site, nor does the donor site require immobilization/splinting.

When vascularized bone flaps are employed by reconstructive surgeons at various locations around the human skeleton, the fibula remains the most common for larger defects (ie, mandibular reconstruction, long bone intercalary defects) or sites requiring structural support afforded by a cylindrical long bone flap (ie, the femur, tibia, or humerus). Because of the frequent incidence of smaller osseous defects or recalcitrant atrophic nonunion in the upper limb, the medial femoral condyle has seen widespread adaptation by reconstructive hand surgeons.

This article will address the use of the corticocancellous medial femoral condyle flap for problematic osseous defects of the tubular bones of the hand (phalanges and metacarpals), the scaphoid waist, and difficult defects of infections or failed wrist fusions. We will also briefly discuss its use in forearm defects of the radius and ulna.

FLAP ANATOMY

The medial femoral condyle is perfused most commonly by osteoarticular periosteal branches of the descending geniculate artery, which arises from the superficial femoral artery in the proximal aspect of the adductor canal. The descending geniculate artery may be absent in 6% of cases. In this instance, these osteoarticular branches covering the periosteum of the medial femoral condyle are fed by the superomedial geniculate artery arising from the popliteal artery. Familiarity with this vascular system enables the surgeon to first identify the periosteal branches, and then follow them proximally to the appropriate source vessel.[14]

The medial femoral condyle flap is often harvested with a skin component. The skin may be harvested using the saphenous artery branch of the descending geniculate artery or the distal cutaneous branches. This enables the surgeon to harvest a longitudinal ellipse of skin over the medial aspect of the thigh. This region may provide generous amounts of skin with while still readily permitting primary closure.[12,15,16]

The descending geniculate artery has a length of 9.1 to 9.9 cm from its origin to the periosteal branches and at its origin has a diameter of 2.1 mm. The average diameter of the associated veins is 1.48 to 1.63 mm. If the flap is harvested utilizing the superomedial geniculate artery, the

surgeon will encounter a vessel whose average length is 4.1 cm with an average diameter of 1.7 mm. The vascular tree and details of its anatomy have been described in detail (Fig. 1).[14,15,17–21]

DEFECTS OF THE PHALANGES

Recalcitrant phalangeal nonunions are most often treated with vascularized bone grafting when the nonunion has previously failed conventional treatments such as autogenous bone grafting. Due to the small size of these defects, the use of the medial femoral condyle is an appealing option. The diameter of the fibula and the very small amount of bone required would make fibular transfer inappropriate for these defects.

If the resection of the nonunion results in an intercalary defect, the corticocancellous segment of the medial femoral condyle would be utilized. This is harvested using either saw or osteotome technique to elevate the cortical bone and the attached underlying cancellous bone. Alternatively, if the phalangeal defect was an atrophic nonunion without bone loss, the pliable medial femoral condyle corticoperiosteal flap may be elevated using an osteotome passed immediately beneath the cortex. This thin cortical bone can be molded (or scored on its deeper surface to enable the appropriate contour to be achieved) and applied as an onlay flap. The author usually utilizes a mid-axial approach to the digit, orients the cortical surface of the MFC on the midaxial surface of the phalanx, applies a plating construct dorsally, and the vascular pedicle is draped proximally. The proximal anastomosis can be performed into the ipsilateral digital artery or draped to the radial artery in the snuffbox if the position of the nonunion and pedicle length will permit. The venous anastomosis is typically performed on the dorsal aspect of the hand. Because of the limitations of the soft tissue envelope around the phalanges, a small skin paddle is typically taken with the MFC flap and inset into the mid-axial incision to permit ease of closure as well as a means of monitoring the microvascular anastomosis via the surface doppler (Fig. 2).

DEFECTS OF THE METACARPALS

Like phalangeal fractures, the use of vascularized bone is typically employed for metacarpal nonunions only after failure of previous cancellous bone grafting.[22–24] In the setting of a single metacarpal nonunion, the flap is typically inset such that the cortical surface is orthogonal to the plating construct. For the small finger, the plating would typically be dorsal and the MFC cortex applied

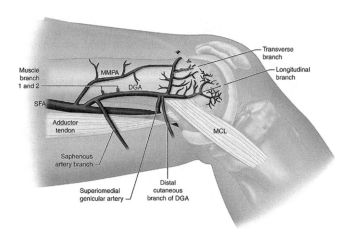

Fig. 1. The descending geniculate artery (DGA) divides into branches to the vastus medialis muscle, skin branches (including the saphenous artery and distal cutaneous artery of the DGA), and articular branches which supply the medial column of the femur.

on the ulnar surface. For the index finger and thumb metacarpals, the plating would be applied dorsally and the cortical bone would be inset radially. For the non-border digits, or for the simultaneous treatment of multiple metacarpals, the MFC flap cortical surface is applied dorsally. In an effort to achieve rigid fixation while not applying compression to the periosteal vessels on the MFC flap, the author has typically applied flexible small caliber plates that can be bent such that screw

fixation can be achieved in the metacarpal defects proximal and distal to the MFC. The plates are contoured dorsally above the level of the periosteum of the intercalary MFC. In the cases of multiple adjacent metacarpals, care should be taken to score the cancellous surface of the MFC flap and bend the flap in such a manner that it recreates the arch of the hand on the coronal plane (**Fig. 3**).

Because of the positioning of the dorsal cortex in these cases, the vascular pedicle is draped

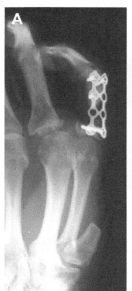
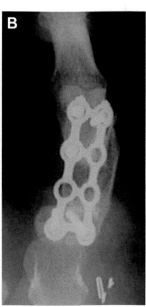
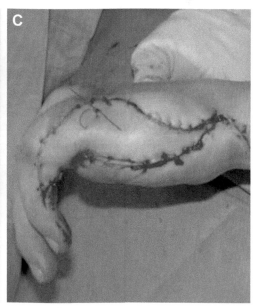

Fig. 2. Example of MFC reconstruction of a phalangeal nonunion. (*A*) Radiograph of ring finger proximal phalangeal nonunion after initial plating and subsequent failed cancellous bone grafting. (*B*) AP radiograph demonstrating healing. The corticoperiosteal MFC was used with the periosteum oriented ulnarly. (*C*) The skin segment was inset on the lateral aspect of the hand. (*From* Assi PE, Giladi AM, Higgins JP. Chapter 18: Medial Femoral Condyle Corticocancellous and Osteochondral Flaps. In: Wiesel SW, Albert T, eds. Operative Techniques in Orthopaedic Surgery. 3rd ed. Lippincott Williams & Wilkins; 2021. p. 3138-3152.; with permission. (Figure 5 in original).)

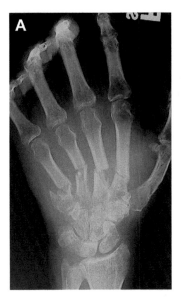

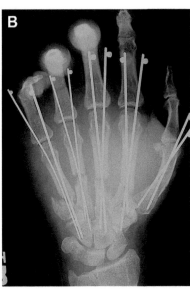

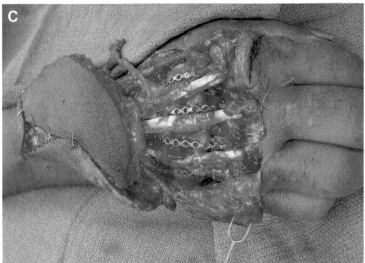

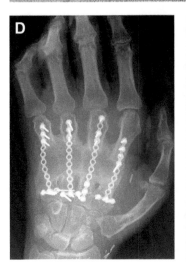

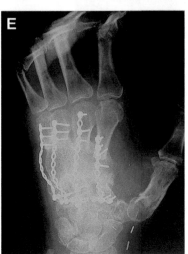

Fig. 3. Example of multiple metacarpal nonunions treated with MFC flap. (*A*) AP radiograph of fixation of five metacarpal fracture sustained from an industrial crush injury. Pin fixation was utilized because of the tenuous appearance of the soft tissue on the dorsal hand. (*B*) Radiographs 4 months after surgery demonstrating the failure of healing of metacarpals 2-5. The poor quality of the dorsal hand skin was felt to be unlikely to heal if conventional plating and cancellous bone grafting was attempted. (*C*) Corticocancellous MFC with skin paddle inset into diaphyseal nonunions of metacarpals 2 to 5. Note that the midline of the bone flap was scored longitudinally and contoured so that the flap recreated the dorsal arch of the palm. (*D*) AP radiograph of hand showing generous healing at the eight osteosynthesis sites. (*E*) Oblique radiograph demonstrating the contoured arch of the plates to avoid contact on the dorsal vascularized periosteum.

into the snuffbox for end-to-side anastomosis into the radial artery and end-to-end anastomosis into surrounding veins. A skin paddle is harvested in conjunction with the MFC flap in these cases and inset along the pathway of the access incision.

SCAPHOID NONUNIONS

The use of the medial femoral condyle corticocancellous flap has become common place in the setting of recalcitrant scaphoid nonunions.[25–28] The flap is applied via a volar approach for waist nonunions where the proximal pole is large enough to preserve. In scaphoid proximal pole nonunions with extremely small or comminuted segments that are deemed non-salvageable, the same vascular pedicle has been utilized to reconstruct the proximal half of the scaphoid using osteochondral medial femoral trochlea flaps. These have been described in detail elsewhere.[22,29–31]

The advantage of the MFC flap for scaphoid waist nonunions is in its ability to provide a corticocancellous segment that is larger than described pedicled vascularized bone flaps for this indication. The size and quality of the osseous segment are very useful in the correction of significantly collapsed scaphoid nonunions with humpback deformity. The scaphoid is approached volarly using an incision along the pathway of the FCR tendon. This approach enables access to the volar scaphoid as well as the radial artery in the distal third of the forearm. The nonunion site is opened, excavated generously and the scaphoid is restored to its appropriate carpal height. This may be done with joysticks or a temporary radiolunate pin applied dorsally (**Fig. 4**). The MFC flap may be harvested simultaneous to the scaphoid nonunion dissection by a second team to minimize operative time. The corticocancellous segment is inserted with the cortical bone facing volarward. Screw fixation is placed retrograde from the distal pole, through the MFC flap, and into the proximal pole. A flap pedicle is draped proximally and end-to-side anastomosis performed into the radial artery as well as venous anastomosis into the adjacent veinae comitante.

This procedure is typically performed without a skin paddle and the skin is loosely closed primarily. This has shown great success in the treatment of difficulty recalcitrant scaphoid nonunions. The author finds this particularly useful in patients that have a significant humpback deformity and are at high risk for surgical failure because of previous instrumentation. Patients are immobilized with 12 weeks of thumb spica casting postoperatively, followed by the confirmation of successful achievement of union with a CT scan.

WRIST DEFECTS

The corticocancellous MFC flap is also very useful in massive carpal defects. Although infrequently encountered, these defects pose a substantial reconstructive challenge in achieving successful wrist arthrodesis. Indications may include previous failed total wrist fusion, traumatic loss of carpal bones, previous osteomyelitis of the wrist joint requiring widespread carpal resection, or failed total wrist arthroplasty with substantial bone loss. These defects are often treated with more conventional cancellous bone grafting as a first-line treatment. However, if the patient has persistent nonunion, the use of the MFC can provide a versatile tool for the treatment of these odd-shaped defects. Use of the fibular flap is difficult because its narrow caliber limits the surgeon's ability to contact various distal osseous targets (ie, multiple metacarpals).

The MFC flap can be harvested as a corticocancellous or onlay corticoperiosteal flap to cover the width and length required to achieve bony union. In these cases, the cortical bone is applied dorsally. The fixation construct required will need to be contoured to protect the dorsal periosteal vessels. If the distal defect extends to the level of the metacarpals (without any remaining carpus), the fixation technique will likely require multiple small plates to bridge the defect and achieve stability of each metacarpal. A skin segment is harvested with the medial femoral condyle and inset to permit closure without tension. The arterial anastomosis is performed either into the radial artery in the snuffbox or the distal volar forearm in an end-to-side fashion (**Fig. 5**).

In these cases, very specific challenges are encountered. If the entirety of the carpus has been lost and fixation is pursued on multiple metacarpals, the surgeon must pay particular heed to ensuring that the rotation of each digit is appropriate. Because of the inherent instability of this defect, the risk of encountering some scissoring of the digits due to malrotation after healing is achieved is substantial.

Because of the size and shape of these defects, additional bone grafting may be helpful. In particularly large defects, the author will harvest the medial femoral condyle flap as a thin pliable corticoperiosteal flap and augment this with additional cancellous autograft, typically harvested from the proximal tibia. The author avoids excessive cancellous bone harvesting from the distal femur with the associated undermining of the support of the condyle. The author has encountered a single case of distal femur pathologic fracture from medial femoral condyle harvest.[32] It is the author's opinion that this risk was created due to the depth

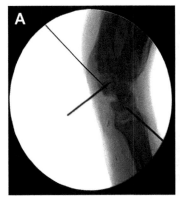
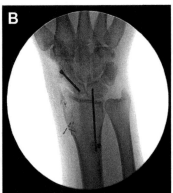
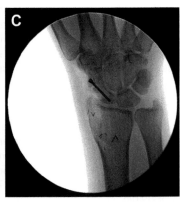

Fig. 4. Intraoperative fluoroscopy demonstrating the correction of scaphoid waist nonunion with collapse using a corticocancellous MFC flap. The scaphoid and lunate are inspected under fluoroscopy for any scaphoid flexion/lunate extension. (*A*) After the reduction of the lunate into neutral posture, an intraoperative radiolunate K wire is placed. Another K wire is used as a joystick in the distal pole for the reduction of the scaphoid and inset of the MFC. (*B*) The defect is filled with the osseous MFC flap and screw fixation is obtained while the radiolunate preserves neutral lunate posture. (*C*) Once scaphoid reconstruction is complete, the radiolunate pin is withdrawn. (*From* Assi PE, Giladi AM, Higgins JP. Chapter 18: Medial Femoral Condyle Corticocancellous and Osteochondral Flaps. In: Wiesel SW, Albert T, eds. Operative Techniques in Orthopaedic Surgery. 3rd ed. Lippincott Williams & Wilkins; 2021. p. 3138-3152.; with permission. (Tech Figure 1C-E in original).)

of the cancellous harvest (rather than the width or length of the cortical harvest).[33–35]

Cases of large wrist nonunion reconstructions are typically approached on a semi-elective basis and performed through an intact skin envelope. A surgeon may be tempted to conclude that no additional skin is needed. It is the author's experience that such a reconstruction will provide a substantial challenge of skin closure and thus harvest of a skin paddle in conjunction with the MFC flap is highly recommended.

FOREARM NONUNIONS

The treatment of radial and ulnar nonunions is addressed in other articles in this publication. A brief commentary on the use of the medial femoral condyle flap for these indications is provided here.

The MFC, while versatile, low morbidity, and clinically effective, should be employed in upper limb long bone nonunions with some specific guidelines. The MFC flap is ideal for onlay corticoperiosteal flap application. It provides a powerful means of correction of nonunion with remarkable osteogenic capability. However, when being used for intercalary defects, it should only be used *when structural bone is not required*. The advent of fixed-angled fixation and locking screw technology has enabled the surgeon to rely on the fixation construct for structural support. However, the surgeon should consider the value of using a stouter structural graft/flap when there is a substantial length of defect that would lead the surgeon to anticipate a prolonged period of healing, or if the site of reconstruction will be

submitted to substantial postoperative stresses (torsional, loading, or varus/valgus stress). This is encountered when the surgeon is faced with intercalary defects of the humerus. The reconstruction may be exposed to substantial multidirectional stress with load forces compounded by the weight and position of the distal arm. This concern is also encountered in cases of massive forearm trauma with intercalary defects of both the radius and ulna. Without the structural support of an intact parallel forearm bone, the reconstruction will be submitted to greater postoperative stress than a single forearm bone intercalary nonunion. These are cases where the surgeon should consider the structural benefit of fibular flap reconstruction.[36]

In smaller defects where the corticocancellous flap will have the support of locking plating constructs and/or an adjacent intact long bone, corticocancellous and intercalary MFC flaps are a useful tool. The author has experience in over 50 cases utilized for long and tubular bones of the extremities and has witnessed rapid bony healing in these cases. However, even years after the reconstruction, the unicortical nature of the MFC flap will not typically achieve the radiodensity of a radius or ulna (where cylindrical cortical surfaces provide a much denser radiographic appearance). Whether due to the stress shielding afforded by the plating constructs, or simply the limited nature of the unicortical flap to hypertrophy, the MFC flap does not typically assume the appearance of a normal radius or ulna.

Like the tubular bones of the hand, the strategy for the application of the MFC corticocancellous

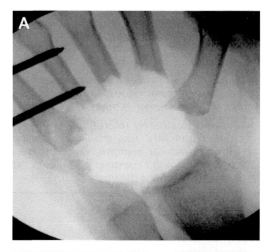

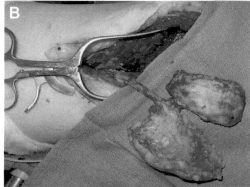

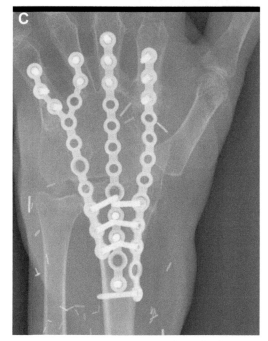

flap to upper extremity long bones is specific to the site. In cases of distal or diaphyseal radius non-unions, the surgeon will most often encounter a previous volar incision and will most likely approach the radius through the same volar approach. When this is performed, the plating is applied volarly and the cortical surface of the MFC is applied orthogonally on the radial column of the radius. The vessel is draped toward the radial artery for end-to-side anastomosis and the skin paddle is typically inset along the same volar incision to provide ease of closure and ability for postoperative monitoring. Because of the configuration of the skin paddle and position of the radial artery, the author finds it easier to harvest an osteocutaneous ipsilateral medial femoral condyle flap as this will result in the skin paddle insetting ulnar to the flap pedicle in the forearm. This will provide ease of positioning of the descending geniculate artery to the radial artery.

In the setting of ulnar shaft nonunion, the surgeon most often encounters a previous incision created on the subcutaneous border of the ulna. This is typically the same incision that is used to re-access the nonunion site. In this setting, a surgeon should consider the planned site of microsurgical anastomosis. The ulnar artery in the proximal half of the forearm is deep to the pronator and becomes relatively inaccessible in the forearm musculature. Thus, the arterial anastomosis is typically performed to the distal ulnar or distal radial artery. The corticocancellous MFC flap is thus inset in such a manner that the pedicle drapes in a distal direction. The skin paddle that is inset will be placed in the longitudinal skin incision along the subcutaneous border of the ulna. In order to have the artery lie volar to the skin paddle and drape appropriately to the distal anastomotic site, selection of the contralateral medial femoral condyle osteocutaneous flap is indicated.

loss of carpal structures. (*B*) Thin, rectangular shaped corticocancellous MFC is harvested from the ipsilateral leg with the large skin paddle to facilitate closure and permit postoperative monitoring. (*C*) X-rays showing consolidation at 12 weeks. Lengthy malleable plates were used to arch over the dorsal MFC periosteum and avoid compression of the periosteal vessels. These plates were used to achieve fixation and osteosynthesis of metacarpals 2-5 and the distal radius. The distal ulna and the thumb metacarpal are purposely maintained free of the fusion mass. (*From* Assi PE, Giladi AM, Higgins JP. Chapter 18: Medial Femoral Condyle Corticocancellous and Osteochondral Flaps. In: Wiesel SW, Albert T, eds. Operative Techniques in Orthopaedic Surgery. 3rd ed. Lippincott Williams & Wilkins; 2021. p. 3138-3152.; with permission. (Figure 6 in original).)

Fig. 5. Example of MFC reconstruction of large bone defect of the wrist. (*A*) Patient transferred to our institution after the radical resection of carpus for osteomyelitis. Fluoroscopic image demonstrates complete

In cases of humeral nonunions, commonly there is a previous lateral brachial incision that is utilized for the nonunion reconstruction. The skin paddle is inset longitudinally into the lateral brachium along the pathway of the incision. However, the anastomosis was performed on the medial aspect of the brachium via a counter incision. Thus, the descending genicular artery pedicle is tunneled medially. This may require that the surgeon create a tunnel through a previous scarred bed or the capsule created by the use of the cement spacer. The microscope is brought onto the field to provide a view of the medial brachial exposure. The vascular pedicle is encountered arising from the depth of the exposure. The microvascular anastomosis is most easily performed in the distal brachium and thus the flap is inset such that the pedicle is draped medially and distally, rather than medially and proximally. This inset of the bone flap in an "upside down" positioning, while counter intuitive, is very helpful in the facilitation of the vascular pedicle and has no impact on the function of the microvascular anastomosis.

Lastly, for the clavicle, the author has found that it is particularly difficult to apply the fixation in any other location than the superficial most aspect of the bone. Likewise, it is difficult to inset the MFC with the cortical surface directed orthogonally. Thus, the author has typically performed these cases by first plating the clavicle in the appropriate position and then applying an onlay corticocancellous malleable MFC flap around the entirety of the clavicle and the plate, typically using additional cancellous graft if needed within this nonunion site. The vessels are typically anastomosed to the thoracoacromial artery and cephalic vein. The skin paddle is applied along the axis of the incision.

SUMMARY

Vascularized bone flaps from the descending genicular artery system are versatile and effective for the use of recalcitrant nonunions from the tubular bones of the hand to the long bones of the upper extremity. Familiarity with the vascular pedicle, various techniques of harvest and inset, and skin paddle harvest and application are essential for the reconstructive surgeon.

CLINICS CARE POINTS

- The MFC flap can provide corticocancellous, corticoperiosteal, and osteocutaneous options for commonly encountered nonunions of the upper extremity.

- The MFC flap has been shown to be effective in the treatment of upper extremity tubular and longbone nonunions as well as scaphoid nonunions.

- The MFC flap provides a unicortical flap that has less structural value than a fibular flap but provides numerous other advantageous.

- The upper extremity reconstructive surgeon utilizing the MFC flap should be familiar with the vascular anatomy, various harvest techniques, and insetting techniques at various locations of the upper limb.

DISCLOSURE

The author has no relevant disclosures.

REFERENCES

1. Kazmers NH, Thibaudeau S, Gerety P, et al. Versatility of the Medial Femoral Condyle Flap for Extremity Reconstruction and Identification of Risk Factors for Nonunion, Delayed Time to Union, and Complications. Ann Plast Surg 2018;80(4): 364–72.
2. Fuchs B, Steinmann SP, Bishop AT. Free vascularized corticoperiosteal bone graft for the treatment of persistent nonunion of the clavicle. J Shoulder Elbow Surg 2005;14(3):264–8.
3. Choudry UH, Bakri K, Moran SL, et al. The vascularized medial femoral condyle periosteal bone flap for the treatment of recalcitrant bony nonunions. Ann Plast Surg 2008;60(2):174–80.
4. Kaminski A, Burger H, Muller EJ. Free vascularised corticoperiosteal bone flaps in the treatment of non-union of long bones: an ignored opportunity? Acta Orthop Belg 2008;74(2):235–9.
5. Muramatsu K, Doi K, Ihara K, et al. Recalcitrant post-traumatic nonunion of the humerus: 23 patients reconstructed with vascularized bone graft. Acta Orthop Scand 2003;74(1):95–7.
6. Del Pinal F, Garcia-Bernal FJ, Regalado J, et al. Vascularised corticoperiosteal grafts from the medial femoral condyle for difficult non-unions of the upper limb. J Hand Surg Eur Vol 2007;32(2):135–42.
7. Doi K, Sakai K. Vascularized periosteal bone graft from the supracondylar region of the femur. Microsurgery 1994;15(5):305–15.
8. De Smet L. Treatment of non-union of forearm bones with a free vascularised corticoperiosteal flap from the medial femoral condyle. Acta Orthop Belg 2009;75(5):611–5.
9. Henry M. Genicular corticoperiosteal flap salvage of resistant atrophic non-union of the distal radius metaphysis. Hand Surg 2007;12(3):211–5.

10. Sakai K, Doi K, Kawai S. Free vascularized thin corticoperiosteal graft. Plast Reconstr Surg 1991;87(2):290–8.

11. Sammer DM, Bishop AT, Shin AY. Vascularized medial femoral condyle graft for thumb metacarpal reconstruction: case report. J Hand Surg Am 2009;34(4):715–8.

12. Pelzer M, Reichenberger M, Germann G. Osteoperiosteal-cutaneous flaps of the medial femoral condyle: a valuable modification for selected clinical situations. J Reconstr Microsurg 2010;26(5):291–4.

13. Cavadas PC, Landin L. Treatment of recalcitrant distal tibial nonunion using the descending genicular corticoperiosteal free flap. J Trauma 2008;64(1):144–50.

14. Iorio ML, Masden DL, Higgins JP. The limits of medial femoral condyle corticoperiosteal flaps. J Hand Surg Am 2011;36(10):1592–6.

15. Iorio ML, Masden DL, Higgins JP. Cutaneous angiosome territory of the medial femoral condyle osteocutaneous flap. J Hand Surg Am 2012;37(5):1033–41.

16. Tremp M, Haumer A, Wettstein R, et al. The medial femoral trochlea flap with a monitor skin island-Report of two cases. Microsurgery 2017;37(5):431–5.

17. Ziegler T, Kamolz LP, Vasilyeva A, et al. Descending genicular artery. Branching patterns and measuring parameters: A systematic review and meta-analysis of several anatomical studies. J Plast Reconstr Aesthet Surg 2018;71(7):967–75.

18. Weitgasser L, Cotofana S, Winkler M, et al. Detailed vascular anatomy of the medial femoral condyle and the significance of its use as a free flap. J Plast Reconstr Aesthet Surg 2016;69(12):1683–9.

19. Hugon S, Koninckx A, Barbier O. Vascularized osteochondral graft from the medial femoral trochlea: anatomical study and clinical perspectives. Surg Radiol Anat 2010;32(9):817–25.

20. Acland RD, Schusterman M, Godina M, et al. The saphenous neurovascular free flap. Plast Reconstr Surg 1981;67(6):763–74.

21. Yamamoto H, Jones DB Jr, Moran SL, et al. The arterial anatomy of the medial femoral condyle and its clinical implications. J Hand Surg Eur Vol 2010;35(7):569–74.

22. Higgins JP, Burger HK. Osteochondral flaps from the distal femur: expanding applications, harvest sites, and indications. J Reconstr Microsurg 2014;30(7):483–90.

23. Wong VW, Higgins JP, Katz RD. Functional reconstruction of subtotal thumb metacarpal defect with a vascularized medial femoral condyle flap: case report. J Hand Surg Am 2014;39(10):2005–8.

24. Hsu CC, Loh CY, Lin YT, et al. The Medial Femoral Condyle Flap for Reconstruction of Intercondylar Pathological Fractures of the Thumb. Plast Reconstr Surg Glob Open 2017;5(2):e1242.

25. Doi K, Oda T, Soo-Heong T, et al. Free vascularized bone graft for nonunion of the scaphoid. J Hand Surg Am 2000;25(3):507–19.

26. Jones DB Jr, Shin AY. Medial femoral condyle vascularized bone grafts for scaphoid nonunions. Chir Main 2010;29(Suppl 1):S93–103.

27. Pulos N, Kollitz KM, Bishop AT, et al. Free Vascularized Medial Femoral Condyle Bone Graft After Failed Scaphoid Nonunion Surgery. J Bone Joint Surg Am 2018;100(16):1379–86.

28. Tsantes AG, Papadopoulos DV, Gelalis ID, et al. The Efficacy of Vascularized Bone Grafts in the Treatment of Scaphoid Nonunions and Kienbock Disease: A Systematic Review in 917 Patients. J Hand Microsurg 2019;11(1):6–13.

29. Higgins JP, Burger HK. Proximal scaphoid arthroplasty using the medial femoral trochlea flap. J Wrist Surg 2013;2(3):228–33.

30. Pet MA, Higgins JP. Long-Term Outcomes of Vascularized Trochlear Flaps for Scaphoid Proximal Pole Reconstruction. Hand Clin 2019;35(3):345–52.

31. Pet MA, Assi PE, Yousaf IS, et al. Outcomes of the Medial Femoral Trochlea Osteochondral Free Flap for Proximal Scaphoid Reconstruction. J Hand Surg Am 2020;45(4):317–26.e3.

32. Son JH, Giladi AM, Higgins JP. Iatrogenic femur fracture following medial femoral condyle flap harvest eventually requiring total knee arthroplasty in one patient. J Hand Surg Eur Vol 2019;44(3):320–1.

33. Katz RD, Parks BG, Higgins JP. The axial stability of the femur after harvest of the medial femoral condyle corticocancellous flap: a biomechanical study of composite femur models. Microsurgery 2012;32(3):213–8.

34. Endara MR, Brown BJ, Shuck J, et al. Torsional stability of the femur after harvest of the medial femoral condyle corticocancellous flap. J Reconstr Microsurg 2015;31(5):364–8.

35. Giladi AM, Rinkinen JR, Higgins JP, et al. Donor-Site Morbidity of Vascularized Bone Flaps from the Distal Femur: A Systematic Review. Plast Reconstr Surg 2018;142(3):363e–72e.

36. Masden DL, Iorio ML, Higgins JP. Comparison of the osseous characteristics of medial femoral condyle and fibula flaps. J Hand Surg Eur Vol 2013;38(4):437–9.

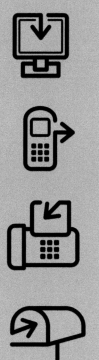